AF669454

A Practical Approach to **ROBOTIC SURGERY**

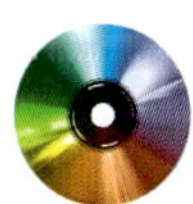

System requirement

- Operating System—Windows Vista or above
- Web Browser—Google Chrome and Mozilla Firefox
- Essential plugins—Java and Flash player
  - Facing problems in viewing content—it may be your system does not have Java enabled.
  - If Videos do not show up—it may be the system requires Flash player or need to manage Flash setting. To learn more about Flash setting, click on the link in the help section.
- You can test Java and Flash by using the links from the help section of the CD/DVD.
- Accompanying CD/DVD ROM is playable only in Computer and not in DVD player. CD/DVD has Autorun function—it may take few seconds to load on your computer. If it does not work for you, then follow the steps below to access the contents manually:
  - Click on my computer
  - Select the CD/DVD drive and click open/explore—this will show list of files in the CD/DVD
  - Find and double click file—launch.html

For more information about troubleshoot of Autorun click on: *http://support.microsoft.com/kb/330135*

DVD Contents

1. **Robotic Demo**
   Ajit Saxena
2. **Robotic Sleeve Gastrectomy**
   Praveen Bhatia
3. **Robotic Transabdominal Preperitoneal with Ventral Hernia Repair**
   Praveen Bhatia
4. **Robotic Rectopexy**
   Praveen Bhatia
5. **Carcinoma Rectum Video**
   Somashekhar SP
6. **Robotic Myomectomy**
   Rooma Sinha
7. **Robotic Hysterectomy with Cholecystectomy**
   Praveen Bhatia
8. **Burch Procedure for Failed Transvaginal Cystocele Repair**
   Ajit Saxena
9. **Vesicovaginal Fistula Repair**
   K Ramesh
10. **Urolithiasis**
    Prem Nath Dogra
11. **Left Robotic Pyeloplasty**
    Ajit Saxena
12. **Ureteric Reimplantation**
    Ajit Saxena
13. **Left Adrenalectomy**
    Gagan Gautam
14. **Robotic Right Adrenalectomy**
    Praveen Bhatia
15. **Radical Prostatectomy**
    Vipul R Patel

A Practical Approach to ROBOTIC SURGERY

Editor

Ajit Saxena
MS (Delhi) FRCS (Edin) FICS MNAMS (Urology) Dip Urology (London)
Senior Consultant Urologist and Andrologist
Indraprastha Apollo Hospitals
New Delhi, India

Foreword

Mahendra Bhandari

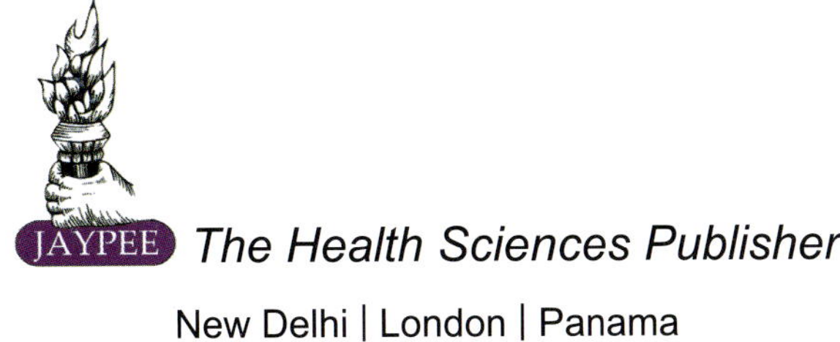

The Health Sciences Publisher
New Delhi | London | Panama

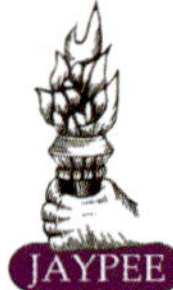

Jaypee Brothers Medical Publishers (P) Ltd.

Headquarters
Jaypee Brothers Medical Publishers (P) Ltd.
4838/24, Ansari Road, Daryaganj
New Delhi 110 002, India
Phone: +91-11-43574357
Fax: +91-11-43574314
E-mail: jaypee@jaypeebrothers.com

Overseas Offices
J.P. Medical Ltd.
83, Victoria Street, London
SW1H 0HW (UK)
Phone: +44- 20 3170 8910
Fax: +44(0) 20 3008 6180
E-mail: info@jpmedpub.com

Jaypee Highlights Medical Publishers Inc.
City of Knowledge, Building 235, 2nd Floor
Clayton, Panama City, Panama
Phone: +1 507-301-0496
Fax: +1 507-301-0499
E-mail: cservice@jphmedical.com

Jaypee Brothers Medical Publishers (P) Ltd.
17/1-B, Babar Road, Block-B, Shaymali
Mohammadpur, Dhaka-1207
Bangladesh
Mobile: +08801912003485
E-mail: jaypeedhaka@gmail.com

Jaypee Brothers Medical Publishers (P) Ltd.
Bhotahity, Kathmandu, Nepal
Phone: +977-9741283608
E-mail: kathmandu@jaypeebrothers.com

Website: www.jaypeebrothers.com
Website: www.jaypeedigital.com

Inquiries for bulk sales may be solicited at: jaypee@jaypeebrothers.com

A Practical Approach to Robotic Surgery

First Edition: **2017**

ISBN: 978-93-86261-26-7

Printed at Sanat Printers

Dedicated to

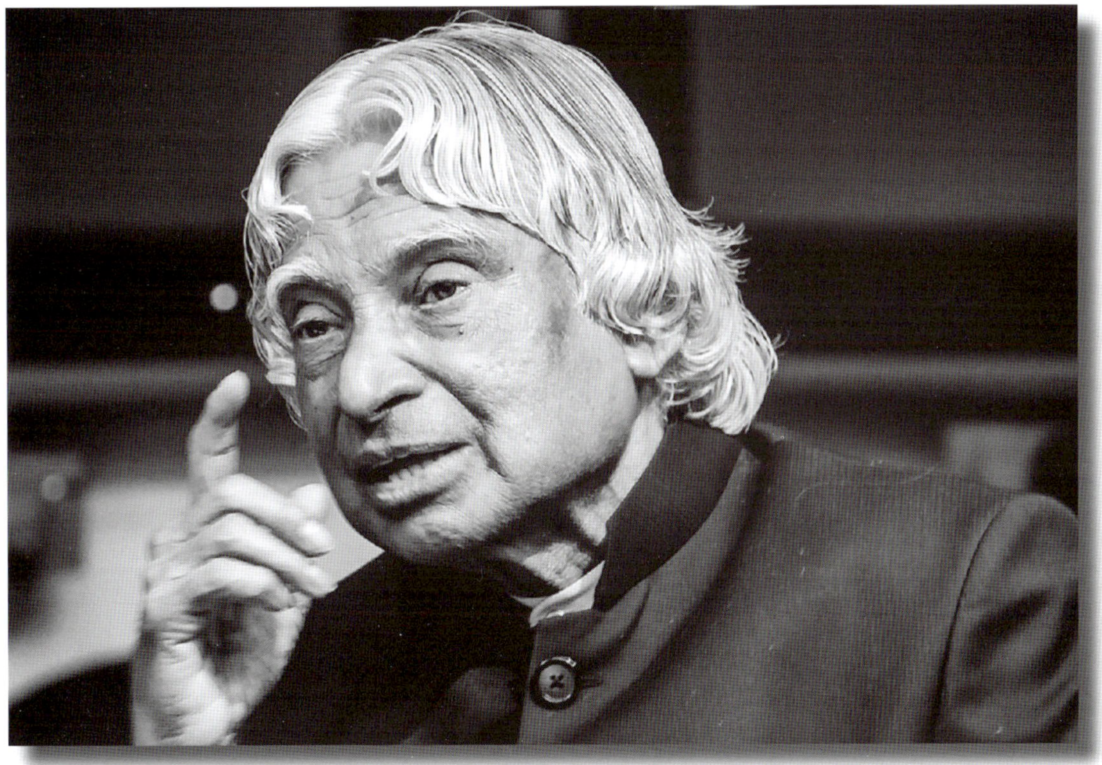

APJ Abdul Kalam
15 October 1931–27 July 2015

A scientist, statesman, poet, visionary, friend
and
above all, a good human being

"Failure will never overtake me if my determination to succeed is strong enough."

—APJ Abdul Kalam

Contributors

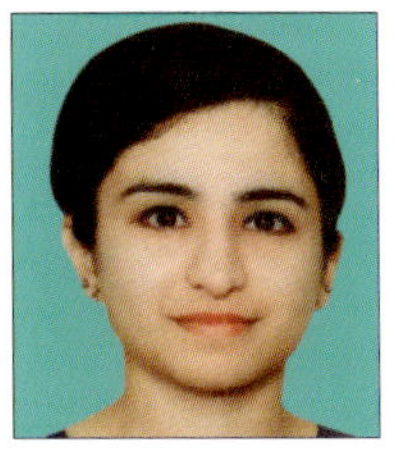

Aditi Midha Masters of Physiotherapy (MPT)
Neuro-Pediatric Physiotherapist
Aktivortho—A German Based Orthopedic and Rehabilitation Centre
New Delhi, India

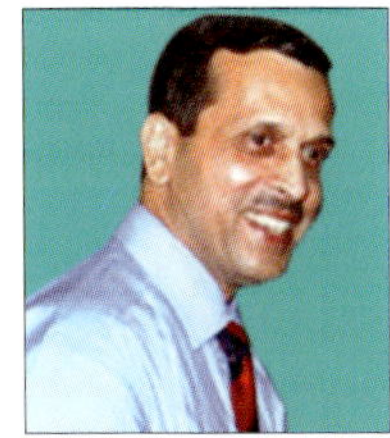

Arvind Kumar MBBS MS (Surgery)
Chairman
Centre for Chest Surgery
Director
Institute of Robotic Surgery
Sir Ganga Ram Hospital
New Delhi, India

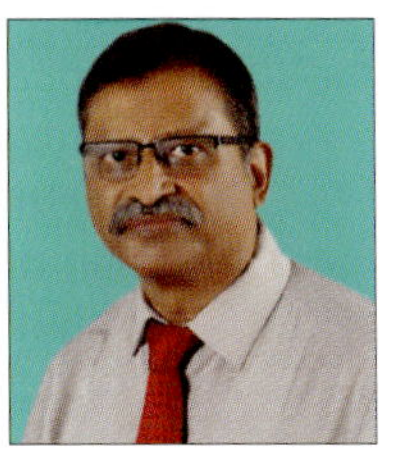

Ajit Saxena MS (Delhi) FRCS (Edin) FICS MNAMS (Urology) Dip Urology (London)
Senior Consultant Urologist and Andrologist
Indraprastha Apollo Hospitals
New Delhi, India

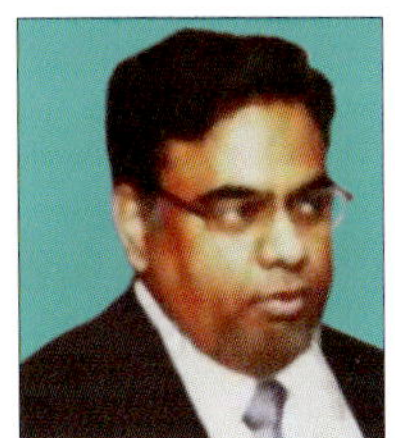

Belal Bin Asaf MBBS MS (General Surgery)
Associate Consultant
Department of Thoracic Surgery
Institute of Robotic Surgery
Sir Ganga Ram Hospital
New Delhi, India

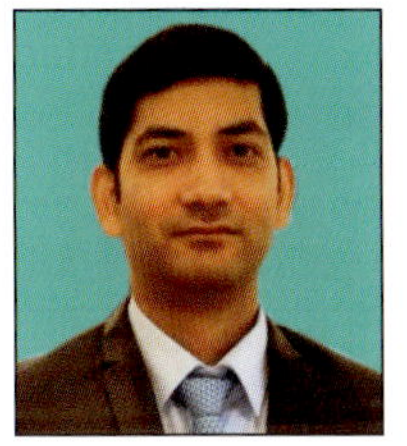

Anand Kumar Yadav MS FMAS FIAGES
Fellow
Institute of Minimal Access
Metabolic and Bariatric Surgery (iMAS)
Sir Ganga Ram Hospital
New Delhi, India

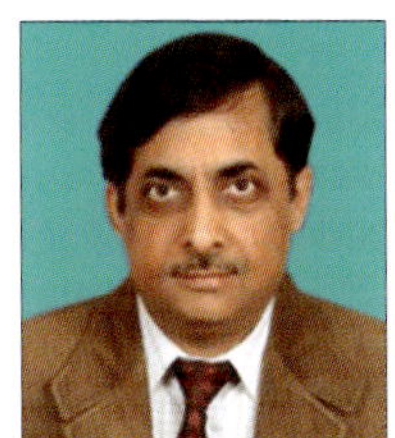

Deepak Govil MBBS MS Postdoctoral Course (PhD)
Senior Consultant
Department of Surgical Gastroenterology
Indraprastha Apollo Hospitals
New Delhi, India

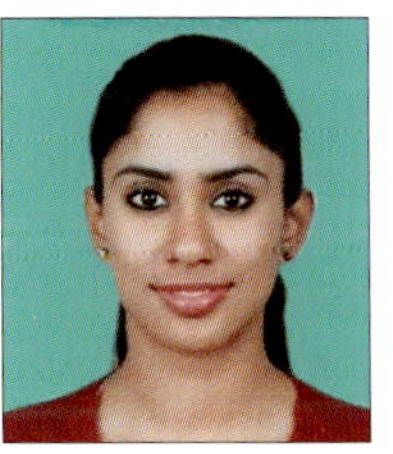

Ankita Srivastava
PG Student
Sri Aurobindo Institute of Medical Sciences
Indore, Madhya Pradesh, India

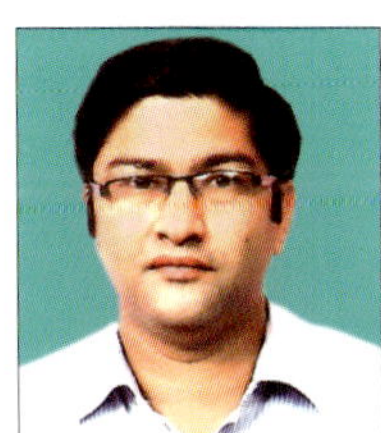

DK Kandpal MS MCh
Consultant
Department of Pediatric Surgery
Indraprastha Apollo Hospitals
New Delhi, India

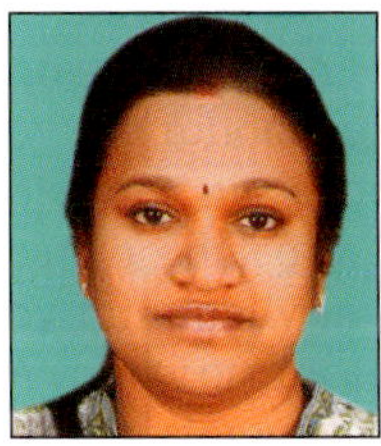

Anupama Rajanbabu MD MRCOG
Professor
Department of Gynecologic-Oncology
Amrita Institute of Medical Sciences
Amrita Vishwavidyapeetham
Kochi, Kerala, India

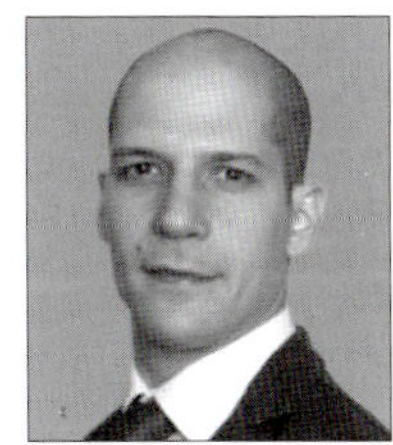

Gabriel Ogaya-Pines
Senior Clinical Fellow
Global Robotic Institute
Celebration Hospital
Florida, USA

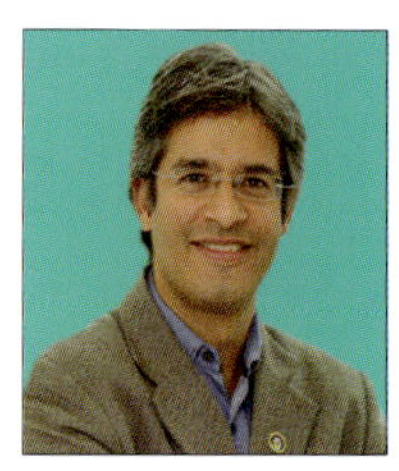

Gagan Gautam MCh
Head
Department of Urologic-Oncology and Robotic Surgery
Medanta—The Medicity
Gurugram, Haryana, India

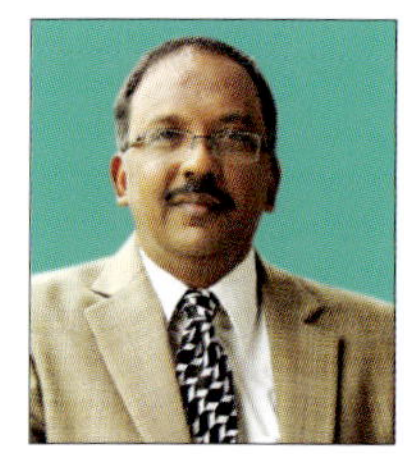

K Ramesh MS FRCS DNB (Urology) FEBU (Fellow of European Board of Urology)
Senior Consultant Urologist and Robotic Surgeon
Apollo Hospitals
Chennai, Tamil Nadu, India

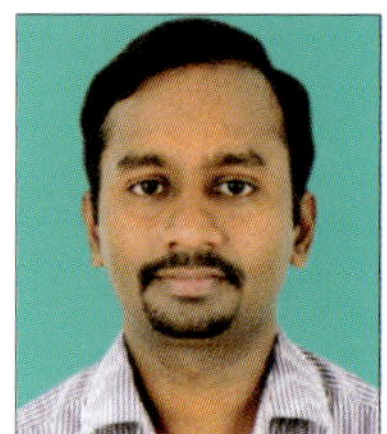

Hariharan Palayapalayam Ganapathi MD
Senior Clinical Fellow
Global Robotics Institute
Florida Hospital Celebration Health
Florida, USA

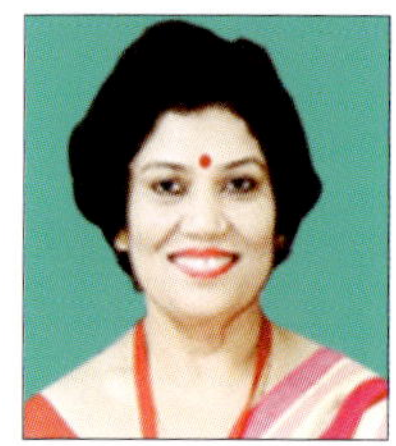

Mala Srivastava FICOG DGO DNB MBBS
Senior Consultant
Sir Ganga Ram Hospital
New Delhi, India

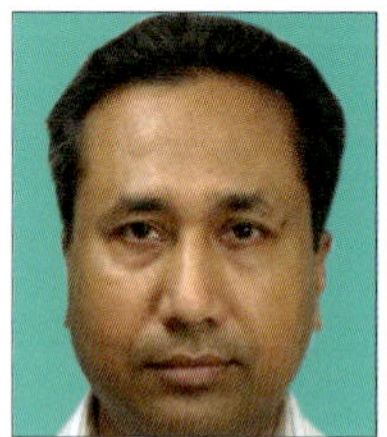

Jaydip Bhadra Roy MBBS FRCS (London) MS
Consultant General Laparoscopic and Robotic Surgeon
Apollo Gleneagles Hospitals
Kolkata, West Bengal, India

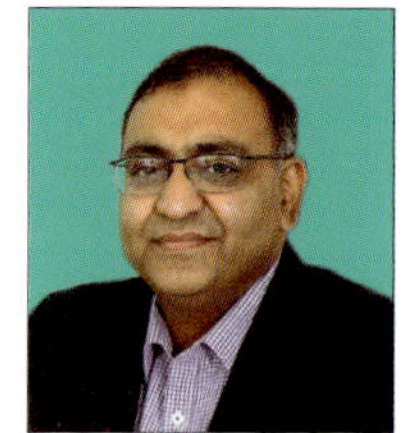

Manu Gupta MBBS MS DNB MCh
Consultant Urological Surgeon
Sir Ganga Ram Hospital
New Delhi, India

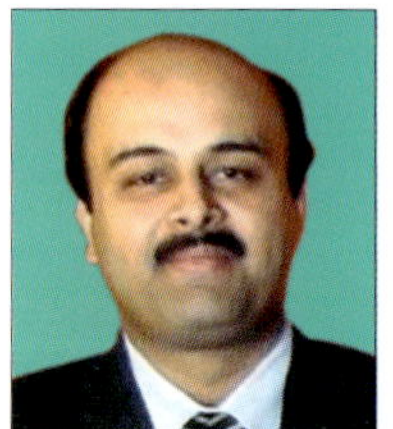

Jyotirmoy Das
Associate Consultant
Department of Anesthesiology
Medanta—The Medicity
Gurugram, Haryana, India

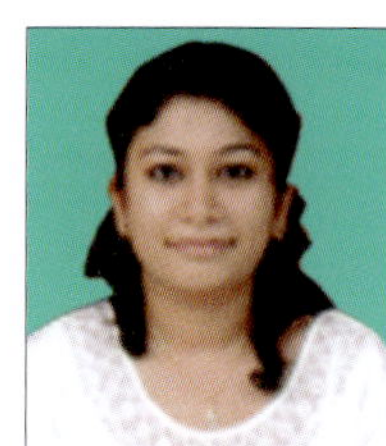

Megha Bhatnagar
Masters in Exercise Physiology and Sports Science
Sports Physiotherapist
Navi Mumbai, Maharashtra, India

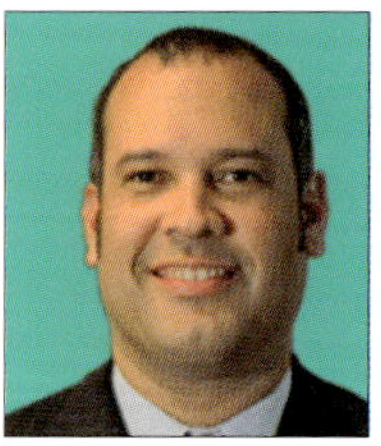

Kenneth J Palmer
Director
University of Central Florida
Director
Global Robotics Institute
Florida Hospital
Florida, USA

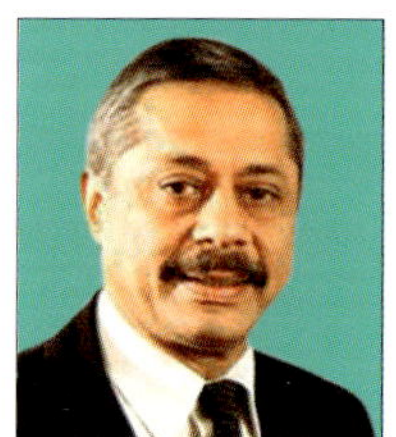

Naresh Trehan
Chairman and Managing Director
Medanta—The Medicity
Gurugram, Haryana, India

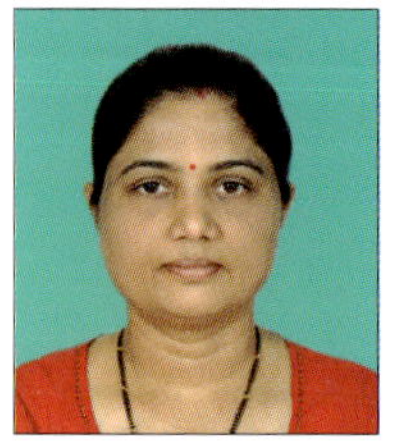

Kiranabala Dash MD
Attending Consultant
Indraprastha Apollo Hospitals
New Delhi, India

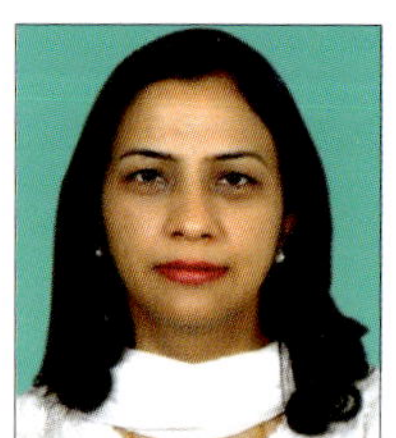

Neelam Suri MBBS MD
Senior Consultant
Obstetrician and Gynecologist
Laparoscopic and Robotic Surgeon
Indraprastha Apollo Hospitals
New Delhi, India

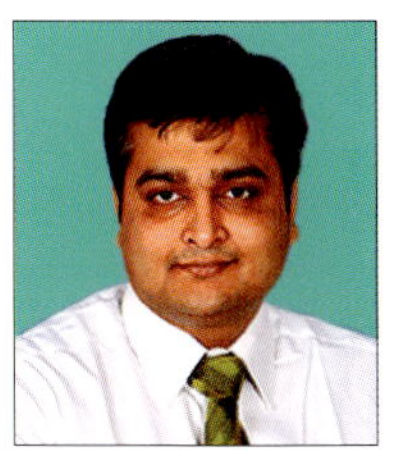

Nitesh Jain MBBS MS (General Surgery) MCh (Urology)
Consultant
Apollo Hospital (Main)
Chennai and Apollo Firstmed Hospital
Chennai, Tamil Nadu, India

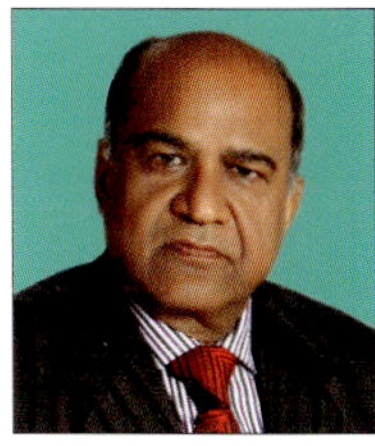

NP Gupta MBBS MS Mch FAMS DSc
Chairman
Academics and Research Division, Urology
Kidney and Urology Institute
Medanta—The Medicity
Gurugram, Haryana, India

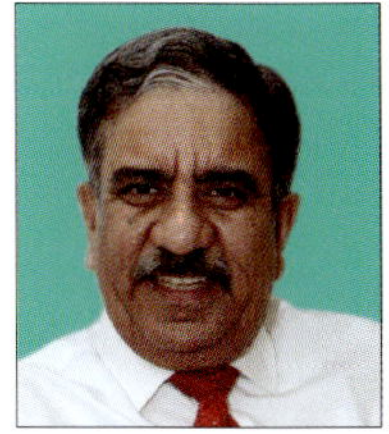

Parveen Bhatia MS FRCS (Eng) FICS FIAGES (Hon) FMAS FIMSA FAIS FALS FCLS
Chairman
Institute of Minimal Access
Metabolic and Bariatric Surgery (iMAS)
Institute of Robotic Surgery (IRS)
Sir Ganga Ram Hospital
New Delhi, India
Consultant Laparoscopic and Bariatric Surgeon
Medical Director
Global Hospital and Endosurgery Institute
New Delhi, India

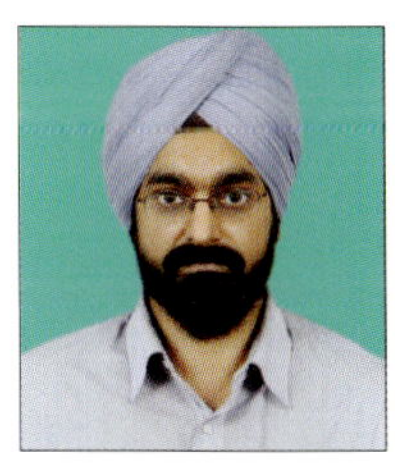

Prabhjot Singh
MS MCh (Urology) DNB (Genitourinary Surgery)
Assistant Professor
Department of Urology
All India Institute of Medical Sciences
New Delhi, India

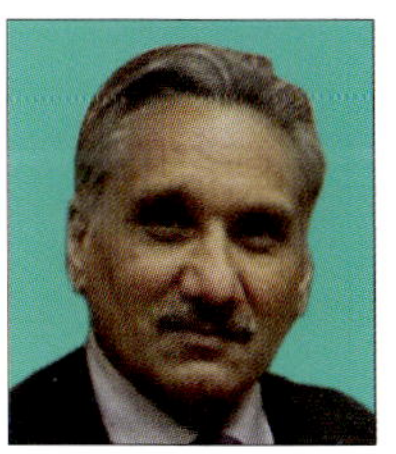

Prem Nath Dogra MCh (Urology)
Professor and Head
Department of Urology
All India Institute of Medical Sciences
New Delhi, India

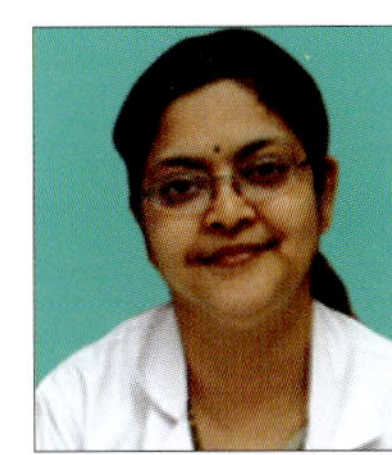

Rooma Sinha MBBS MD DNB MNAMS
Senior Consultant
Department of Minimally Invasive Gynecology and Robotic Surgery
Apollo Health City
Hyderabad, Telangana, India

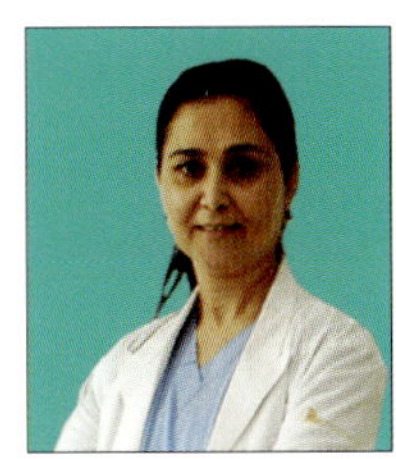

Sabhyata Gupta MD (Gynecology)
Director
Department of Gynecology and Gynec–Oncology
Medanta—The Medicity
Gurugram, Haryana, India

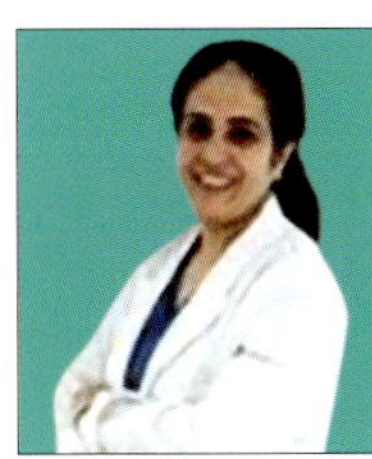

Sangeeta Khanna
Associate Director
Institute of Critical Care and Anesthesiology
Medanta—The Medicity
Gurugram, Haryana, India

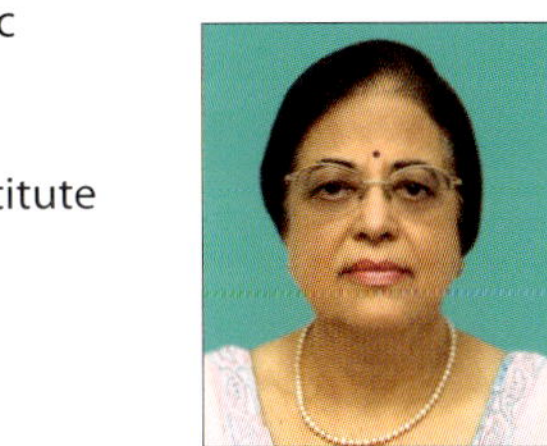

SB Khanna MD
Senior Consultant
Indraprastha Apollo Hospitals
New Delhi, India

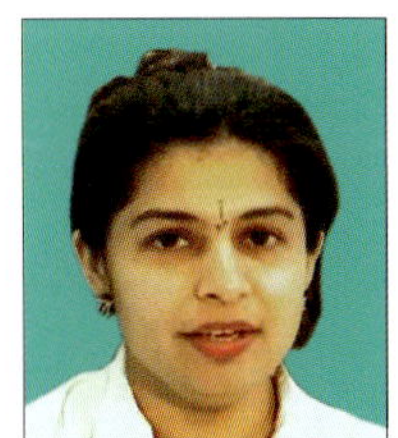

Shradha Chaudhari
Consultant Gynecologist
Medanta—The Medicity
Gurugram, Haryana, India

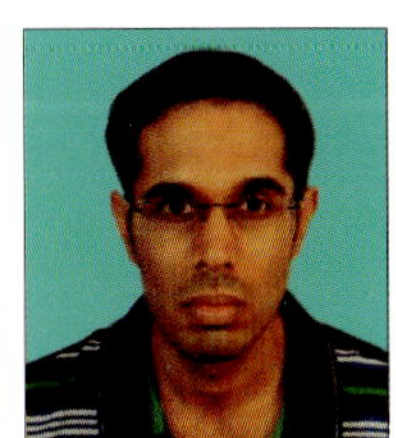

Siddharth Yadav MS
Senior Resident
Department of Urology
All India Institute of Medical Sciences
New Delhi, India

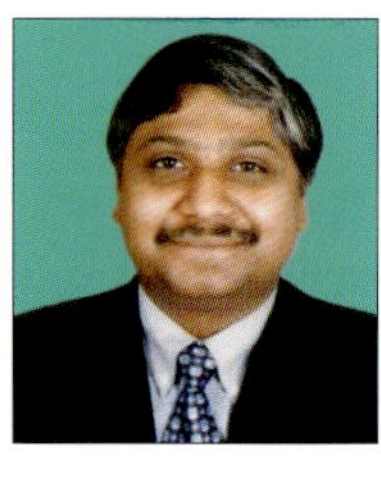

SK Chowdhary FRCS FACS MCh
Consultant Pediatric Urologist
Director, Pediatric Surgical Sciences
Indraprastha Apollo Hospitals
New Delhi, India

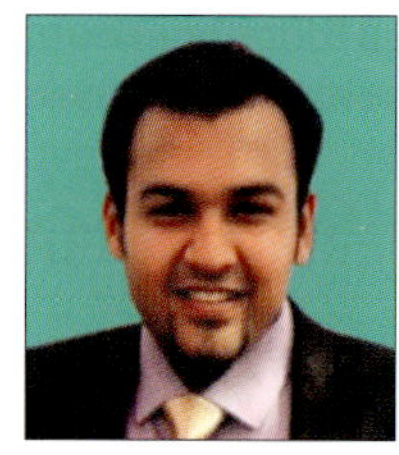

Vachan Hukkeri MBBS MS (General Surgery)
Registrar, DNB GI Surgery
Department of Surgical Gastroenterology
Indraprastha Apollo Hospital
New Delhi, India

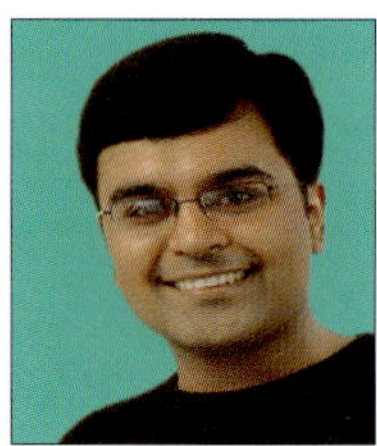

Sohrab Arora MCh Urology and Kidney Transplant (SGPGI Lucknow) (Gold Medalist)
Senior Fellow—Minimally Invasive Urology
Medanta Kidney and Urology Institute
Medanta—The Medicity
Gurugram, Haryana, India

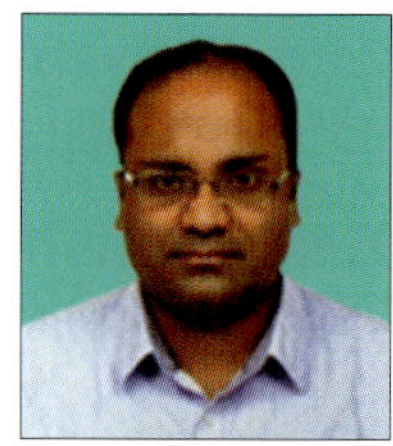

Varun Mittal MBBS MS Mch DNB
Senior Fellow
Minimal Invasive and Robotic Urology
Kidney and Urology Institute
Medanta—The Medicity
Gurugram, Haryana, India

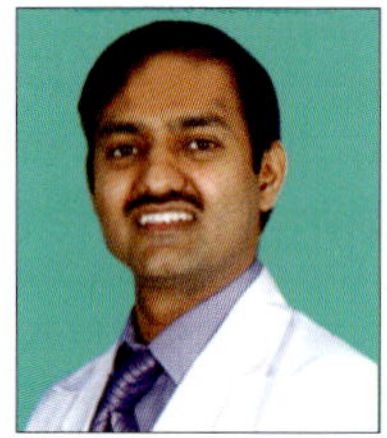

Somashekhar SP MS MCh (Onco) FRCS (Edin)
Chairman and Head
Department of Surgical Oncology
Manipal Health Enterprise
Consultant Surgical and Gynec–Onco and Robotic Surgeon
Manipal Comprehensive Cancer Centre
Manipal Hospital
Bengaluru, Karnataka, India

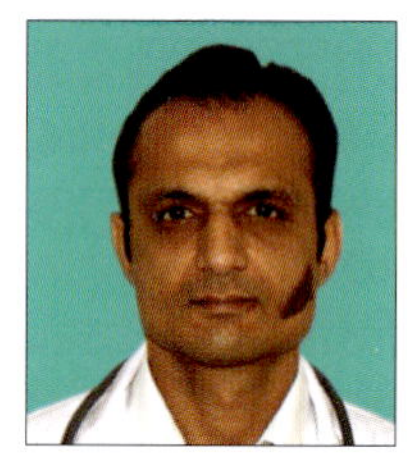

Vinay Mahendra FRCS (Urology) FRCS (Glasgow) MCh (Urology) DNB (Urology) MS (General Surgery)
Senior Consultant Urologist
Laparoscopic, Robotic Urological Surgeon and Renal Transplant Surgeon
Apollo Gleneagles Hospitals
Kolkata, West Bengal, India

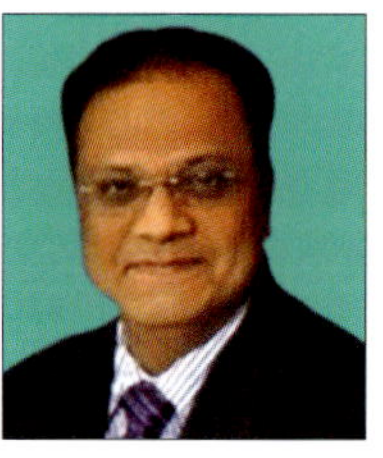

Sudhir Rawal MBBS MS MCh DNB
Director, Surgical Oncology
Chief of Uro-Gyne Surgical Oncology
Rajiv Gandhi Cancer Institute and Research Centre
New Delhi, India

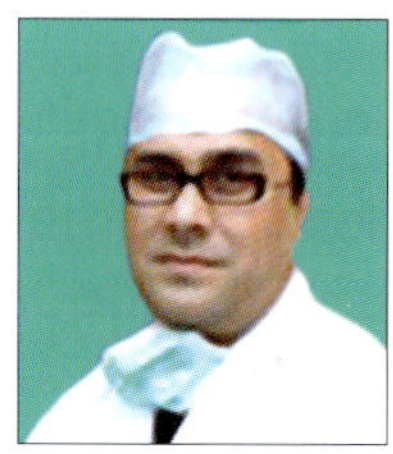

Vipin Tyagi DNB (Urology and Transplant Surgery)
Consultant Urologist
Robotic Surgeon and Kidney Transplant Surgeon
Department of Urology and Kidney Transplant Surgery
Sir Ganga Ram Hospital
New Delhi, India

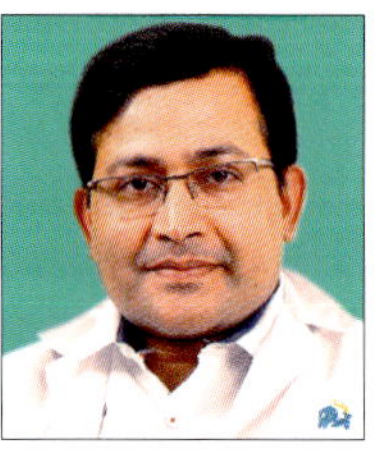

Tridibes Mondal MBBS MS (General Surgery) DNB
Consultant
Apollo Gleneagles Hospitals
Kolkata, West Bengal, India

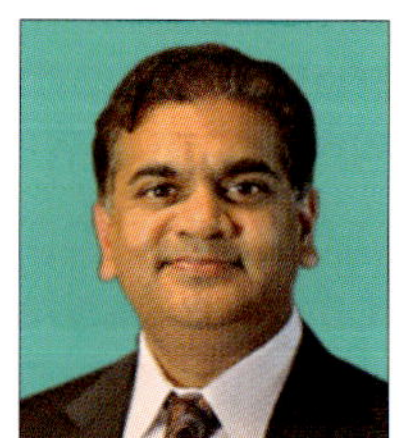

Vipul R Patel MD FACS
Medical Director, Global Robotics Institute
Florida Hospital
Florida, USA

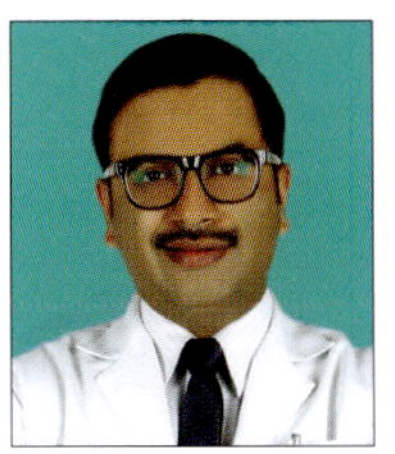

Vivek Bindal
MS MRCS (Glasgow) DNB FNB (MAS) MNAMS FACS
Consultant and Coordinator (Robotic Surgery)
Institute of Minimal Access
Metabolic and Bariatric Surgery (iMAS) and
Institute of Robotic Surgery (IRS)
Sir Ganga Ram Hospital
New Delhi, India

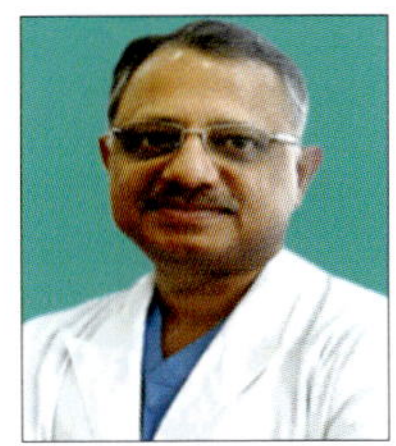

Yatin Mehta MBBS MD
Associate Director
Institute of Critical Care and Anesthesiology
Medanta—The Medicity
Gurugram, Haryana, India

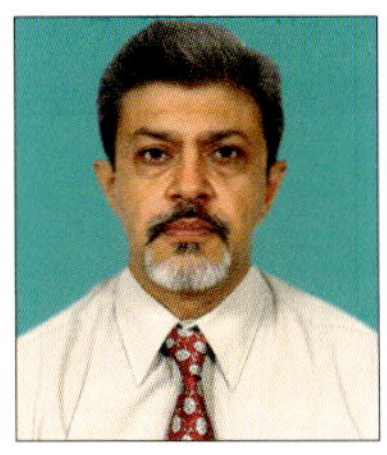

Vivek Tandon MBBS MS Mch
Senior Consultant
Laparoscopic and General Surgery
Indraprastha Apollo Hospitals
New Delhi, India

Foreword

It was the summer of 1995, I was ready to leave for Jaipur by road with a friend of mine. While getting into the rear seat of the car, I found a young gentleman already sitting in the car. My friend introduced this smart young gentleman to me as a urologist from Delhi, who was accompanying us to the same conference at Jaipur we were to attend. Within minutes, we were already mutually comfortable, conversing with each other. Soon, I learnt that he was a practicing urologist in Delhi who had returned to India a few years ago after extensive training in urology in the United Kingdom. My fellow passenger's confidence and passion for urology was obvious on his face. Our conversation was so intense that we were totally unaware of how busy and choked the highway was. Our 5-plus hours journey to Jaipur turned into a timeless event. When we stopped over for lunch at the midway, our fascinating conversation continued uninterrupted. Suddenly, we realized that we were already in Jaipur. This was my first meeting with Ajit Saxena. It was the beginning of a durable friendship and mutual professional regard for each other which has extended for the past several years. In Ajit, I found an enthusiastic urologist dedicated to his patients—and to top it up, a compassionate man inside. Even with his aging—and his nagging professional schedule—one could not combat his creativity and enterprising nature. I recall that each time I met him, I found him reinventing himself.

Just a few months ago, he compiled a series of interviews with senior urologists whom he identified to have played significant roles in establishing urology. I had to face him sitting on a hot seat in a studio environment—answering his pointed questions. His latest mission is to publish this book. *A Practical Approach to Robotic Surgery* is perhaps the first book authored by Asian authors. Myself having also been in the business of editing and publishing over the past four decades, I fully understand the onerous task of editing a multi-author book. This has heightened my respect for Ajit even more—as if there was any scope to do so.

The history of robotic surgery in India dates back to the visionary Dr Naresh Trehan installing the first *da Vinci* robot at the Escorts Heart Institute, in 2001, and using it for cardiac surgical applications. Following this, other cardiac surgery programs installed robots in different institutions in Asia. Ajit is to be credited for persuading Dr Trehan to grant him permission to organize the very first urology workshop in robotic surgery with live surgical demonstrations at the Escorts Heart Institute.

The Vattikuti Foundation (VF) rolled out its mission in India in 2010, by establishing four multispecialty robotic surgery institutes: one each in Delhi, Mumbai, Bengaluru and Hyderabad. The goal of the VF mission was to revive and foster robotic surgery in Asia. The Foundation had inherited 7 poorly performing robotic surgery programs. When the surgical robots were used, mainly they were called on to perform cardiac and urological procedures.

At the time of my writing this Foreword, robotic surgery has come a long way in the field of multispecialty robotic surgery. We now have 35 plus, and growing, installations. In 2015, Indian surgeons performed a total of 4000 procedures in 8 specialties. To date, 190 trained robotic surgeons are involved in using the robot. It is also important to note that Asian surgeons located the world over, have become the leaders in all forms of robotic surgery.

Asia is at the threshold of growth in the field of robotic surgery. Because of this, I believe, it is the most opportune time to publish a book on robotic surgery—written about Asian patients—by Asian surgeons. The need for such a book is acutely felt, as a large number of young surgeons are beelining to take it up as a career. Ajit has taken the yoke of responsibility for training our next generation surgeons to help fill in this void.

As the editor, he has been fortunate to find some of the top Indian surgical talent—who have built in their expertise in their respective specialties. He has deservedly invited them to contribute their hard-earned experience to this effort.

The book is complete in all aspects, having 7 sections: Robot and Surgery, General Surgery, Thoracic and Vascular Surgery, Gynecology, Urogynecology, Pediatric Urology and, Adult Urology. The chapter on Ergonomics is especially designed to assist the hospitals which are desirous of establishing robotic surgery—from square one.

I congratulate Dr Ajit Saxena for undertaking the arduous task of editing this very important and timely book. It is my sincere hope that this will be just the first milestone on his path of editing. I am confident he will continue updating the contents of this book periodically, keeping pace with the unprecedented growth of robotic surgery worldwide.

I sincerely hope that this book will be a useful companion not only to the growing Indian surgical fraternity but also globally—irrespective of their specialty—as they continue on their journey to surgical excellence. Furthermore, I hope it serves as a guide in their sincere efforts to give their very best to all patients. The contents of this book reinforce what the Vattikuti Foundation embarked on only a few years ago—and continue to this day. I thank Dr Saxena immensely for that.

Mahendra Bhandari
MS MCh (Urology) FAMS FNA SC DSc (Hon) MBA
Director
Robotic Surgery Education and Research
Vattikuti Urology Institute
Henry Ford Hospital
Detroit, USA
CEO
Vattikuti Foundation

From the Editor's Desk

The rules must change…

When we were students, the dictum was 'big surgeons make big incisions'. Barely two decades later, with the advent of first laparoscopy and, now, have robotic surgery, the entire concept has been changed. With these technological advancements, even the biggest of surgery can be done through smallest of incision. Thus, in the new millennium, the dictum must be revised as 'bigger the surgeon, smaller the incision'. The rules must change…

Another feature that has changed with the advent of robot, is the recognition of the ureter as a gateway to retroperitoneal and pelvic surgery. Beginners in robotic surgery will be well advised to identify the ureter as it crosses the bifurcation of common iliac artery at the pelvic brim.

This is the easiest structure to identify even in the most obese person. Squeeze the structure with a pair of non-tooth forceps to confirm the ureter by its wriggly movements. Trace the ureter upwards, and it leads one to the renal hilum. Trace the ureter downwards from the pelvic brim and it leads you to the urinary bladder. In the females, the ureter provides a solid landmark for ovarian and uterine vessels. These vessels can be safety ligated once the ureter is identified.

In short, in the current-day robotic surgery for retroperitoneal and pelvic structures, robotic surgeons will be well advised to spend an extra time in identifying the ureter and tracing it prior to embarking on surgery of the diseased tissue. Tracing the ureter after identifying it initially and respecting the relations of various structures especially pertaining to the large vessels, will go a long way in preventing catastrophic complications. The rules must change…

Preface

'From Mars to India' was the caption we used for the first-ever robotic surgery workshop held in this giant subcontinent. The year was 2005 and the surgeon was a jolly young chap by the name of Vipul Patel. Thanks to his midas touch, the conference transpired like a dream and is remembered to this date as one of the memorable seminars.

It took almost ten years for the robot to gain a foothold on Indian soil, and one of the chapters, in this book, traces the development of robotic surgery globally.

As regards the book, I am excited because the best of Asian talent has put the best foot forward to contribute toward this venture. A unique feature of the book is that all the authors are from Asia and that each chapter ends with the author's now-significant experience.

The book has been divided into seven sections encompassing the major specialties using the robot. Section 1 is a 'must-read' not only because it deals with the historical landmarks, but also because it emphasizes the importance of ergonomics in robotic surgery. Do go through it; it is particularly relevant for the younger generation. The small pointers tucked throughout the primary chapter might prolong your surgical career by leaps and bounds. Also included are anesthesia details, which underscore the vital role anesthetists play in the overall early recovery of the patient.

Finally, this book comes with a high-definition DVD visual demonstration, which will be a delight for the beginner and veteran robotic surgeon alike.

It is my dream to see India as the hub of robotic tourism in the immediate future...and a vision of a robotic surgeon performing surgery, sitting anywhere on earth, on persons living in outer space in the near future!

In the end, if you have any suggestion/comment, please do not hesitate to write to me at *ajitsaxena@hotmail.com*.

Friends, together we can do it!

Ajit Saxena

Obituary

K Subramaniam, who was widely known as 'KS', was instrumental in taking the benefits of robotic surgery, a cutting-edge technology, to a host of surgeons and hospital administrators in India. He diligently created tie-ups with a wide range of institutions to fulfil the dream of taking India to the next level of surgery. KS put into place a series of programs that helped more and more hospitals acquire robotic systems, and also assisted surgeons get trained and certified in robotics to help create immensely successful robotic centers.

KS also painstakingly set up the functions of an organization and a team that could support the sales and service and technical maintenance required to seamlessly run da Vinci robotic surgery systems installed across the length and breadth of the country. At the organizational level, KS was an inspirational leader who led by example. Indeed, he was a powerhouse of energy who would always find solutions to any problem and drive execution with great passion and zeal.

The robotic surgery fraternity knew him as an ever-active, hardworking workaholic and as a soft compassionate man who would make friends for life in an interaction of a few minutes, while at the same time, with a straightforward approach and a code of integrity—a man who always promised what he could deliver. The vacuum created by his loss shall remain.

KS will always be remembered as a leader, a great friend and a good human being.

RIP

Acknowledgments

First of all, I am grateful to my publishers, who not only gave me a long rope but also contributed actively in making this 'one of its kind' book possible.

I am grateful to Dr Praveen Bhatia, and his team for contributing most of the top quality, edited videos that come to you on a DVD with this book.

I would be failing in my duty if I do not thank my team, Ms Swati Thapar, Mr Anuj Ahuja, Ms Shuchita Singh, Mr Amit Rana and Ms Chandani Alaudhin, for their untiring efforts. I sincerely thank my wife Dr Neeta, who has become a virtual robotic surgeon in her untiring effort to get the book published on schedule. My thanks also go to my two lovely daughters Pooja and Roopa, who lifted my spirits when the chips were down.

Contents

Section 1: Robot and Surgery

1. Robotic Surgery: Past, Present and Future 3

Naresh Trehan

Past 3
Present 3
Future of Robotic Surgery 5

2. Ergonomics 6

Megha Bhatnagar, Aditi Midha

Impact on Musculoskeletal System 6
Muscular Load and Disorders 6
Challenges in the Operation Room 7
Appropriate Posture 7
Need for Exercise and Physical Activity 7
Postural Advice to Counter Effects of Work 8
Quick Fit Break that Can Help! 8

3. Immunofluorescence and Robotic Surgery 10

Vivek Bindal, Anand Kumar Yadav

Clinical Applications of Immunofluorescence Imaging in General Surgery 11
Other Applications in Robotic Surgery 14
Future Applications 14

4. Anesthesia 17

Sangeeta Khanna, Jyotirmoy Das, Yatin Mehta

Preoperative Preparation 17
Intraoperative Management 17
Patient Positioning 18
Few Systemic Considerations in Steep Trendelenburg Position 19
Anesthesia for Transoral Robotic Surgery 20
Robot-assisted Minimally Invasive Renal Transplantation 20
Robot-assisted Esophagectomy 21

Section 2: General Surgery

5. Robot-assisted Sleeve Gastrectomy 27
Parveen Bhatia, Vivek Bindal, Anand Kumar Yadav
Surgical Procedure 27
Review of Literature 31
Discussion 31

6. Robot-assisted Roux-en-Y Gastric Bypass 33
Parveen Bhatia, Vivek Bindal, Anand Kumar Yadav
Advantages of Robotic Roux-en-Y Gastric Bypass 33
Surgical Techniques 34
Perioperative Care 37
Robotic RYGB: Current Status and Future 38

7. Robotic Surgery for Benign Colorectal Diseases 40
Deepak Govil, Vivek Tandon, Vachan Hukkeri, Satyaprakash Jindal, Adithya GK
Right Hemicolectomy 40
Transverse Colectomy 41
Left and Sigmoid Colectomy 42
Total Proctocolectomy with Pouch Ileo-anal Anastomoses 43
Rectopexy 43

8. Carcinoma Rectum 47
Somashekhar SP
Laparoscopic Surgery in Rectal Cancer 47
Preoperative Preparation and Precautions 48
Anesthesia 48
Robotics in Rectal Cancer 50
Short-term Clinical Outcomes 50
Indian Experience 52
Ongoing Trials 52

9. Robotic Surgery for Bile Duct Tumors 55
Vivek Bindal, Anand Kumar Yadav
Surgical Treatment 55
Palliative Surgery 59
Liver Transplantation 59
Postoperative Outcomes 59

Section 3: Thoracic and Vascular Surgery

10. Thymus 63

Arvind Kumar, Belal Bin Asaf

Robotic Surgery for Thymus and Anterior Mediastinum **63**

Preoperative Preparation and Precautions for Patients Undergoing Thymectomy **63**

Anesthesia and Position **64**

Port Placement **65**

Docking **65**

11. Lung Resection 68

Belal Bin Asaf, Arvind Kumar

Indications **68**

Preoperative Preparation and Precautions **68**

Anesthesia and Positioning **68**

Port Placement **68**

Docking **69**

Steps of Surgery **69**

Postoperative Care **70**

Complications and Their Management **70**

12. Esophagectomy 72

Arvind Kumar, Belal Bin Asaf

Preoperative Preparation and Precautions **72**

Anesthesia and Positioning **72**

Port Placement **73**

Steps of Surgery **73**

Postoperative Care **73**

13. Vascular Surgery 76

Arvind Kumar, Belal Bin Asaf

Anesthesia and Positioning **76**

Status of Robotic Aortic Surgery **77**

Section 4: Gynecology

14. Myomectomy 81

Rooma Sinha, Madhumati S, B Rupa

Preoperative Assessment and Role of Magnetic Resonance Imaging **82**

Role of Intrauterine Manipulation **82**

Port Placement, Positioning and Docking **82**
Techniques to Reduce Blood Loss **83**
Hysterotomy **84**
Enucleation **84**
Suturing Techniques **85**
Adhesion Prevention **86**
Fibroid Retreival **86**
Hybrid Technique **86**

15. Challenges in Robotic Myomectomy 88
Kiranabala Dash, SB Khanna
Preoperative Preparation and Precautions **88**
Anesthesia and Port Placement **88**
Steps of Surgery **89**

16. Robotics in Benign Gynecology 92
Mala Srivastava, Ankita Srivastava
Surgical Evolution is Nothing New **92**
Indications **93**
Hysterectomy **93**
Myomectomy **94**
Tubal Reanastomosis **94**
Sacrocolpopexy **95**
Endometriosis **96**
Vesicovaginal Fistula **97**
Cervical Cerclage **98**

17. Sentinel Node Mapping in Gynecological Cancers 101
Anupama Rajanbabu
Background **101**
Technique of Sentinel Lymph Node Mapping using Indocyanine Green **101**
Learning Curve **103**

18. Robotic Staging Surgery for Endometrial Cancer 105
Anupama Rajanbabu
Preoperative Evaluation and Preparation **105**
Patient Positioning **105**
Uterine Manipulator **106**
Port Placement **106**
Docking **107**
Instrument Placement **108**

Cautery Settings 108
Surgical Technique 108
Hysterectomy 109
Pelvic Lymphadenectomy 109

19. Endometrial Cancer and Cervical Cancer 111
Sabhyata Gupta, Shradha Chaudhari
Pretreatment Evaluation 111
Surgical Staging Overview 111
Routes of Surgery 111
Comparison of Robotic Route with Other Routes 113
Robotic Surgery in Cervical Cancers 114
Robot-assisted Radical Hysterectomy 114
Comparison of Robotic Route to Laparoscopy and Open Route 115

20. Ovarian Cystectomy 117
Neelam Suri
Preoperative Evaluation 117
Surgical Approach 118
Specific Considerations 119
Suturing in Ovarian Surgery 123

Section 5: **Urogynecology**

21. Vesicovaginal Fistula Repair 127
Nitesh Jain, K Ramesh
History and Physical Examination 127
Investigations 127
Repair of Vesicovaginal Fistula 127
Tips and Tricks 129

Section 6: **Pediatric Urology**

22. Pediatric Urology: The First Hundred Cases 133
DK Kandpal, SK Chowdhary
Starting the Pediatric Robotic Program 133
Pyeloplasty for Pelviureteric Junction Obstruction 134
Ureteric Reimplantation for Refluxing/Obstructed/Ectopic Ureters, Retrocaval Ureter 135
Partial Nephrectomy/Hemi-nephroureterectomy/Nephroureterectomy for Complex Renal Anomalies 136
Augmentation Cystoplasty with Ureteric Reimplantation 136

Section 7: Adult Urology

23. Radical Prostatectomy 141

Hariharan Palayapalayam Ganapathi, Kenneth J Palmer, Gabriel Ogaya-Pines, Travis Rogers, Vipul R Patel

Preoperative Preparation 141

24. Role of Pelvic Lymphadenectomy in Robot-assisted Radical Prostatectomy 148

Varun Mittal, NP Gupta

Lymphatic Drainage of Prostate 148

Imaging for Lymph Node Involvement 148

Indications of Pelvic Lymphadenectomy 150

Extent of Pelvic Lymphadenectomy 151

Survival Benefit with Pelvic Lymphadenectomy 152

Complications Associated with Pelvic Lymphadenectomy 152

Robot-assisted Pelvic Lymphadenectomy; Current Status 153

25. Radical Cystoprostatectomy 157

Sudhir Rawal

Patient Selection 157

Preoperative Preparation 157

Robotic Radical Cystectomy 158

Postoperative Care 159

Technical Tips and Tricks 160

Complications 160

Evidence 161

26. Partial Nephrectomy 162

Ajit Saxena

Patient Selection 162

Preoperative Preparation 162

Technique 163

Robotic Partial Nephrectomy (RPN) 165

Postoperative Care 166

Technical Tips and Tricks 166

Complications 167

Evidence 168

27. Donor Nephrectomy 169

Vinay Mahendra, Jaydip Bhadra Roy, Tridibes Mondal

Preoperative Investigations 169

Surgical Steps 169

28. Adrenalectomy 172
Sohrab Arora, Gagan Gautam
Patient Selection 172
Work-up and Preoperative Preparation 173
Technique 173
Postoperative Care 177
Technical Tips and Tricks 178
Complications 178
Evidence 178

29. Urolithiasis: Expanding the Horizons of Robotic Surgery 180
Siddharth Yadav, Prabhjot Singh, Prem Nath Dogra
Robotic Stone Surgery 180
Robotic Renal Stone Surgery 181
Steps of Surgery 183
Robotic Ureterolithotomy 185
Steps of Surgery 186
Postoperative Care 187
Outcomes, Complications and Management 187

30. Pyeloplasty 190
Manu Gupta
Diagnosis of Pelvi-ureteric Junction (PUJ) Obstruction 190
Indications for Robot-assisted Surgery 190
Treatment 190
Robot-assisted Pyeloplasty 191
Operation Theater Ergonomics 191
Technique 191
Results 192
Different Surgical Techniques 192
Discussion 193

31. Ureteric Reimplantation 195
Vipin Tyagi
Indications 195
Type of Ureteric Reimplantation 195
Preoperative Evaluation and Preparation 195
Operating Room Configuration and Patient Positioning 196
Trocar Placement 196
Psoas Hitch 197
Boari Flap 197
Postoperative Management 197
Complications 197

Index 199

Hello Mr Robot

The only robotic system so far available is the da Vinci Surgical System (Intuitive Surgical, Mountain View, California, United States).

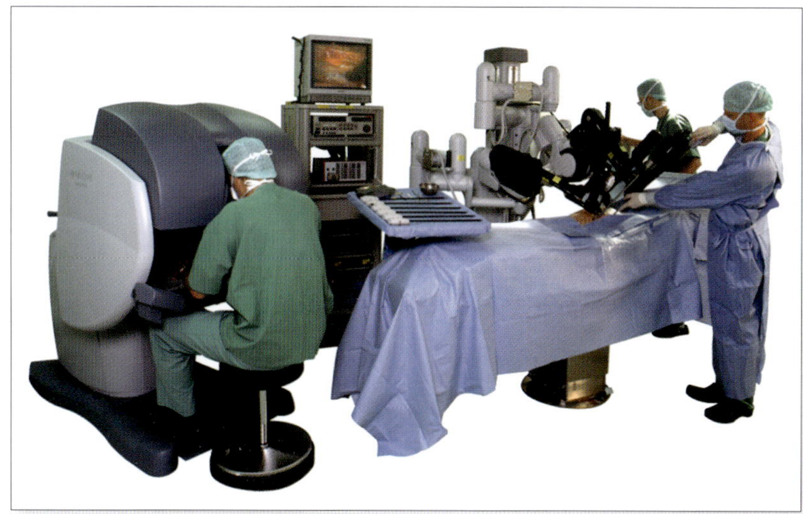

This consists of a console at some distance from the patient where the surgeon sits while operating, and the robotic cart with its three or four robotic arms, which is in close proximity to the patient. Various instruments attached to the robotic arms, are inserted into the patient through small incisions. The console provides a magnified high-definition three-dimensional view of the operating field through a stereo endoscope fitted to one of the robotic arms, whose visual field and angle of vision are adjustable. The surgeon manipulates two-finger joysticks (finger and wrist movements) at the console while watching the surgical field through the visual system. Movements of the surgeon's hands are transmitted through the robot to the robotic arms, so that equivalent but scaled movements of the surgical instruments are made within the surgical field. The instruments have 7 degrees of movement freedom and hand tremor is filtered out. The da Vinci system appears able to overcome many of the problems that characterize laparoscopic resection. Initially, the three-dimensional high-definition camera is under the direct control of the surgeon, and the double optical system makes consistently clear vision more likely. Furthermore, the tremor-filtered, multiple-degree-of-movement instruments, which can be scaled relative to the surgeon's hand movements, permit more precise dissection in narrow spaces and render the more difficult steps of the operation easier. Tissue retraction with the robot is also easier, since the third arm can be used as a fixed retractor, and is always manipulated by the surgeon. These potential advantages within the narrow space of the pelvis have been shown to be translated into concrete advantages for robotic radical prostatectomy, and in our opinion, the excellent ergonomics and precise dissection offered by the robotic system can be helpful in colorectal surgery also for vessel ligation and flexure mobilization amongst other surgeries. This is why there is a standardized 'fully robotic' technique for left colon and rectal resection. The robot allows for 7 degrees of motion versus the limited 4 degrees of motion in laparoscopy.

SECTION 1

Robot and Surgery

- **Robotic Surgery: Past, Present and Future**
  Naresh Trehan
- **Ergonomics**
  Megha Bhatnagar, Aditi Midha
- **Immunofluorescence and Robotic Surgery**
  Vivek Bindal, Anand Kumar Yadav
- **Anesthesia**
  Sangeeta Khanna, Jyotirmoy Das, Yatin Mehta

CHAPTER

1

Robotic Surgery: Past, Present and Future

Naresh Trehan

INTRODUCTION

Robotic surgery and robotically assisted surgical procedures are newer technological developments in the field of minimally invasive surgical procedures, which enhance the capability of a surgeon. A surgeon can control the robotic instruments directly by a remote manipulator like telemanipulator or through the computer during any minimal invasive robotic surgery.

Robotic surgeries carry higher accuracy, small incision, less blood loss, decreased pain and early healing. Major advances in robotic surgery now offer three-dimensional view of surgical field with magnification.

During robotic surgeries, the surgeon need not have to stand throughout the duration of procedure and will not get tired easily. The hand tremors can be filtered out by the robot. The surgical robotic system can work continuously and easily used by different surgical teams in shifts.

The da Vinci system is a surgical robot which is Food and Drug Administration (FDA) approved. Robotic surgeries on the heart, gastrointestinal tract, kidney, urethra, prostate can be carried out using the da Vinci system.

The US FDA has also approved Zeus surgical system, which has three robotic arms. The Automated Endoscopic System for Optimal Positioning (AESOP) Robotic System is a robotic arm which can respond to voice commands and hold endoscope.

Robotic surgery is evolving as a significantly promising newer technology and considered revolutionary by many. However, this emerging field of robotic surgery has been sometimes, criticized by considering the facts that robots are expensive and market driven.

PAST

The earliest robotic surgery dates back to 1983 when orthopedic robotic surgery was conducted with the help of robot named the "Arthrobot". A robot called PUMA 560 was used for neurosurgical biopsy in 1985. At Imperial College, London, a robotic surgery on prostate was conducted in 1985 by the robotic system PROBOT. PROBOT was specifically designed for transurethral resection of prostate. Another robotic system named ROBDOC was designed to assist hip replacement surgeries in 1992.

Various organizations such as Intuitive Surgical and Computer Motion made more development of systems associated with robotic surgeries. They introduced da Vinci Surgical System and ZEUS robotic surgical systems.

The da Vinci Surgical System consists of three components. They are console for the surgeon, robotic cart containing four arms (one for the camera and other three arms for instruments) and a high definition three-dimensional vision system.

Towards the end of 1980s the minimally invasive surgery (MIS) or minimal access surgery became famous and revolutionized the concept by inserting the instruments in body by making small incisions.

In 1990s, the laparoscopic revolution happened and many surgical procedures were changed from traditionally done open surgeries to minimal access procedures. Even though there was decrease in collateral surgical trauma, there were inherent problems which included difficult wrist articulation, no tremor filtration, fulcrum effects, loss of three dimensional vision and poor ergonomics. Many of these were eliminated when robotic surgery evolved and made a transit from laparoscopy. Robotic surgery slowly emerged as effective procedure which could address the limitations of laparoscopic operations.

PRESENT

Clinical Applications

Robotic surgery has been conducted for many male and female patients for varieties of indications in different age groups. In pediatric patients, robotic surgery may be beneficial for Kasai procedure in biliary atresia, choledochal cyst repair and tumor excisions and reconstructive procedures in thoracic or abdominal region.

In gynecological surgeries, the Robotic procedures had shown good results in patients who had undergone hysterectomy and myomectomy. Robotic surgery has been considered beneficial in cases of tubal reconstruction and pelvic reconstruction procedures.

In general surgery, robotic surgery has been applied for antireflux procedures, cholecystectomy, gastroplasty surgery for obesity, hernia repair and colorectal procedures. Robotic surgery is mostly suitable for conditions affected in one quadrant of the abdomen, which has challenging access.

Robotic surgery is considered advantageous in urological procedures, which are minimally invasive. Better outcomes in robotic surgery have been seen in patients who had undergone robotic radical prostatectomy, robotic radical cystectomy, pyeloplasty, partial or complete nephrectomy and ureteral reimplantation.

In cardiovascular surgeries with robotic assistance, encouraging results have been shown in patients who had undergone robotic-assisted coronary bypass grafting and mitral valve repair.

In otorhinolaryngology, patients requiring transoral oncologic resections of tumors in the area of pharynx or larynx have benefited from robotic surgery.

Current Robotic Surgery Set-up and Technique

Commonly used surgical robot is the da Vinci surgical system which is approved by the FDA since 2000. The da Vinci robotic surgical platform uses four overhead arms. The da Vinci robotic instruments have longer shafts and the endoscope which has a camera built into its distal tip **(Fig. 1.1)**.

The da Vinci Xi system follows a standardized approach for positioning of the robot over the camera port and then targeting of the camera is done before docking of the remaining robotic ports. The robotic camera easily fits into the 8 mm trocar which allows its insertion into any of the four robotic arms.

The Zeus system consists of a surgeon control console and three table-mounted robotic arms. The robotic arms present on right and left side can replicate the right and left arm of the robotic surgeon. The third arm is a voice-controlled robotic endoscope used for better visualization (AESOP).

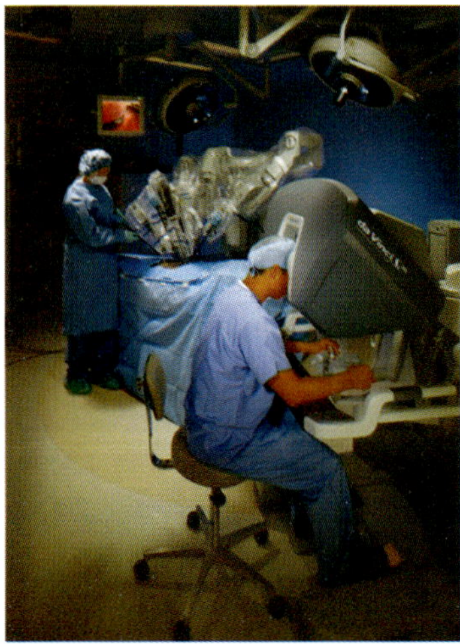

Fig. 1.1: da Vinci robotic surgery set-up

Current Robotic Systems

Many robotic systems had been approved by the US FDA for specific surgeries. ROBODOC was used in past to core out femur during hip replacement operation. The Zeus and the da Vinci system had been used by several surgical disciplines which include gallbladder surgeries, cardiac valve repair, radical prostate surgery, reversing the tubal ligations, gastro-intestinal operations, nephrectomy, and renal transplant. Day-by-day many institutions are procuring these robotic systems to perform many types of surgery including coronary artery grafting with less morbidity.

Robotic surgeries are highly beneficial in cases of intra-abdominal microsurgery where manipulations are done in very small spaces. Since early 2000 general surgical interventions such as esophageal and pancreatic surgery were done with the help of da Vinci device. Currently commonly done cardiac surgeries are septal defect repairs, valve repairs and coronary artery bypass. Robotic colorectal surgeries are being done in many of malignant colon and rectal lesions. There is better visualization of pelvic nerves during robotic surgery and less chance of nerve injury by which many postoperative complications of impotence or incontinence are avoided. In urology, robotic surgeries are most popular. Robotic surgical procedures are mostly done for surgery of kidney, prostate and urinary bladder cancers due to difficultly in accessing the anatomical structures.

Current Robotic Surgery Advantages

The robotic systems recently available have instruments which offer higher degrees of freedom to enhance the surgeon's capacity to manipulate. Robotic systems are designed to compensate tremors by hardware or software filters.

The robotic system can reduce the fulcrum effect by making the instrument manipulations intuitive and avoids twists or turns from awkward position.

Currently robotic surgery has proven itself to be of significant value, particularly in inaccessible places in comparison to conventional procedures. Robotic surgeries are safe operations with decreased morbidity. Robotic surgeries had given significant benefits to patients by decreased blood loss and transfusions, less pain, short hospital stay of patients and faster recovery. The minimally invasive robotic approach has slowly becoming a standard of care for many small size tumors.

Robotic surgeries involve the use of a sophisticated robotic device (known as the da Vinci Surgical Robotic System) with wristed instrumentation to permit the surgeon to dissect while controlling these instruments from a surgeon console externally.

Most of the recent advantages in robotic surgeries ensure its development and continued expansion. Currently, the sophisticated control and multiple degrees of freedom provided by Zeus and da Vinci systems offer greater mobility and no tremor without any compromise in visual field.

Evidence

A study by Cadiere et al. evaluated the feasibility of robotic surgeries in 146 patients. Robotic surgeries were done with help of a da Vinci robot, which included thirty-nine antireflux operations, fortyeight cholecystectomies, twenty-eight tubal re-anastomoses, ten gastroplasties in obese patient, three inguinal hernia repairs, three intrarectal operations, two hysterectomies, two cardiac operations, two prostatectomies, two AV fistulas, one lumbar sympathectomy, one appendectomy, one laryngeal exploration, one varicocele procedure, one endometriosis and one neosalpingostomy. The study found that the robotic surgeries will be most effective in abdominal microsurgery or for manipulations in small spaces.[1]

Damiano et al. had conducted a multicenter clinical trial on robotic-assisted coronary artery bypass grafting. The study had 32 patients scheduled for primary coronary surgery who underwent endoscopic anastomosis of the left internal thoracic artery to left anterior descending artery. Two-month follow up revealed a graft patency of 93%. The study had opined that robotic-assisted coronary bypass grafting as feasible procedure.[2]

In a study Mohr et al. used the da Vinci system to conduct coronary artery bypass graft procedure on 131 patients and repair of diseased mitral valve on 17 patients. They concluded that robotic systems can be used safely in patients to perform robotic cardiac surgery.[3]

FUTURE OF ROBOTIC SURGERY

Many people imagine that robotics is all about automation. In future robotic systems, there might be chance for a surgeon to program the procedure and simply supervise while the robot performs the surgery.

The robotic surgical procedures are expected to play crucial roles in future. Hence there should be emphasis on training of robotic surgery in residency or postgraduation courses for surgeons in academic centers.

There are advances happening in robotic surgery in areas of new tissue anastomosis procedures, improved robotic instruments and digitally integrating the existing robotic technologies in many disciplines of surgery.

In future, there is a possibility that there could be fusion of images from CT scan or MRI during surgery and before surgery to help the surgeon to identify the pathology and dissect.

In future, the data can be stored to rehearse any complex robotic operation and make long distance consultation and assessments. The advances in computer graphics (CG) and simulation technology aided by computers will take robotic surgeries to a new level.

Next generation of robotic technology will involve non-contact tools during navigating or intervention. The robotic surgery will be scarless in future with help of laser scalpel. Mobile robots may be introduced in future for monitoring postoperative condition of a patient.

REFERENCES

1. Cadierre GB, Himpens J. Feasibility of robotic laparoscopic surgery: 146 cases. World J Surg. 2001;25:1467-77.
2. Damiano RJJr, Tabaie HA, Mack MJ, et al. Initial multicenter clinical trial of robotically assisted coronary artery bypass grafting. Ann Thorac Surg. 2001;72:1263-8.
3. Mohr FW, Falk V, Diegeler A, et al. Computer-enhanced "robotic" cardiac surgery: experience in 148 patients. J Thorac Cardiovasc Surg. 2001;121:842-53.

BIBLIOGRAPHY

1. Ahmed K, Khan MS, Vats A, Nagpal K, Priest O, Patel V, Vecht JA, Ashrafian H, et al. Current status of robotic assisted pelvic surgery and future developments. International Journal of Surgery. 2009;7(5):431-40.
2. Ballantyne GH, Moll F. The da Vinci telerobotic surgical system: the virtual operative field and telepresence surgery. Surg Clin North Am. 2003;83:1293-304.
3. Ballantyne GH. The pitfalls of laparoscopic surgery: challenges for robotics and telerobotic surgery. Surg Laparosc Endosc Percutan Tech. 2002;12:1-5.
4. Camarillo DB, Krummel TM, Salisbury JK. Jr Robotic technology in surgery: past, present, and future. Am J Surg. 2004;188(4A Suppl):2S-15S.
5. Chauhan S, Coelho RF, Kalan S, Satava RM, Patel VR. Evolution of robotic surgery: past, present, and future. In: Patel VR (Ed). Robotic Urologic Surgery. 2nd edition. London: Springer-Verlag; 2012. pp. 3-10.
6. Gomez G. Sabiston Textbook of Surgery. 17th edition. Philadelphia, Pa: Elsevier Saunders; 2004. Emerging Technology in Surgery: Informatics, Electronics, Robotics.
7. Jeong W, Kumar R, Menon M. Past, present and future of urological robotic surgery. Investigative and Clinical Urology. 2016;57(2):75-83. doi:10.4111/icu.2016.57.2.75.
8. Lanfranco AR, Castellanos AE, Desai JP, Meyers WC. Robotic Surgery: A Current Perspective. Annals of Surgery. 2004;239(1):14-21. doi:10.1097/01.sla.0000103020.19595.7d.
9. Mohr FW, Falk V, Diegeler A, et al. Computer-enhanced "robotic" cardiac surgery: experience in 148 patients. J Thorac Cardiovasc Surg. 2001;121:842-53.
10. Morris B. Robotic Surgery: Applications, limitations, and impact on surgical education. Medscape General Medicine. 2005;7(3):72.
11. Satava RM. How the future of surgery is changing: robotics, tele-surgery, surgical simulators and other advanced technologies. J Chirurgie. 2009;5:311-25.

CHAPTER

2

Ergonomics

Megha Bhatnagar, Aditi Midha

INTRODUCTION

Robot-assisted surgery (RAS) is minimally invasive surgery which is very technically demanding and needs a lot of concentration to perform the task. Though, RAS has reduced the physical stress on the surgeon that is associated with an increased prevalence of musculoskeletal pain and injury as compared to laproscopic surgery; further ergonomic integration is required in the operating room to improve efficiency, safety and comfort of the operating team.[1]

Ergonomics is mainly derived from two Greek words, 'ergo' means work and 'noma' means law of systems.[2] Ergonomics is an applied science concerned with designing tools and procedures which maximize efficiency and safety.[3] Human muscle and physical activities, fatigue and somatic performance, work station design, hand tool design, product design, occupational health, psychology and cognitive ergonomics, anthropometry and kinesiology, human computer interaction, interface design, manual material handling, work/rest schedules, aesthetics and environmental ergonomics form some main parts of ergonomics scope.[4] If these ergonomic principles are not optimally used, surgeons experience physical discomforts during and after the surgeries. Sensorial ergonomics, manipulation and visualization can improve precision, dexterity and confidence while providing physical comfort for surgeons. These can together improve outcome and reduce stress.[5] Proper instrument and operating theatre designs are critical to avoid human error during RAS.[6] Surgeons performing need to hold static postures for long hours. It has been demonstrated that static postures are more disabling and harmful than dynamic one because the muscles and tendons from lactic acid and toxins when held in static posture.[7]

IMPACT ON MUSCULOSKELETAL SYSTEM

It is hypothesized that the Robotic surgical systems may help resolve some musculoskeletal disorders if the ergonomics are utilized to its optimal level. The chief surgeon is seated at the console away from the patient in a much more ergonomic posture than the traditional patient side surgeon. The finger-tip controls allow intuitive rather than fulcrum type control over the laproscopic instruments, thereby reducing the fatigue in the upper extremity and neck. The complex surgical tasks like suturing are made easier by Endo-wrist technology which allows an overall 7 degrees of freedom as compared to 4 degrees of freedom for laproscopy. The 3D stereoscopic vision with enhanced magnifications and motion scaling of surgeon's hand movements down to site of operation is another advantage.[8]

Many musculoskeletal pain and injuries were associated with laproscopic sugery by Hemat et al. in 2001. Neck, back, forearm, shoulder and eye strains were among the common complains.[9] These factors can increase the overall fatigue of the surgeon and restrict the number of procedures that can be comfortably performed by a single surgeon in a given operative session. Similar problems can also be seen in surgeons using the Robotic surgical systems if they do not use the ergonomic freedom provided optimally.

MUSCULAR LOAD AND DISORDERS

The most common method of evaluating the muscular load is electromyography (EMG). Lundervold[10] used EMG to investigate activity in patients with so called 'occupation myalgia.' 'Occupation myalgia' was defined as pain in muscles overstrained as a result of unvaried static work. A number of people using visual display units (VDU) characterized by low level of muscle activities, especially in the trapezius and no safe lower limit of muscle activity might exist.[11] Low static contractions during work may result in a recruiting pattern in which only type I muscle fibers are used and this may lead to selective motor unit fatigue and damage. This can lead to further disorders of the neck and shoulder.[12] A study proved that non-neutral postures of the neck (i.e flexion or extension), shoulder (i.e. flexion and abduction) are found to be associated with neck/shoulder/hand/arm disorders.[13,14] Extreme position of wrist may increase the risk factor for musculoskeletal disorders of hand and wrist like carpal tunnel syndrome.[15,16] Repetitive work also increases the risk of musculoskeletal symptoms in wrist and forearm.[15] A combination of high repetitiveness in fingers and wrist, the static loading imposed on the thumb to grip console, the prolonged extension and ulnar deviation of the wrist for long durations can give rise musculoskeletal disorders like tendonitis, tenosynovitis, trigger finger, epicondylitis, De Quervain's syndrome etc. In a critical review of epidemiologic evidence for work related musculoskeletal disorders of neck, upper extremity and low back, it may be concluded that static work postures are worse than heavy weight lifting dynamic working postures.[15] Thus, we can conclude that recognition, evaluation and correction of work stations and environment is very important in order to provide comfort while working for long hours. Thereby, increasing efficiency and reducing the risk of injury.

CHALLENGES IN THE OPERATION ROOM

Surgery is a high stress task performed by a team. Medical interventions may be performed in sitting or standing for long hours. There may be some physical loads due to static work, repetitive movements, bending or twisting, compensated environment like difficulty to reach for instruments or poor visual ergonomics, muscular tension due to tiring sounds, working long hours and lack of fluid intake. Psychological strain is another aspect which one has to continuously deal with while in the operation room. Research indicates that repetitive movements carried in a stressful environment more than double the risk of pain and injury.[17]

APPROPRIATE POSTURE

Chief Surgeon: At Console (Fig. 2.1)

From an ergonomic perspective, a surgeon at the Console when seated must sit at a supported chair having a backrest to support the natural curvature of the spine. The top of the viewing chamber should be at or below the eye level so that the resting position of the eyes is at roughly 30° down from horizontal. Elbows must be held close by the side of the body at roughly 90° such that the joystick that is to be used for surgery is not too far from the elbow. An added feature to form the robot is the forearm support to rest the arms. This is crucial at the same time must be kept in mind that hands ought to move from the support in order to relieve pressure. The sitting should be ideal ie buttocks back into the seat, thighs resting on the seat such that the hips-knees and ankles maintain a 90-90-90° angle with respect to each other.

Assistant Surgeon (Fig. 2.1)

The bedside surgeon must be seated in a more or less parallel angle to the bed and the monitor/screen placed directly in front of him at a minimum distance of 8–10 feet for better viewing and reduced eye strain.

NEED FOR EXERCISE AND PHYSICAL ACTIVITY

Our bodies are said to be healthy if they are able to maintain their various functions. This capacity of the body is maintained by the optimal quantity of movement, weight and recovery. Physical activity and exercise help to create a reserve capacity relative to the work demands and at the same time also reduces the risks of having the Musculoskeletal disorders. As an additive effect, exercise releases endorphins in the brain which create a rejuvenated state of mental well-being and thus psychological relaxation. The hallmark of a healthy performance is variations, along with a fine balance of work, rest and recovery.[17]

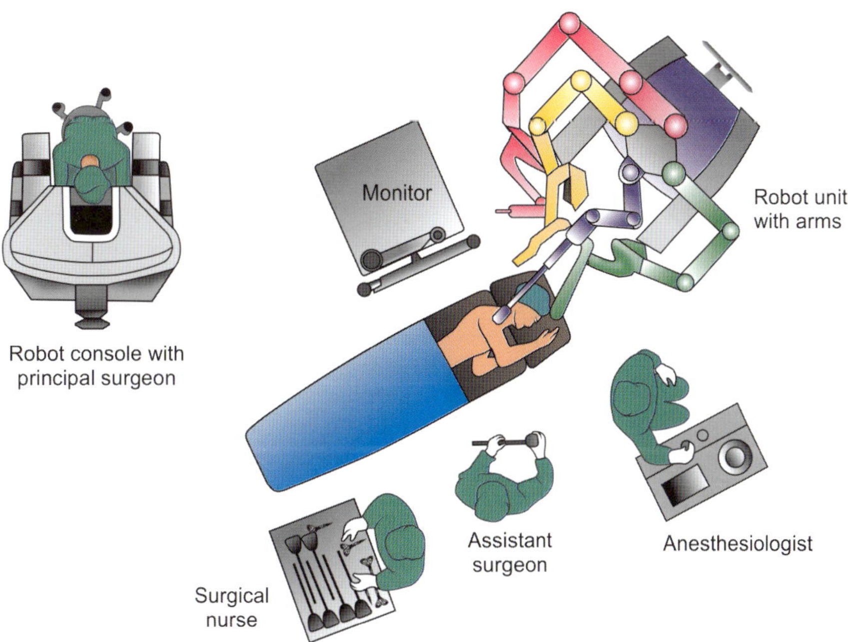

Fig. 2.1: Placement of robot and units for appropriate posture (right lung resections)

POSTURAL ADVICE TO COUNTER EFFECTS OF WORK

The three common ergonomic errors in surgeon posture are: forward head position, improper shoulder elevation, and pelvic girdle asymmetry. Postural reset and motion strategies are explained to help the surgeon learn techniques to counterbalance the sustained and awkward positions common during surgery that lead to muscle fatigue, pain, and degenerative changes.[18]

It is imperative that one takes a break and release all the tension in the body. With the emergence of the new-age Robot having a special feature to walk away from the console and have a coffee or tea break, it becomes all the more approachable to some of the exercises. In general practice, it is not unknown that surgeries can last anytime beyond 2 hours, multiplied by the surgeries one may need to conduct for the day. It is only wise that a reminder is set on the calendar or otherwise to do a break or do some stretches every 30 minutes to one hour as also recommended by the Michigan State University. Walking for a few minutes is a great way to unwind as it creates movement at different joints.

QUICK FIT BREAK THAT CAN HELP!

To relieve the stress from the hands and wrist, a simple stretch of pulling the wrist back and down and holding for 10–30 seconds can work wonders.

Another savior exercise is for the back, where one can simply sit up straight and do a scapular set where the scapula are retracted or pinched to hold the shoulder blades together and relaxed.

To take the tension off the muscles on the side of the neck, sit up straight and lift the sternum up. Hold hand on one side of the chair and lean away the body to the other side, dropping the head to the opposite side as well. Now place a hand on top of the head to gently guide the movement to the opposite side. Hold this stretch for 10–20 seconds and repeat on the other side.

To stretch the muscles at back of the neck, tuck in the chin rotate head to 45° and then bend the neck to the opposite side maintaining a stretch. Make sure that the chin is not poking out. To avoid too much stretch, overpressure at the head can be avoided.

For the lower body, one very good exercise is the glut set where one simply needs to squeeze the gluteal muscles together while seated on the chair. This exercise makes one go up and down in the chair and from there rocking the pelvis forward and backward can make sure to loosen the thigh circulation to the area one is sitting on. It can help to take care of the pain experienced from long hours of sitting.

Hamstring muscles can be stretched while sitting on the edge of the seat up and tall, straighten out one leg and pull the toes in and out to feel at stretch behind the thighs and at the calf. To feel the stretch better, simply lean forward in the seat from the trunk and feel the stretch going all the way down to the leg. The stretch can be held for 10–30 seconds and done for the other side.

Another hip stretch that may be performed is crossing the leg over to the opposite knee to feel it in the back pocket area. One can either pressure on the folded knee to so that it is pushed towards the ground or one can lean forward from the trunk and the stretch can be held for 10–30 seconds. Repeat the stretch for the other side.

To do the above exercise more dynamically, after pushing down on the knee, bring it up towards the torso in a way to hug the knee and do 10–15 repetitions.

Next, stand up and hold the console balance, place one foot on the back of the chair, from a straight position, bend on the leg one is standing on, to feel a stretch on the front of the bent leg. Stabilize the pelvis by squeezing the gluteal muscles and draw the belly-button/tummy in.

To stretch the shoulders and back in one go, place both the hands in front on the arm rest, roll back in the wheeled seat. Now try to elongate the arms to reach forward as much as possible and sliding the hips back. So the stretch is through the arms and triceps, latissimus dorsi, shoulder but no pinching pain at the topside of the shoulder. This can be modified by side bending onto one way and repeating the other way to get a stretch more for the back including along Quadratus lumborum muscle.

In addition to the above, to ease off the effects of long standing as experienced by the OT Technician and OT Nurse, it is best recommended to stretch the calf muscles against the wall, in attempt to push it away. With wider arm span the inward rounded posture can be stretched open too.

CONCLUSION

Prevention is better than cure. One must exercise 30. Preferably 45-60 minutes of regular physical activity at a level corresponding to a brisk walk. The activity may be paced over shorter periods. These exercises must be planned and structured in a way that incurs optimal physical function. Physical functions include certain aspect of fitness namely cardiovascular, breathing, muscle strength and endurance, body composition and mobility. The psychological stability is as important as the physical one. Physical inactivity, insufficient recovery after long shift hours, lack of sleep, incorrect diet and stress all reduce our immunity levels. It is mandatory to drink fluids both which training and in between surgical procedures. Losing too much fluid reduces performance and the risk of injury increases.[17]

Correct ergonomics is a learned and practiced behavior. It is suggested that consideration of operating room setup, proper posture, and practices of postural resets are necessary components for a longer, healthier, and pain-free surgical career.[18]

REFERENCES

1. Supe AN, et al. J Minim Acess Surg. 2010 Apr;6.
2. Phesant S. Body space: Anthropometry, Ergonomics and the Design of Work, 2nd edition. London: Taylor & Francis, 2003.
3. Ergonomics for Dental Students [Internet]. American Dental Association; 2011 [cited 2103Dec22). Available from:http://

www.richmondinstitute.com/wpcontent/uploads/2012/03/Ergonomics-for-Dental-Students-2011.pdf
4. Naeini H, Mosaddad S. The Role of Ergonomics Issues in Engineering Education. Procedia—Social and Behavioral Sciences. 2013;102:587-90.
5. Stylopoulos N, Rattner D. Robotic Ergonomics. SCNA. 2003 (pubmed)
6. Berguer R, Smith W. An ergonomic comparison of robotic and laparoscopic technique: the influence of surgeon experience and task complexity. J Surg Res. 2006;134(1):87-92.
7. Berguer R. Ergonomics in laproscopic surgery. 2nd edition.
8. Elhage O, Challacombe B, Murphy D, Khan M, Dasgupta P. The Evolution and Ergonomics of Robotic-assisted Surgical Systems. ISBN. 2007;978-3-902613-04(2):648.
9. Hemal AK, Srinivas M, Charles AR. Ergonomic problems associated with laparoscopy. J Endourol. 2001;15(5):499-503.
10. Lundervold A. Occupation myalgia. Electromyographic investigations. Acta Psychiatr Neurol Scand. 1951;26:359-69.
11. Westgaard RH, Winkel J. Guidelines for occupational musculoskeletal load as a basis for intervention: a critical review. Appl Ergon. 1996;27:79-88.
12. Hagberg M. Occupational musculoskeletal stress and disorders of the neck and shoulder: a review of possible pathophysiology. Int Arch Occup Environ Health. 1984;53:269-78.
13. Tittiranonda P, Burastero S, Rempel D. Risk factors for musculoskeletal disorders among computer users. Occup Med. 1999;14:17-38.
14. Marcus M, Gerr F, Monteilh C, et al. A prospective study of computer users: II. Postural risk factors for musculoskeletal symptoms and disorders. Am J Ind Med. 2002;41:236-49.
15. Bernard BP (Ed). Musculoskeletal Disorders and Workplace Factors: A Critical Review of Epidemiological Evidence for Work-Related Musculoskeletal Disorders of the Neck, Upper Extremity, and Low Back, 2nd edition. Cincinnati: National Institute for Occupational Safety and Health (NIOSH),1997.
16. Liu CW, Chen TW, Wang MC, et al. Relationship between carpal tunnel syndrome and wrist angle in computer workers. Kaohsiung J Med Sci. 2003;19:617-23.
17. Kerstin Mandler. Ergonomics in the operating room, Molynlycke Healthcare Brochure, 2013.
18. Rosenblatt PL, McKinney J, Adams SR, Ergonomics in the operating room: protecting the surgeon. J Minim Invasive Gynecol. 2013;20(6):744.

CHAPTER

3

Immunofluorescence and Robotic Surgery

Vivek Bindal, Anand Kumar Yadav

INTRODUCTION

Information about the operative field is one of the most desired aspects of surgery in any given procedure from a surgeon's perspective. Minimally invasive surgery has increased the need for better visualization techniques because of the reduced amount of direct feedback from tissues that the surgeon usually gets in open surgery. Immunofluorescence imaging technology combines the three-dimensional high definition view, and many such details in robotic surgery, which are otherwise not available to the surgeon.

Immunofluorescence imaging enables the use of electromagnetic spectrum between 700 nm and 1,000 nm, which is invisible to the human eye, and along with fluorescent tracers produces fluorescence, thus helping in identification. Immunofluorescence spectrum has many advantages: it is invisible to the robotic camera, so it does not change the appearance of the surgical field unless the camera is activated to view the spectrum. It is nonionizing and has a decent tissue penetration (up to 5 mm), without any unfavorable effect on the tissue. As image acquisition takes only a few milliseconds, this technique provides real-time guidance during a procedure.[1]

Immunofluorescence imaging technique requires a contrast agent containing a molecule, called a fluorophore which on excitation by a immunofluorescence light source emits fluorescent light. Depending on the application, a targeting ligand directs the fluorophore to the structure under study. Visualization of the tissue is based on the signal of the contrast agent in the region of interest relative to the background signal, known as signal-to-background ratio (SBR). The only immunofluorescence fluorophores that are registered with the Food and Drug Administration (FDA) and the European Medicines Agency (EMA) for clinical use are indocyanine green (ICG) and methylene blue (MB).[1]

On illumination with immunofluorescence light, protein-bound ICG emits light that peaks at approximately 840 nm **(Fig. 3.1)**.[2] This fluorescence property of ICG was revealed in detail back in the 1970s, and the clinical application of real-time fluorescence imaging using ICG started in the early 1990s in the field of ophthalmology with fundus angiography.[3] This application of imaging was extended to surgery as an intra-operative navigation tool of lymphatic flow, sentinel lymph node mapping, determining blood flow during coronary artery bypass grafting, and identifying cerebral aneurysms for clipping.[4-7] ICG is safe to use, with rare complications.[8,9]

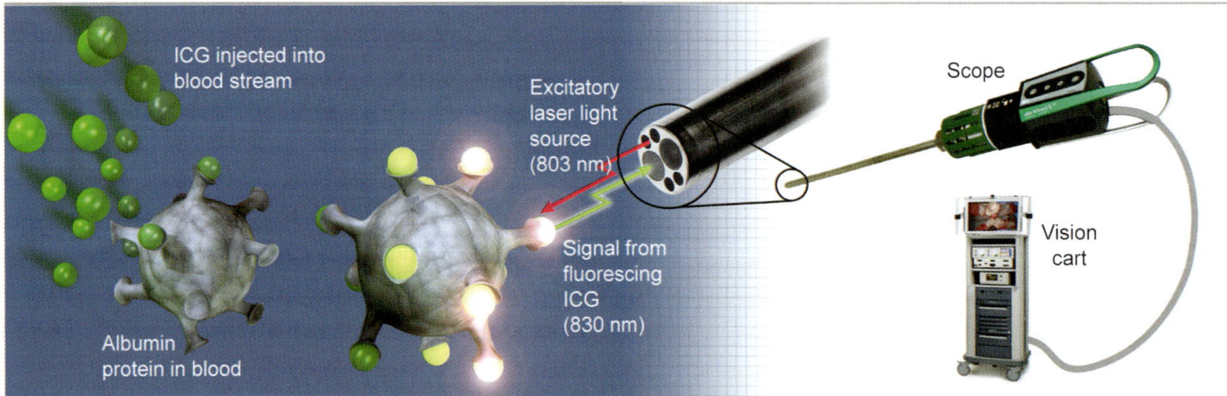

Fig. 3.1: The da Vinci Si surgical system integrated fluorescence imaging capability providing real-time, image-guided identification of key anatomical landmarks using near-infrared technology. Copyright © [2016] Intuitive Surgical, Inc

Clearance of the ICG in intravascular circulation happens rapidly by liver and much gets excreted in bile in particular. During laparoscopy procedure and robotic surgical procedures ICG is utilized mostly as fluorophore. By 2011 the Fluorescence Imaging Vision System got integrated in robotic platform like Da Vinci. After that there has seen a rapid expansion in most of the fields of the robotic surgery due to the critical role of immunofluorescence-ICG imaging. To date, there are many publications available as papers in scientific literature on various roles and responsibilities of fluorescence imaging in robotic procedures. However, there is limitation in experience as the technology is considered relatively new and few medical centers have initiated the use of this technique. The major operations where immunofluorescence-ICG is utilized are general surgery, urologic surgical procedures, thoracic and gynecologic robotic surgeries.[10-15]

Since 120 years methylene blue (MB) has been used for several medical procedures. When dilution happens to an extent which makes it nearly undetectable to normal human eyes, Methylene blue turns out to emit fluorophore at ≈700 nm.[16] This is known as 'unquenching' phenomena. At higher concentration, emission of fluorescence from methylene blue has intermolecular re-absorption which on dilutions, turns out unquenched. Methylene blue gets metabolized by both hepatic and renal tissues equally, allowing the imaging of both bile duct and ureters.

Identifying the cancers in real-time by utilizing fluorescence probes has recently become a very active field of research. Dye agents like methylene blue and indocyanine green (ICG) are considered as nonspecific immunofluorescence contrast agents. Novel immunofluorescence fluorescent probes are being developed to permit targeted imaging. To target a tumor cell the fluorophores are conjugated to any of the tumor specific ligand like tumor-specific antibody, nano body, small peptides. Alternatively they could be activated by enzymatic cleavage for fluorescence activity.[17]

CLINICAL APPLICATIONS OF IMMUNOFLUORESCENCE IMAGING IN GENERAL SURGERY

Following intravenous administration of ICG, in between 5 s and 60 s, initially arteries are seen following which veins can be visualized **(Fig. 3.1)**. This phase lasts only for few minimum seconds, but extra dose of ICG can be injected if required. The maximum recommended dose for an adult is 2 mg/kg with high toxicity margin.[8,9] Later, micro perfusion of organs and tissues gets more evident, followed by the lymphatic channels and neural anatomical structures. After nearly 45–60 minutes ICG gets accumulated in the hepatic tissues and secreted in bile, and hence can be used to assess liver and bile duct. Immunofluorescence imaging has many significant advantages in robotic surgery for various surgical operations. It can be used while dissecting a blood vessel or lymph node and it can help in identification of blood perfusion and hence viability of tissue before doing an anastomosis. It can help in identifying an anatomical structure or any lesion which needs resection (e.g. tumors) or protected (e.g. bile duct) **(Figs 3.2 and 3.3)**. Researchers are now making efforts to enable the targeted imaging, which in future will be able to change the way robotic procedures are performed.

Immunofluorescence imaging's used in various clinical applications are summarized in **Table 3.1**.

Biliary Imaging

In general surgery, ICG fluorescence can be used for identifying the biliary anatomy which is considered very

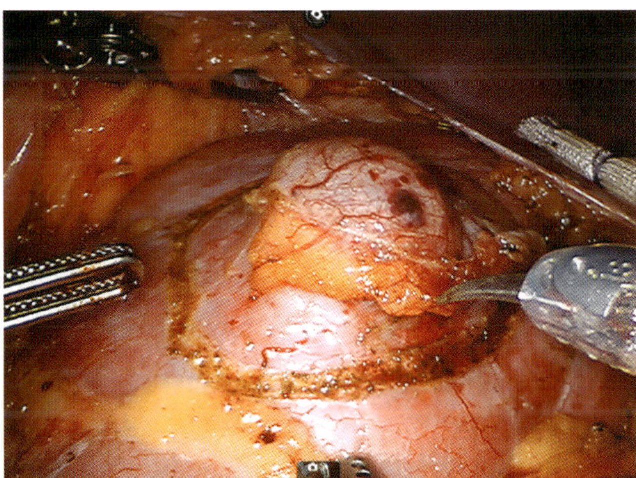

Fig. 3.2: Normal 3D HD illumination mode during da Vinci® Partial Nephrectomy. Firefly fluorescence imaging endoscope view before activation: Renal parenchyma. Copyright © [2016] Intuitive Surgical, Inc

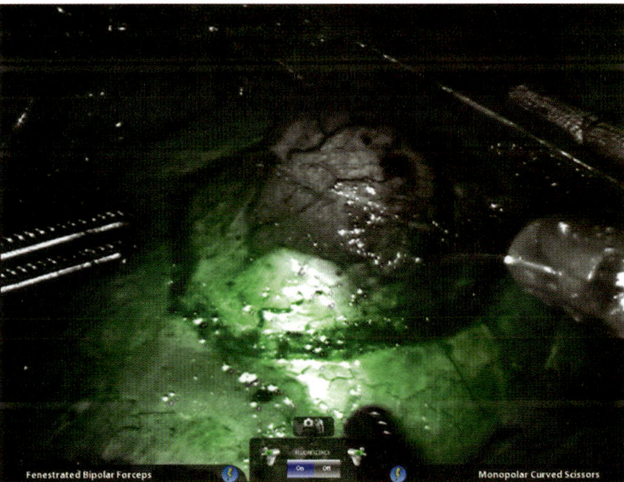

Fig. 3.3: Assessing parenchymal perfusion during tumor excision in FireFly™ fluorescence imaging mode during da Vinci® partial nephrectomy. Firefly fluorescence imaging endoscope view after activation: Renal parenchyma. Copyright © [2016] Intuitive Surgical, Inc

Table 3.1: Clinical applications of immunofluorescence in robotic surgery

Imaging in robotic surgery	
Biliary imaging: Fluorescent cholangiogram	Example: Extrahepatic biliary ducts during cholecystectomy and hepatectomy
Vascular imaging:	
• Anatomy of blood vessels	Example: Hepatic artery during hepatectomy, splenic artery and vein during distal pancreatectomy
• Organ and tissue perfusion	Example: Recognizing vital tissue during gastrointestinal anastomosis, renal perfusion after transplant
• Blood flow	Example: After vascular anastomosis
Lymphatic channels: Lymph node identification	Example: Sentinel lymph node in endometrial cancer
Specialized tissue:	
• Nerve identification • Parathyroid identification	Example: Phrenic nerve during thymectomy, inferior hypogastric plexus during pelvic dissection, recognition of parathyroids during thyroidectomy
Identification of lesions, based on their vascular and metabolic pattern	Example: Well- vs poorly differentiated HCC, neuroendocrine lesions, angiomas

important application. Immunofluorescence imaging helps in reducing the risk of biliary duct injuries in cholecystectomy. ICG permits better visibility of the extra-hepatic biliary ducts in real time, thereby allowing a constant monitoring by 'nonradiographic' cholangiogram. Using the immunofluorescence-ICG during a robotic cholecystectomy procedure had been described as to how the ICG fluorescence had capabilities to help in identifying an aberrant biliary side branch from hepatic segment VI to common hepatic duct during robotic procedure. The side branch could be preserved with success, and postoperative biliary leaks were avoided.[18] Other reputable authors have also published their experiences and confirmed the advantage of the technique.[19,20] Buchs et al. initially reported their assessments following 12 robotic cholecystectomies with immunofluorescence-ICG at single site. The cystic duct, common bile duct and common hepatic duct (CD, CBD, CHD) were visualized with success prior to dissections in Calot's triangle area among 91.7%, 50%, 33% of the cases, respectively. Following the surgical dissection, the visualization rates for the three anatomical structures were 100%, 83.3%, 66.7%.[19] Spinoglio et al. had published their evaluations after completion of 45 cases of robotic cholecystectomy with immunofluorescence-ICG at a single site, with successful visualization of three main biliary anatomical structures at a rate of 97% following dissection of Calot's triangle.[20] Daskalaki et al. had reported their results after 184 cases of robotic cholecystectomies where cholangiography had ICG fluorescent as an agent.[10] The overall rate of visualization for the cystic, common hepatic and common bile was 97.8%, 94%, 96.1%, respectively. Visualization rates of biliary structures in complex cases, like acute cholecystitis and patients with obesity were analyzed independently. In the first group, the CD, CBD, CHD were identified with success among 91.6%, 79.1%, 79.1% of patients respectively. In the second group of patients the visualization rates were 97%, 94%, 95%. The near-infrared light had the penetration ability of approximately 5–10 mm,[21,22] managing issues like presence of inflammation and obese patients that might potentially affect visualization of anatomical structures. It is important to note that, there were no biliary duct injury or any allergic reaction to ICG in any of these published series of articles. Immunofluorescence-ICG might improve the outcome of cholecystectomies, by replacing the usual X-ray method of cholangiograms, with no significant increase in operation time and with minimum risk of any adverse effect due to the dye.

Identification of the vascular and biliary structures during complex procedures such as hepatic resections and pancreaticoduodenectomies by immunofluorescence imaging allows a more precise and accurate dissection, potentially decreasing the risk of intraoperative complications.

Vascular Imaging

Identification of arteries and veins is one of the most interesting applications of the indocyanine green. Identifications of normal anatomical structures and/or recognition of the variations of anatomical structure in real-time decreases the risk of inadvertent injuries to nearby vascular elements. This can be considered as a substantial improvement, in any simple cholecystectomy operation (where vascular structures identification could reduce the risks of inadvertent injury of anomalous and accessory blood vessels), as well as in any complex situations of liver or pancreas resection (where identifying and dissecting any major blood vessel is a critical step to successful completion of the procedure).

Recently, immunofluorescence-ICG had been utilized in urology for clamping of selective arterial blood vessel (often referred to as 'firefly') in procedures like robotic partial nephrectomy **(Figs 3.4 and 3.5)**. Borofsky et al. published their first assessment in 34 patients of zero-ischemia robotic partial nephrectomies (RPNs) and opined that this imaging technique helps in super-selective arterial clamping methods, resulting in better functional outcomes.[23]

Organ and Tissue Perfusion

Evaluation of tissue perfusion is another important application of immunofluorescence imaging. Partial ischemia may lead to anastomotic leaks, which is a dreaded complication. Many a times the color demarcation is not precise and the Doppler scan may require specific probes which may show artifacts like poor contact or interphase. Adequately done ICG microperfusion assessment in colorectal operations and

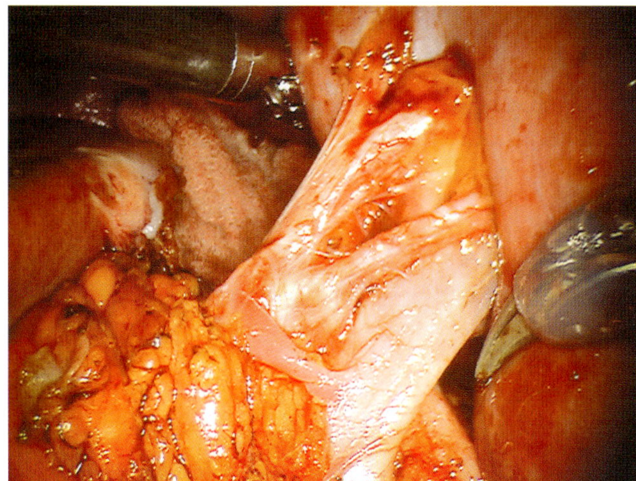

Fig. 3.4: Normal 3D HD illumination mode (view of renal hilum) during da Vinci® partial nephrectomy. Firefly fluorescence imaging endoscope view before activation: Renal hilum. Copyright © [2016] Intuitive Surgical, Inc

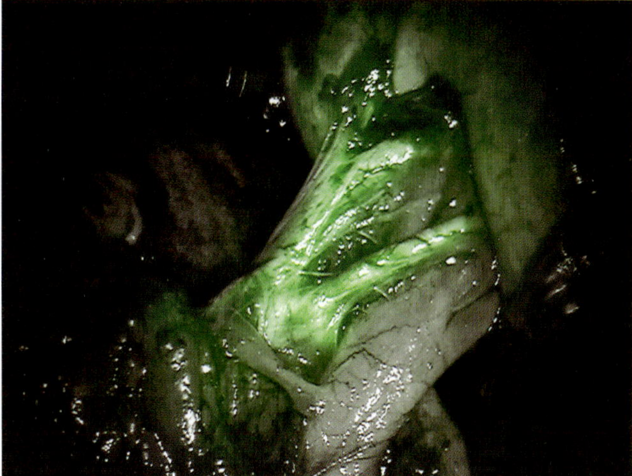

Fig. 3.5: Vessel identification in FireFly® fluorescence imaging mode (view of renal hilum) during da Vinci® partial nephrectomy. Firefly fluorescence imaging endoscope view after activation: Renal hilum. Copyright © [2016] Intuitive Surgical, Inc

esophageal surgeries provides real time recognition of viable tissue and operating surgeons may be able to revise their line of resection, if required, and therefore can perform safe anastomosis. Jafari et al. had first evaluated the anastomotic tissue perfusion at the time of robotic low anterior resection (RLAR).[24] The authors had carried out a retrospective case control analysis to find whether immunofluorescence-ICG can reduce the rate of anastomotic leaks following procedures like RLAR. A 12% decrease of overall risks for anastomotic leaks was reported in the immunofluorescence-ICG group.[24] Other relevant clinical studies also confirmed the effectiveness of the technique in evaluation of the bowel perfusion.[25-27] Hellan et al. had reported about 40% rate of changing the point of bowel or gastrointestinal tract transection following fluorescent imaging.[26] Many more studies are required to know whether this translates in a decrease of true incidences of anastomotic leaks, but the preliminary reports appear promising. It has been reported that a prospective multicentric trial is ongoing, in an effort to find out the real impact of immunofluorescence-ICG procedure in changing the point of bowel transection at the time of left-sided colorectal resections.[11] Immunofluorescence imaging with the help of ICG could be used to check blood flows and perfusion in solid organ. Example of this kind application could be used in robot-assisted renal transplant procedures. Following the completion of a vascular anastomosis, ICG can also assess the blood flow through the anastomosed blood vessel and the perfusion of the transplanted organ like kidney.[28]

Lymph Node and Nerve Identification

Immunofluorescence imaging helps in mapping of the possible of lymph nodes and identification of any sentinel lymph node. This application can be specifically useful in cancer surgery, allowing highly selective lymphadenectomy with better precision. In laparoscopic surgical procedure it is being successfully utilized in the cases of GI and colorectal cancers.[29,30] In robotic surgeries, it has recently been used for the purpose of mapping lymph nodes and sentinel lymph node identification in cancers of endometrium and cancer cervix. Rossi et al. had first reported their evaluation of 20 cases who received cervical injection of ICG.[13] They had reported success rate of 88% in procedures like detection of SLN. They had concluded that this type of imaging procedure is reliable for SLN detection and mapping of lymph nodes during early stages of endometrial cancer and cancer of cervix. The same authors had recently published that cervical ICG injection is of higher efficiency in comparison to the hysteroscopic endometrial injection in identifying SLN, with similar distribution of anatomical lymph nodes.[31] Holloway et al. had reviewed the identification rates of SLN in patients suffering from endometrial cancer who also had robotic staging, compared immunofluorescence-ICG procedure with colorimetric imaging procedure using isosulfan blue (ISB).[32] They had reported that immunofluorescence-ICG was much useful while identifying bilateral SLNs and metastasis of lymph nodes, with 77% versus 97% identification rates of bilateral pelvic or aortic SLNs utilizing procedures ISB and ICG respectively.

Few drawbacks of immunofluorescence-ICG in cases of colorectal surgeries, reported by some authors especially in patients of tattooed lesion and mapping of lymph nodes.[11] There were details of excess or inadequacy in diffusion of colorant around tumor location, spreading within the abdomen cavity and resulting in visualization failure of the lymph nodes, specifically after neoadjuvant radiotherapy of cancers of rectum.[11]

Identifying nerves could be one more application of interest for immunofluorescence imaging which can be explored in future as novel procedure when highly selective contrast agents are available. Detection of nerves and its plexuses may facilitate in better dissection and prevent inadvertent nerve injury, improving postoperative outcome. Surgical procedures like prostatectomy (prostatic nerve), colorectal surgeries (inferior hypogastric nerve plexus), thyroid surgery (detection of recurrent laryngeal nerve) and thymus surgery (phrenic nerve) are considered as the better examples.

Wagner et al. had reported their assessments with 10 cases of unilateral right robotic thymectomy utilizing immunofluorescene-ICG to detect the contralateral pericardiophrenic neurovascular bundle (PNB).[14] They had success rates of 80% while visualizing the PNB, mostly from left sided pleural view. No injury happened to the PNB. The authors reported that this technique can provide maximum tissue resection and reduce the nerve injuries.

Identification of Lesions

The normal and cancerous tissue parenchyma has many differences in their hemodynamic and metabolic physiological properties, also the difference in ICG excretions in biliary mechanism helps in identification of various lesions from the surrounding normal tissues.

Hepatocellular carcinoma (HCC) is an example for these kind of properties. There are many study groups who had reported the different varieties of fluorescent patterns in cases of well differentiated hepatocellular carcinoma, poorly differentiated hepatocellular carcinoma, colorectal cancers with metastases.[33-35] In cases of well differentiated hepatocellular carcinomas the ICG uptake is well preserved, but the biliary excretion is mostly impaired, hence they have appearance of uniform fluorescent lesions. Poorly differentiated hepatocellular carcinomas and colorectal cancer metastases, on the contrary, have the appearance of hypofluorescent lesions enclosed by a fluorescent ring, due to presence of biliary excretion disorder of the surrounding tissues which is getting compressed by tumor mass. In our total understanding, immunofluorescence-ICG had been more useful in identifying hepatocellular cancers, hemangioma, pheochromocytoma and small neuroendocrine pancreatic tumors.

Manny et al. reported a case series of three robotic partial adrenalectomies where immunofluorescence-ICG was used to confirm the identification of masses from normal adrenal tissues, which in turn will promote parenchyma sparing resections.[36]

OTHER APPLICATIONS IN ROBOTIC SURGERY

Ureteral Stricture Identification

Currently, the indications for immunofluorescence-ICG procedure have expanded to intraoperative localization of strictures in ureter. Lee et al. had published 7 cases of robotic ureteroureterostomy procedure for stricture.[37] ICG was given intraureterally to delineate the ureter and an extra intraureteral dose was administered to identify the healthy ureteral tissues from the devitalized tissues, allowing safe repair. Reconstruction of the upper urinary tract appears to be a likely newer indication for immunofluorescence-ICG procedure. In a separately conducted study on 40 patients who underwent robotic pyeloplasty surgery, ureteral implantation and ureteroureterostomy with ICG, radiological and symptomatic improvement following the procedure was 100%.[12]

ICG in Cases of Total Endoscopic Robotic-assisted Procedures for Coronary Artery Bypass

A probable future application of immunofluorescence-ICG had been reported by Hassan et al.[38] In a canine model they had identified internal mammary artery, characterized the coronary anatomy and checked patency of the anastomoses during robotic coronary bypass.

Segmentectomy in Early Stages of Lung Cancers

Pardolesi et al. reported a novel technique to identify the intersegmental planes at the time of robotic anatomic segmentectomy for smaller sized early stage lung cancers.[15] The ICG was administered intravenously following the division of bronchus, vein and artery of target segment. The results showed green coloration of the perfused parenchymal tissue where the target segment remained uncolored. The authors had also reported the excellent demarcation of the segment to be excised, facilitating the segment transection.

FUTURE APPLICATIONS

New technologies are emerging for improving immuno-fluorescence imaging procedures.[39] Scientists had been working on newer techniques to overcome the limitation of low tissue penetration and also to improve the fluorescent signals.[40,41]

The most revolutionary future applications can be *in vivo*, real time tumor identification and its characterization. Specific targeting ligand or monoclonal antibodies which are conjugated to near-infrared fluorophores may allow real time molecular diagnosis and identification of the cancer masses during surgical operation. Recently Metildi et al. reported a clinical study where the tumors of pancreas in orthotopic mice were labeled with fluorescent anticarcinoembryonic antigen antibodies. Fluorescence guided laparoscopy operation resulted in decreased local and distant recurrence rates and extended duration of median disease free survival as compared to bright light laparoscopic surgery.[42,43] It is expected that in future the major progress in immunofluorescence imaging will be with better software for image processing (subtraction and fusion imaging), estimate a quantitative evaluation of blood flow (speed) and patterns of perfusions (architectures).

CONCLUSION

Near-infrared fluorescent imaging with ICG is one of the latest innovations in the field of surgery. This is a safe and non-invasive technique without any radiation hazard. Currently its main applications in the robotic general surgical procedures are real-time visualization of biliary anatomical structures and evaluation of anastomosis site perfusion during various gastrointestinal surgeries and colorectal operations. Although there are only a few clinical studies present, in the literature, the reported assessments are encouraging. In recent future, it is expected that these applications of technology will provide real time *in vivo* microscopy that can be a valuable asset during minimally invasive oncologic surgical procedures. This can be considered as initial phase of a new era in surgical field. As newer technological innovations grow, so will the multiple indications of immunofluorescence imaging procedure. Further clinical research and trials are required to understand the real value of immunofluorescence imaging procedure and expand its indications.

REFERENCES

1. Verbeek FP, van der Vorst JR, Schaafsma BE, Hutteman M, Bonsing BA, van Leeuwen FW, et al. Image-guided hepatopancreatobiliary surgery using near-infrared fluorescent light. Journal of Hepato-biliary-pancreatic Sciences. 2012;19(6):626-37. Epub 2012/07/14.
2. Landsman ML, Kwant G, Mook GA, et al. Light-absorbing properties, stability, and spectral stabilization of indocyanine green. Journal of Applied Physiology. 1976;40(4):575-83. Epub 1976/04/01.
3. Guyer DR, Puliafito CA, Mones JM, Friedman E, Chang W, Verdooner SR. Digital indocyanine-green angiography in chorioretinal disorders. Ophthalmology. 1992;99(2):287-91. Epub 1992/02/01.
4. Ogata F, Azuma R, Kikuchi M, et al. Novel lymphography using indocyanine green dye for near-infrared fluorescence labeling. Annals of Plastic Surgery. 2007;58(6):652-5. Epub 2007/05/25.
5. Kitai T, Inomoto T, Miwa M, et al. Fluorescence navigation with indocyanine green for detecting sentinel lymph nodes in breast cancer. Breast Cancer. 2005;12(3):211-5. Epub 2005/08/20.
6. Rubens FD, Ruel M, Fremes SE. A new and simplified method for coronary and graft imaging during CABG. The Heart Surgery Forum. 2002;5(2):141-4. Epub 2002/07/13.
7. Raabe A, Nakaji P, Beck J, Kim LJ, Hsu FP, Kamerman JD, et al. Prospective evaluation of surgical microscope-integrated intraoperative near-infrared indocyanine green videoangiography during aneurysm surgery. Journal of Neurosurgery. 2005;103(6):982-9. Epub 2005/12/31.
8. Marshall MV, Rasmussen JC, Tan IC, Aldrich MB, Adams KE, Wang X, et al. Near-Infrared Fluorescence Imaging in Humans with Indocyanine Green: A Review and Update. Open Surg Oncol J. 2010;2(2):12-25. Epub 2010/01/01.
9. Alford R, Simpson HM, Duberman J, Hill GC, Ogawa M, Regino C, et al. Toxicity of organic fluorophores used in molecular imaging: literature review. Molecular Imaging. 2009;8(6):341-54. Epub 2009/12/17.
10. Daskalaki D, Fernandes E, Wang X, Bianco FM, Elli EF, Ayloo S, et al. Indocyanine Green (ICG) Fluorescent Cholangiography During Robotic Cholecystectomy: Results of 184 Consecutive Cases in a Single Institution. Surgical Innovation. 2014. Epub 2014/03/13.
11. Marano A, Priora F, Lenti LM, Ravazzoni F, Quarati R, Spinoglio G. Application of fluorescence in robotic general surgery: review of the literature and state of the art. World Journal of Surgery. 2013;37(12):2800-11. Epub 2013/05/07.
12. Bjurlin MA, Gan M, McClintock TR, Volpe A, Borofsky MS, Mottrie A, et al. Near-infrared fluorescence imaging: emerging applications in robotic upper urinary tract surgery. European Urology. 2014;65(4):793-801. Epub 2013/10/09.
13. Rossi EC, Ivanova A, Boggess JF. Robotically assisted fluorescence-guided lymph node mapping with ICG for gynecologic malignancies: a feasibility study. Gynecologic Oncology. 2012;124(1):78-82. Epub 2011/10/15.
14. Wagner OJ, Louie BE, Vallieres E, et al. Near-infrared fluorescence imaging can help identify the contralateral phrenic nerve during robotic thymectomy. The Annals of Thoracic Surgery. 2012;94(2):622-5. Epub 2012/07/24.
15. Pardolesi A, Veronesi G, Solli P, et al. Use of indocyanine green to facilitate intersegmental plane identification during robotic anatomic segmentectomy. The Journal of Thoracic and Cardiovascular Surgery. 2014. Epub 2014/04/01.
16. Tanaka E, Chen FY, Flaumenhaft R, Graham GJ, Laurence RG, Frangioni JV. Real-time assessment of cardiac perfusion, coronary angiography, and acute intravascular thrombi using dual-channel near-infrared fluorescence imaging. The Journal of Thoracic and Cardiovascular Surgery. 2009;138(1):133-40. Epub 2009/07/07.
17. Luo S, Zhang E, Su Y, et al. A review of immunofluorescence dyes in cancer targeting and imaging. Biomaterials. 2011;32(29):7127-38. Epub 2011/07/05.
18. Calatayud D, Milone L, Elli EF, et al. ICG-fluorescence identification of a small aberrant biliary canaliculus during robotic cholecystectomy. Liver International: Official Journal of the International Association for the Study of the Liver. 2012;32(4):602. Epub 2012/02/02.
19. Buchs NC, Hagen ME, Pugin F, Volonte F, Bucher P, Schiffer E, et al. Intraoperative fluorescent cholangiography using indocyanin green during robotic single site cholecystectomy. The International Journal of Medical Robotics + Computer Assisted Surgery: MRCAS. 2012;8(4):436-40. Epub 2012/06/01.
20. Spinoglio G, Priora F, Bianchi PP, Lucido FS, Licciardello A, Maglione V, et al. Real-time near-infrared (Immunofluorescence) fluorescent cholangiography in single-site robotic cholecystectomy (SSRC): a single-institutional prospective study. Surgical Endoscopy. 2013;27(6):2156-62. Epub 2012/12/29.
21. Houston JP, Thompson AB, Gurfinkel M, et al. Sensitivity and depth penetration of continuous wave versus frequency-domain photon migration near-infrared fluorescence contrast-enhanced imaging. Photochemistry and photobiology. 2003;77(4):420-30. Epub 2003/05/08.
22. Ishizawa T, Kaneko J, Inoue Y, Takemura N, Seyama Y, Aoki T, et al. Application of fluorescent cholangiography to single-incision laparoscopic cholecystectomy. Surgical endoscopy. 2011;25(8):2631-6. Epub 2011/03/23.
23. Borofsky MS, Gill IS, Hemal AK, Marien TP, Jayaratna I, Krane LS, et al. Near-infrared fluorescence imaging to facilitate super-selective arterial clamping during zero-ischaemia robotic partial nephrectomy. BJU international. 2013;111(4):604-10. Epub 2012/12/21.
24. Jafari MD, Lee KH, Halabi WJ, Mills SD, Carmichael JC, Stamos MJ, et al. The use of indocyanine green fluorescence to assess

anastomotic perfusion during robotic assisted laparoscopic rectal surgery. Surgical Endoscopy. 2013. Epub 2013/02/14.

25. Bae SU, Baek SJ, Hur H, Baik SH, Kim NK, Min BS. Intraoperative near infrared fluorescence imaging in robotic low anterior resection: three case reports. Yonsei Medical Journal. 2013;54(4):1066-9. Epub 2013/05/28.
26. Hellan M, Spinoglio G, Pigazzi A, et al. The influence of fluorescence imaging on the location of bowel transection during robotic left-sided colorectal surgery. Surgical Endoscopy. 2014;28(5):1695-702. Epub 2014/01/05.
27. Bianchi PP, Pigazzi A, Choi GS. Clinical Robotic Surgery Association Fifth Worldwide Congress, Washington DC, 3-5 October 2013: Robotic Colorectal Surgery. Ecancermedicalscience. 2014;8:385. Epub 2014/02/01.
28. Tzvetanov I, Giulianotti PC, Bejarano-Pineda L, Jeon H, Garcia-Roca R, Bianco F, et al. Robotic-assisted kidney transplantation. The Surgical Clinics of North America. 2013;93(6):1309-23. Epub 2013/11/12.
29. Kelder W, Nimura H, Takahashi N, Mitsumori N, van Dam GM, Yanaga K. Sentinel node mapping with indocyanine green (ICG) and infrared ray detection in early gastric cancer: an accurate method that enables a limited lymphadenectomy. European Journal of Surgical Oncology: The Journal of the European Society of Surgical Oncology and the British Association of Surgical Oncology. 2010;36(6):552-8. Epub 2010/05/11.
30. Cahill RA, Anderson M, Wang LM, Lindsey I, Cunningham C, Mortensen NJ. Near-infrared (immunofluorescence) laparoscopy for intraoperative lymphatic road-mapping and sentinel node identification during definitive surgical resection of early-stage colorectal neoplasia. Surgical endoscopy. 2012;26(1):197-204. Epub 2011/08/20.
31. Rossi EC, Jackson A, Ivanova A, et al. Detection of sentinel nodes for endometrial cancer with robotic assisted fluorescence imaging: cervical versus hysteroscopic injection. International Journal of Gynecological Cancer: Official Journal of the International Gynecological Cancer Society. 2013;23(9):1704-11. Epub 2013/11/02.
32. Holloway RW, Bravo RA, Rakowski JA, James JA, Jeppson CN, Ingersoll SB, et al. Detection of sentinel lymph nodes in patients with endometrial cancer undergoing robotic-assisted staging: a comparison of colorimetric and fluorescence imaging. Gynecologic Oncology. 2012;126(1):25-9. Epub 2012/04/18.
33. Ishizawa T, Bandai Y, Ijichi M, Kaneko J, Hasegawa K, Kokudo N. Fluorescent cholangiography illuminating the biliary tree during laparoscopic cholecystectomy. The British Journal of Surgery. 2010;97(9):1369-77. Epub 2010/07/14.
34. Ishizawa T, Fukushima N, Shibahara J, Masuda K, Tamura S, Aoki T, et al. Real-time identification of liver cancers by using indocyanine green fluorescent imaging. Cancer. 2009;115(11):2491-504. Epub 2009/03/28.
35. Kokudo N, Ishizawa T. Clinical application of fluorescence imaging of liver cancer using indocyanine green. Liver Cancer. 2012;1(1):15-21. Epub 2012/06/01.
36. Manny TB, Pompeo AS, Hemal AK. Robotic partial adrenalectomy using indocyanine green dye with near-infrared imaging: the initial clinical experience. Urology. 2013;82(3):738-42. Epub 2013/07/19.
37. Lee Z, Simhan J, Parker DC, Reilly C, Llukani E, Lee DI, et al. Novel use of indocyanine green for intraoperative, real-time localization of ureteral stenosis during robot-assisted ureteroureterostomy. Urology. 2013;82(3):729-33. Epub 2013/08/31.
38. Hassan M, Kerdok A, Engel A, et al. Near infrared fluorescence imaging with ICG in TECAB surgery using the da Vinci Si surgical system in a canine model. Journal of Cardiac Surgery. 2012;27(2):158-62. Epub 2012/03/01.
39. Schaafsma BE, Mieog JS, Hutteman M, van der Vorst JR, Kuppen PJ, Lowik CW, et al. The clinical use of indocyanine green as a near-infrared fluorescent contrast agent for image-guided oncologic surgery. Journal of Surgical Oncology. 2011;104(3):323-32. Epub 2011/04/16.
40. Gioux S, Mazhar A, Cuccia DJ, Durkin AJ, Tromberg BJ, Frangioni JV. Three-dimensional surface profile intensity correction for spatially modulated imaging. Journal of Biomedical Optics. 2009;14(3):034045. Epub 2009/07/02.
41. Themelis G, Yoo JS, Soh KS, et al. Real-time intraoperative fluorescence imaging system using light-absorption correction. Journal of Biomedical Optics. 2009;14(6):064012. Epub 2010/01/12.
42. Metildi CA, Kaushal S, Luiken GA, et al. Advantages of Fluorescence-Guided Laparoscopic Surgery of Pancreatic Cancer Labeled with Fluorescent Anti-Carcinoembryonic Antigen Antibodies in an Orthotopic Mouse Model. Journal of the American College of Surgeons. 2014. Epub 2014/04/29.
43. Metildi CA, Kaushal S, Hardamon CR, Snyder CS, Pu M, Messer KS, et al. Fluorescence-guided surgery allows for more complete resection of pancreatic cancer, resulting in longer disease-free survival compared with standard surgery in orthotopic mouse models. Journal of the American College of Surgeons. 2012;215(1):126-35; discussion 35-6. Epub 2012/05/29.

CHAPTER

4

Anesthesia

Sangeeta Khanna, Jyotirmoy Das, Yatin Mehta

INTRODUCTION

One of the primary building blocks for a successful robotic surgery program is a robust and experienced team of anesthesia providers. The meticulous steps of patient preparation, positioning, operating room ergonomics, robot orientation and docking have to be practiced, improvized and resurrected multiple times for the best results in terms of surgical outcome and to reduce unacceptable nonsurgical complications. Protocolization should be stressed upon to bring more objectivity and avoid errors of omission. It also requires foresightedness, vigilance, coordination and close communication between the team members.

PREOPERATIVE PREPARATION

Routine preoperative assessment is the same as for any other major surgery dictated by the patient's age and comorbidities. A good understanding of the altered oculocerebral and cardiopulmonary physiology in extreme patient positioning with the additional burden of pneumoperitoneum is crucial. Special preoperative considerations which should be addressed are shown in **Table 4.1**.

INTRAOPERATIVE MANAGEMENT

Intraoperative monitoring generally involves electrocardiogram (ECG), noninvasive blood pressure, pulse

Table 4.1: Specific preoperative considerations for robot-assisted surgeries

Pre-existing morbidity/ Consideration	*Preoperative optimization/protocol*
Intracranial pathology	• History of arteriovenous malformation, recent history of cerebrovascular event, possible breach of blood brain barrier by cerebral tumor are relative contraindications for robotic pelvic surgery • Raised intracranial tension (ICT) intraoperatively can compromise cerebral perfusion and lead to deterioration in cerebral function
Intraocular pathology	• Raised intraocular pressure (IOP) can lead to retinal ischemia and artificial lens displacement if recently placed • Glaucoma is a relative contraindication to robotic pelvic surgery
Cervical spine pathology	• Spinal pathologies like spinal cord compression due to vertebral fracture or prolapsed intervertebral disc can lead to further deterioration in neurological function following prolonged extreme positioning • Proper patient counseling is essential along with optimization of pathology if possible. The entire team of surgeons and anesthetists should arrive at a consensus on the optimal patient position in such a compromized situation
Lung condition	Chronic obstructive pulmonary disease, restrictive lung pathologies can increase the risk of alveolar damage during positive pressure ventilation. Lung bullae can rupture when airway pressure rises during robotic pelvic surgery. Patients should be counseled for the need of conversion to open surgery, insertion of chest tubes or postoperative ventilatory support in intensive care unit if the need arises
Cardiac status	Cardiac conditions like low ejection fraction, intracardiac shunt, valvular pathologies and pulmonary hypertension are relative contraindications due to extreme patient positioning with pneumoperitoneum
Renal function	Pneumoperitoneum reduces renal blood flow and glomerular filtration rate. Chronic kidney disease patients may show a possible transient rise in markers like serum creatinine
Joint pathology	Safe patient positioning requires a meticulous history and examination for any joint pathologies or movement restrictions. Final positioning should be dictated by preoperative demonstration of safe range of movements
Obesity	Obesity and increased body mass index patients are at an increased risk of difficult airway, position-related injuries, high airway pressures and recovery-related morbidities. Proper planning is a must to address all these issues

oximetry, temperature, urine output, airway pressure, end-tidal CO_2 ($EtCO_2$) and gas analysis. Insertion of central venous and arterial catheter are dictated by the nature of surgery and the preoperative functional status of the patient. The number and caliber of intravenous cannula should be planned before hand especially for pelvic surgeries as securing an intravenous access is difficult intraoperatively. Body temperature has to be monitored and maintained in robotic surgeries. This can be achieved by use of forced warm air blankets, fluid warming devices and low flow anesthesia. Adequate muscle relaxation is required[1] to avoid inadvertent patient movement while the robot is docked and hence use of an infusion of muscle relaxant is highly recommended. The carina to tube tip distance decreases during pneumoperitoneum in steep Trendelenburg position (STP). So, auscultation for bilateral equal air entry and vigilant monitoring of airway pressure and $EtCO_2$ curve is mandatory. Loss of lung isolation during one lung anesthesia can occur intraoperatively and can be detected by fiberoptic bronchoscopy. Maintaining peak airway pressure within the conventional range of 40 cm H_2O can be challenging in robotic pelvic surgeries with pneumoperitoneum. As permissive hypercarbia is not practiced because of the risk of raising the intracranial tension (ICT), allowing a higher level of peak airway pressure in such surgeries may be warranted. When volume control (VC) and pressure control (PC) modes were compared to achieve equivalent tidal volumes during robotic pelvic surgery, it was observed that PC yields better compliance and lower airway pressures without any statistically significant difference in hemodynamics.[2] Minute ventilation may need to be increased by nearly 50% to maintain normal $PaCO_2$ levels. High levels of positive end expiratory pressure in a titrating manner can be utilized as a recruitment maneuver. Although controversial as a surrogate marker of intravascular volume, a key principle that we routinely follow if a central line is in place is to measure the baseline CVP during supine position and note the values during Trendelenburg and pneumoperitoneum and thereafter, compare the trend keeping these baseline values as reference. The other option although restricted by its high cost is the use of dynamic parameters like stroke volume variation (SVV) as a guide of fluid status as it has been shown that SVV is not influenced by patient position and pneumoperitoneum.[3]

Perioperative thromboprophylaxis is an area of controversy in robotic surgery. Although the risk benefit ratio between bleeding and risk of thrombosis should guide us in the final decision making, following a protocol based on International standards like American College of Chest Physicians guideline[4] would help to prevent confusion. The less controversial adjuncts like sequential pneumatic compression devices should always be applied.

Tables 4.2 and 4.3 depict some of the intraoperative considerations in robotic surgery.

Table 4.2: Considerations due to the robot itself

Characteristic	*Challenges*
Bulky machine parts	• Operating room (OR) space constraints: Good OR ergonomics is helpful • Patient accessibility is reduced • Two IV cannulae, long anesthesia circuit and tubings are necessary • A robotic surgery should not be started with a single intravenous cannula no matter how well it is functioning
Heavy robotic arms	• Injury to the patient or surgical assistant is a real possibility[5] • Meticulous planning while positioning the patient is essential to prevent injury • Patient's face, thigh and arm need to be protected by adequate padding • Close communication with the surgeon is essential throughout the procedure
Once docked robot stands like a fixed tower over the patient	Any movement of the patient or the operating table is prohibited when the robot is docked

Table 4.3: Special surgical requirements

Dark operating room: 'Situational awareness' is compromised
One lung anesthesia for robot-assisted thoracic surgery (RATS) procedures: Risk of tube migration and loss of lung isolation is a possibility
Suspension laryngoscopy for transoral robotic surgery (TORS) procedures: It can be hemodynamically deleterious
Use of pneumothorax or capnothorax: Discussed further

PATIENT POSITIONING

Robot-assisted surgeries often require extreme non-physiological positioning for prolonged period. For pelvic surgeries, patient is kept in low lithotomy with STP position (angulation of at 25–45°,[6] **Fig. 4.1A**). Risk of patient sliding, nerve injury and pressure damage are quite frequent. Meticulous care is necessary to prevent injury to the neurovascular bundles. Proper padding/cushions over pressure points should be used to avoid tissue damage and nerve impingement. For kidney and upper ureter surgery, patient is kept in the lateral flank position **(Fig. 4.2)** with the point of breaking the table between the costal margin and anterior superior iliac spine. The anesthesiologist should ensure proper placement of axillary roll, pillows and cushions below the head to prevent cervical spine extension and care of the dependent eye and pressure points. Bolsters on the back and safety straps over the hip and thorax can ensure a secured patient in the lateral position. For thoracic procedures patient needs to be positioned in the lateral position or supine with arm abducted **(Fig. 4.1B)** and operating room (OR) table rotated 180° away from the anesthesia machine.

To prevent patient sliding towards the head end during STP, various devices have been used. Egg crate mattress, foam mattress, bean bag immobilizers, shoulder rest are some of them. In the absence of these materials, simple leucoplast can be used for a moderately tight 'Figure of 8' strapping **(Fig. 4.1A)** done with the upper loops placed at the angle of

Figs 4.1A and B: Patient position for (A) Robotic pelvic surgery; (B) Mediastinal surgery

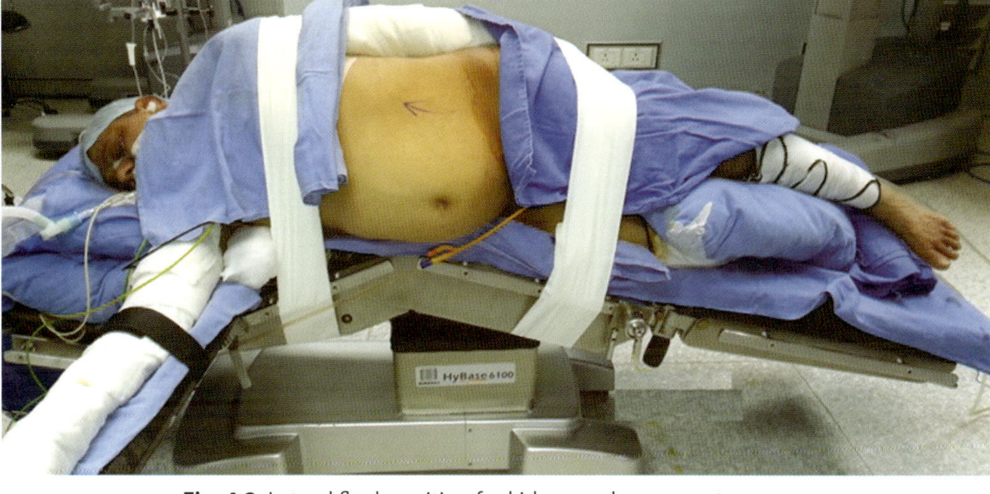

Fig. 4.2: Lateral flank position for kidney and upper ureter surgery

the shoulder and the lower loops just above the costal margin avoiding excessive pressure over the breasts. Lithotomy position can be maintained with the use of padded stirrups with lift assist function. These prevent damage to the head of fibula and peroneal nerve and also help in intraoperative repositioning of the legs. A 'trial run' of the final table position should be done before cleaning and draping to check for any strain on monitoring cables, circuit, intravenous tubings and any cardiorespiratory compromise.

FEW SYSTEMIC CONSIDERATIONS IN STEEP TRENDELENBURG POSITION

Cerebral Circulation and Intracranial Tension

In STP, cerebral perfusion increases with a corresponding decrease in venous outflow. This may lead to an increase in intracranial pressure if rescue measures are not initiated promptly. The increase in cerebral blood flow is dependent on the mean blood pressure beyond the autoregulatory range and the partial pressure of carbon dioxide in the arterial blood ($PaCO_2$). Moreover, central venous pressure is raised because of the positioning and creation of pneumoperitoneum. The driving pressure determining brain perfusion, the cerebral perfusion pressure (CPP) is the difference between mean arterial pressure (MAP) and the central venous pressure (CVP) or intracranial pressure, whichever is higher.[7] Kalmar et al.[5] has shown that CPP and regional brain tissue oxygenation are more or less maintained during laparoscopic surgery in STP. However, MAP should be maintained in the normal autoregulatory range.

Ocular Considerations

Pneumoperitoneum in STP has been shown to cause ocular hypertension as high as 13 mm Hg above the baseline.[8,9] Although reversible, if maintained for a long period of time, it can lead to ocular complications ranging from conjunctival edema, corneal damage, lens dislocation, retinal detachment and ischemic optic neuropathy causing postoperative visual loss (POVL).[10] Severe corneal ulceration and conjunctival burns have been reported following reflux of gastric acid onto the face while operating in STP. Proper sealing of eyelids with preferably transparent dressing is a must. Maintaining the mean ocular perfusion pressure (MOPP) which is the difference between MAP and intraocular pressure, above 50 mm Hg[11] is important for retinal integrity and avoiding the devastating complication of POVL. Duration of surgery and end tidal CO_2 levels are the two independent factors of intraocular hypertension in laparoscopic surgery in Trendelenburg position.[8]

Issues with Dependent Part Venous Drainage

Trendelenburg position may impair venous drainage from the upper half of the body and can lead to significant edema of head and neck region including cerebral edema. Patient's head should be kept in the neutral position throughout the procedure to facilitate venous drainage. Presence of peri-orbital edema should alert the anesthetist of the possibility of concomitant airway edema. One has to be careful before tracheal extubation in the presence of airway edema.

Nerve Injury

The most commonly injured nerve in lithotomy position is the common peroneal nerve followed by femoral and sciatic nerves. It has been observed that every hour spent in lithotomy position increases the risk of lower limb motor neuropathy by 100%.[12] Reports of brachial plexus injury are plenty during robot-assisted pelvic surgery (the neck bearing the weight of the dependent head for a prolonged period while the trunk is strapped to the table) and RATS thymectomy (following abduction of the left upper limb to accommodate the robotic arm, **Fig. 4.1B**). Hyperabduction of the extremity should be avoided.

Kidney Perfusion and Glomerular Filtration Rate

Pneumoperitoneum above 10 mm Hg has been shown to reduce renal blood flow and glomerular filtration rate transiently.[13,14] Direct compression of the renal parenchyma[15] or renal vein or artery vasoconstriction (mediated by vasopressin, catecholamines, endothelin I, angiotensin II[16]) may affect renal function adversely during pneumoperitoneum. Intra-abdominal pressure of 20 mm Hg can reduce the glomerular filtration rate by almost 25% by an impaired renal perfusion gradient.

Limb Hypoperfusion

Prolonged lithotomy and Trendelenburg position increases the risk of lower limb hypoperfusion[17] and deep venous thrombosis. The "well leg compartment syndrome"[18] is the result of decreased perfusion to the elevated legs combined with the compromised venous drainage due to faulty lower limb positioning and high intra-abdominal pressure. This manifests as lower limb pain, rhabdomyolysis and possibly myoglobinuria with deterioration of renal function which is unacceptable especially in robotic renal transplantation. Risk factors are prolonged surgery (>4 hours), obesity, muscular legs, hypotension and STP.

Postoperative Considerations

Recovery from anesthesia can be delayed because of the need for maintenance of proper depth of anesthesia while the robot is docked. Although not well established, brain edema might set in during prolonged Trendelenburg position causing unpredictable reversal and emergence delirium. Shorter acting agents like desflurane or sevoflurane can shorten the recovery time. Majority of the robotic surgeries per se do not require elective postoperative ventilation. The 'cuff leak test' should be performed before extubation and use of nasopharyngeal airway as an adjunct is extremely useful in the postoperative period. Postoperative pain is usually managed with intravenous nonsteroidal anti-inflammatory drugs (NSAIDs) and paracetamol as it is a minimally invasive surgery. Corneal and conjunctival edema is self-limiting and does not require treatment.

Considerations in Robotic-assisted Thoracic Surgery (Figs 4.3A and B)

Apart from positioning issues and one lung anesthesia in RATS, capnothorax may be created during one lung anesthesia for RATS and coronary revascularization. Careful insufflation of CO_2 under conditions of low pressures <8 mm Hg and low flow <1 L/minute[19] is generally considered safe during thoracic surgery. **Table 4.4** depicts some of the deleterious effects of capnothorax.

In case of hemodynamic instability, capnothorax should be released immediately with resumption of two lung ventilation if deemed necessary. External defibrillation should be attempted only when capnothorax is released.

ANESTHESIA FOR TRANSORAL ROBOTIC SURGERY (FIG. 4.4)

Transoral robotic surgery (TORS) directly avoids the need for mandibulectomy or sometimes tracheostomy and gives the surgeon an unparalleled 3 dimensional endoscopic vision. OR table needs to be rotated 180° away from the anesthetist as the robotic patient cart towers above the patient's head. Continuous suspension laryngoscopy, limited access, airway sharing, risk of loss of airway, etc. are considerations that need to be addressed proactively.

ROBOT-ASSISTED MINIMALLY INVASIVE RENAL TRANSPLANTATION (FIGS 4.5A AND B)

Started in India in 2013, minimally invasive renal transplantation with regional hypothermia is gradually receiving worldwide acceptance. Apart from the routine considerations for robotic pelvic surgeries, additional issues with intra-abdominal ice slush,[20] fluid restriction, maintenance of cardiovascular stability in the face of metabolic acidosis and restriction in volume infusion[21] till the time of vascular anastomosis. Robot docks between the legs of the patient while he lies in low lithotomy and moderate 20° Trendelenburg position.

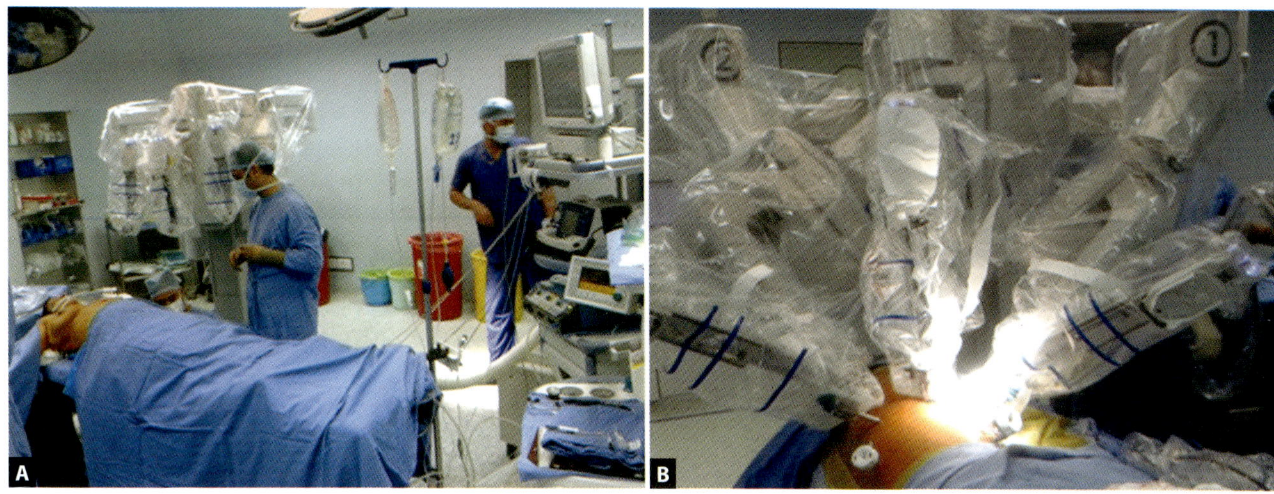

Figs 4.3A and B: (A) Patient's and table's head end may be 180° away from the machine; (B) Lateral decubitus position with single lung ventilation for lobectomies

Table 4.4: Deleterious effects of capnothorax

Increase	*Decrease*
Heart rate, central venous pressure	Dynamic lung compliance
Cerebral blood flow, intracranial pressure	Preload and compliance of the heart
Peak airway pressure, intrathoracic pressure	Functional residual capacity of the dependent ventilated lung

ROBOT-ASSISTED ESOPHAGECTOMY

One lung anesthesia with double lumen tube is instituted along with insertion of invasive lines. The patient lies in the lateral decubitus position with arm 180° extended touching the head. Then the patient is tilted till the patient is near prone. The robot docks from the side. Care should be taken to avoid risk of brachial plexus and ocular injury. In transhiatal approach robot docks from the head end while the patient stays supine with neck tilted to the opposite side.

Robot-assisted Liver Surgery

Patient is positioned in semilithotomy reverse Trendelenburg to supine position slightly tilted to the left. The table is rotated 180° away from the anesthesia machine and robot docks from the cephalic end.

Practical Tips and Tricks

A few pearls in the anesthetic management of robotic-assisted surgeries are:

- The patient is subjected to a dynamic hazardous situation. Repeated checkups and vigilance for robotic parts coming in close proximity to the patient, head and neck position, face area, cable and tubings, etc. are important.
- The final determining factor for barotrauma due to high airway pressure is the transalveolar or transpulmonary pressure (difference between the alveolar pressure and intrapleural pressure) rather than the peak airway pressure. During positive pressure ventilation in STP with pneumoperitoneum, intrathoracic pressure also increases and maintains the transalveolar pressure within a normal range. We have observed that a higher than usual peak airway pressure of 40–45 mm Hg is well tolerated by the patient.
- In case of sudden cardiorespiratory compromise, robot needs to be undocked and patient's position normalized. Routine undocking drills and dry runs should be practised as an institutional protocol.[22]
- Robot can malfunction in the middle of operation. So, anesthesia as well as surgical consent should always take laparoscopic and open surgery consent.
- Operating table remote should be in the switch off mode to prevent accidental activation leading to patient movement.

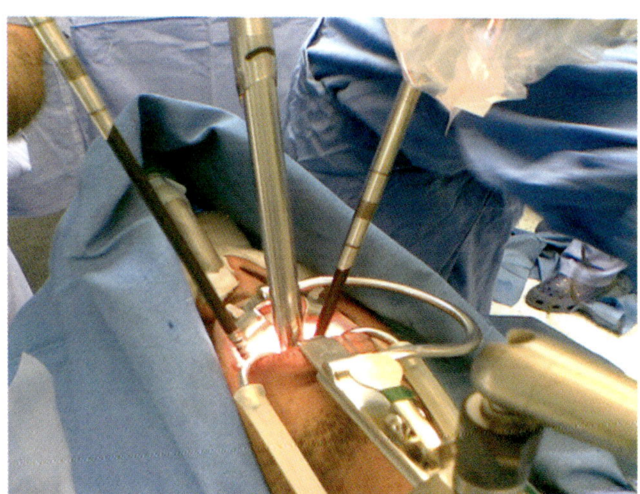

Fig. 4.4: Transoral robotic surgery

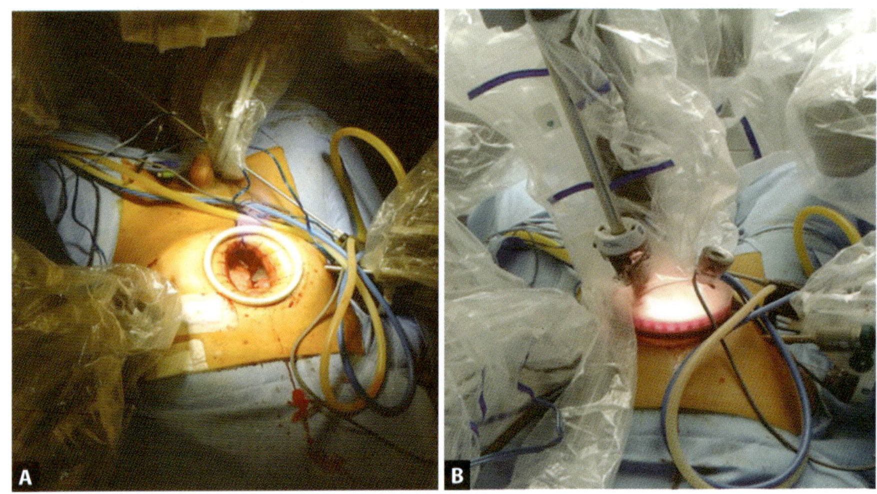

Figs 4.5A and B: (A) Incision for kidney insertion; (B) Robotic arms going through the Gelport

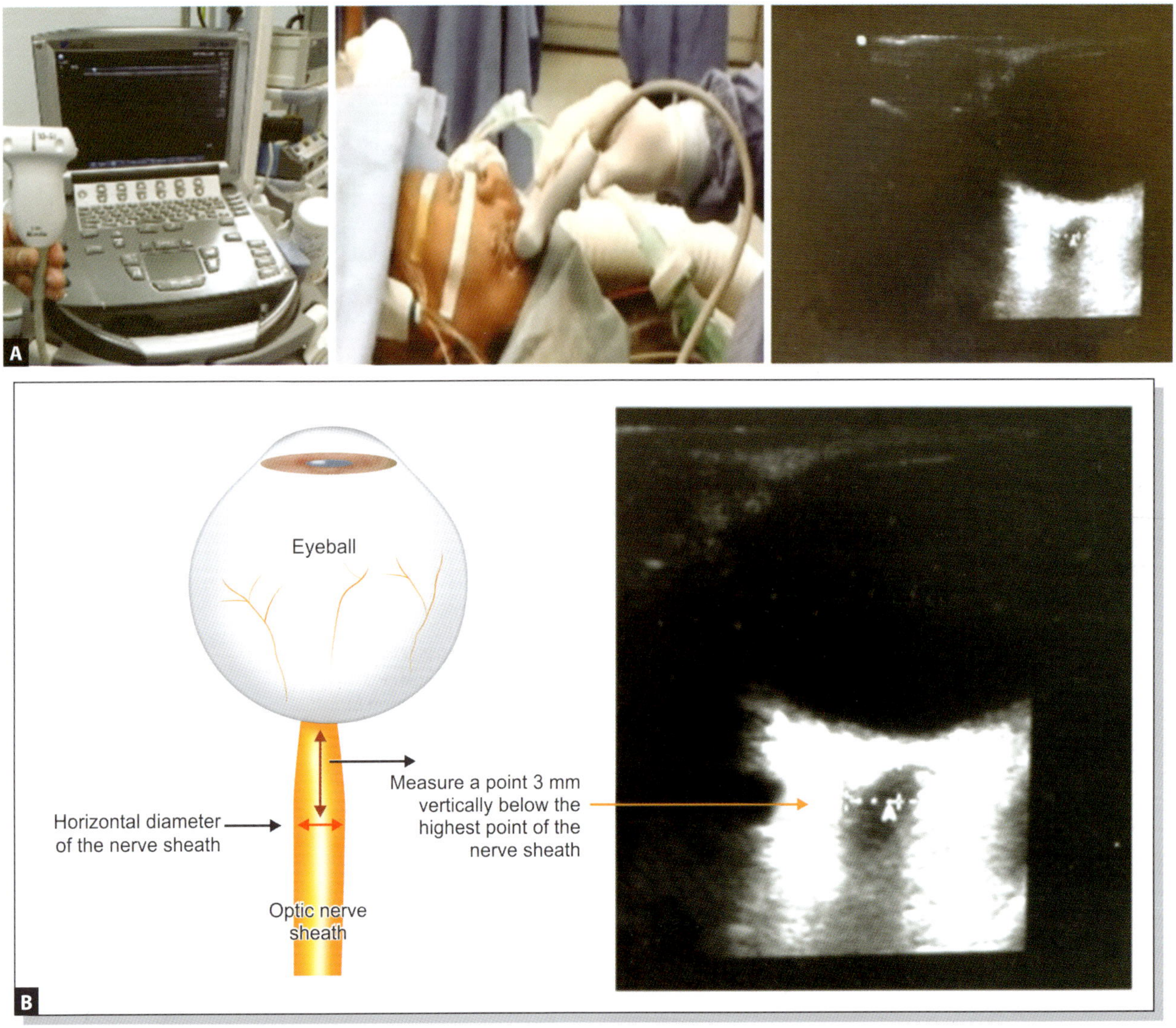

Figs 4.6A and B: (A) Optic nerve sheath diameter measurement for intraoperative ICT estimation; (B) Technique of optic nerve sheath diameter measurement

- Intraoperative fluid management in robotic pelvic surgeries needs special mention. In order to reduce the incidence of dependent edema in the head and neck region and diuresis-related problem during urethral anastomosis, fluid is restricted till the patient is repositioned back to normal supine position. It has been shown conclusively that restricted fluid therapy has no adverse outcome and is well tolerated by the patient.[23]
- Stomach decompression and aspiration of stomach content via an orogastric or nasogastric tube is recommended to prevent ocular surface injuries.
- Ocular protection by use of transparent film dressings over the closed lids is a well-accepted practice.
- Change in ICT can be estimated by portable on site ultrasonic measurement of the optic nerve sheath diameter **(Figs 4.6A and B)** at various time durations and prophylactic measures should be initiated if necessary.[24]

CONCLUSION

As the number of surgical specialties resorting to robot assisted procedures increases, there will be a corresponding increase in newer challenges for the anesthesiologist. Taking into consideration the rapidity with which the technology is spreading and the improved accessibility to the best health care thanks to the health insurance policies, we can safely say that surgical robotics will be the norm rather than the exception for most surgeries. So, it is imperative that we understand the unique demands and challenges involved and try to practice and formulate anesthetic protocols and guidelines specially meant for robot-assisted surgical procedures.

REFERENCES

1. Das J, Khanna S, Goswami D, Kapoor PK, Mehta Y. Monitoring of neuromuscular blockade by pulse oximetry tracing: A simple modification of mechanomyographic and acceleromyographic principles. J Anaesthesiol Clin Pharmacol. 2011;27(3):424-5.
2. Eun Mi Choi, Sungwon Na, Seung Ho Choi, Jiwon An, Koon Ho Rha, Young Jun Oh. Comparison of volume-controlled and pressure-controlled ventilation in steep Trendelenburg position for robot-assisted laparoscopic radical prostatectomy. Journal of Clinical Anesthesia. 2011;23(3):183-8.
3. Darlong V, Kunhabdulla NP, Pandey R, Chandralekha, Punj J, Garg R, Kumar R. Hemodynamic changes during robotic radical prostatectomy. Saudi J Anaesth. 2012;6(3):213-8.
4. GH Guyatt, Elie A Akl, Mark Crowther, David D Gutterman, Holger J Schuünemann and for the American College of Chest Physicians Antithrombotic Therapy and Prevention of Thrombosis Panel. Executive Summary: Antithrombotic Therapy and Prevention of Thrombosis, 9th edition. American College of Chest Physicians Evidence-Based Clinical Practice Guidelines. Chest. 2012;141(Suppl 2):7S-47S. doi:10.1378/chest.1412S3.
5. Kalmar AF, Foubert L, Hendrickx JF, et al. Influence of steep Trendelenburg position and CO2 pneumoperitoneum on cardiovascular, cerebrovascular, and respiratory homeostasis during robotic prostatectomy. Br J Anaesth. 2010;104(4):433-9.
6. Gupta K, Mehta Y, Jolly AS, Khanna S. Anaesthesia for robotic gynaecological surgery. Anaesth Intensive Care. 2012;40(4):614-21.
7. Munis JR, Lozada LJ. Giraffes, siphons and starling resistors. Cerebral perfusion pressure revisited. J Neurosurg Anesthesiol. 2000;12:290-6.
8. Awad H, Santilli S, Ohr M, Roth A, Yan W, Fernandez S, Roth S, Patel V. The effects of steep trendelenburg positioning on intraocular pressure during robotic radical prostatectomy. Anesth Analg. 2009;109(2):473-8.
9. Kakar PN, Das J, Roy PM, Pant V. Robotic invasion of operation theatre and associated anaesthetic issues: a review. Indian J Anaesth. 2011;55(1):18-25
10. Roth S. Perioperative visual loss: what do we know, what can we do? Br J Anaesth. 2009;103(Suppl 1):i31-i40..
11. Zheng Y, Wong TY, Mitchell P, Friedmn DS, He M, Aung T. Distribution of Ocular Perfusion Pressure and its relationship with Open angle glaucoma: the Singapore Malay Eye Study. Invest. Ophthalmol. Vis Sci. 2010;1(7):3399-404.
12. Warner MA, Martin JT, Schroeder DR, et al. Lower extremity motor neuropathy associated with surgery performed on patients in a lithotomy position. Anesthesiology. 1994;81:6-12.
13. Demyttenaere S, Feldman LS, Fried GM. Effect of pneumoperitoneum on renal perfusion and function: a systematic review. Surg Endosc. 2007;21:152-60.
14. Nishio S, Takeda H, Yokoyama M. Changes in urinary output during laparoscopic adrenalectomy. BJU Int. 1999;83:944-7.
15. Chiu AW, Azadzoi KM, Hatzichristou DG, Siroky MB, Krane RJ, Babayan RK. Effects of intra-abdominal pressure on renal tissue perfusion during laparoscopy. J Endourol. 1994;8:99-103.
16. Gudmundsson FF, Viste A, Myking OL, Bostad L, Grong K, Svanes K. Role of angiotensin II under prolonged increased intraabdominal pressure (IAP) in pigs. Surg Endosc. 2003;17:1092-7.
17. Halliwill JR, Hewitt SA, Joyner MJ, Warner MA. Effects of various lithotomy positions on lower-extremity blood pressure. Anesthesiology.1998;89(6):1373-6.
18. Simms MS, Terry TR. Well leg compartment syndrome after pelvic and perineal surgery in the lithotomy position. Postgrad Med J 2005;81:534-6.
19. Harris RJ, Benveniste G, Pfitzner J. Cardiovascular collapse caused by carbon dioxide insufflations during one-lung anaesthesia for thoracoscopic dorsal sympathectomy. Anaesth Intensive Care. 2002;30:86-9.
20. Das J, Kumar S, Khanna S, Mehta Y. Re: Mani Menon, Akshay Sood, Mahendra Bhandari, et al. Robotic kidney transplantation with regional hypothermia: a step-by-step description of the Vattikuti Urology Institute–Medanta Technique (IDEAL Phase 2a). Eur Urol. 2014;65:991-1000.
21. Sood A, GHosh P, Jeong W, Khanna S, Das J, Bhandari M, Kher V, Ahlawat R, Menon M. Minimally invasive kidney transplantation: Perioperative considerations and key 6-month outcomes. Transplantation. 2015;99:316-23.
22. Khanna S, Das J, Kumar S, Mehta Y, Ahlawat R. Being "intuitive": Starting a comprehensive multispecialty robotic surgery programme. OA Robotic Surgery. 2014;2(1):8.
23. Giorgio Della Rocca, Luigi Vetrugno, Gabriella Tripi, Cristian Deana, Federico Barbariol and Livia Pompei. Liberal or restricted fluid administration: are we ready for a proposal of a restricted intraoperative approach? BMC Anesthesiology. 2014;14:62 doi:10.1186/1471-2253-14-62.
24. Khanna S, Das J, Kumar S, Mehta Y. Perioperative noninvasive assessment of intracranial tension by ultrasonographic monitoring of optic nerve sheath diameter: our experience. Int J Periop Ultrasound Appl Technol. 2013;2(3):118-21.

SECTION 2

General Surgery

- **Robot-assisted Sleeve Gastrectomy**
  Parveen Bhatia, Vivek Bindal, Anand Kumar Yadav
- **Robot-assisted Roux-en-Y Gastric Bypass**
  Parveen Bhatia, Vivek Bindal, Anand Kumar Yadav
- **Robotic Surgery for Benign Colorectal Diseases**
  Deepak Govil, Vivek Tandon, Vachan Hukkeri, Satyaprakash Jindal, Adithya GK
- **Carcinoma Rectum**
  Somashekhar SP
- **Robotic Surgery for Bile Duct Tumors**
  Vivek Bindal, Anand Kumar Yadav

CHAPTER

5

Robot-assisted Sleeve Gastrectomy

Parveen Bhatia, Vivek Bindal, Anand Kumar Yadav

INTRODUCTION

With rise in the prevalence of obesity, the field of bariatric surgery is witnessing an ever increasing demand. Obesity along with comorbidities such as type 2 diabetes, hypertension, increased triglycerides and hypercholesterolemia and sleep apnea has become the leading cause of death worldwide.[1] Bariatric surgery has proven to be most safe and effective in treating this disease.[2] Sleeve gastrectomy (SG) is a restrictive bariatric surgical procedure and the most common procedures performed nowadays.[3,4] In 1988, Doug Hess performed the first sleeve gastrectomy as part of duodenal switch (DS).[5] Excellent weight loss was seen in this procedure in 1997 by Anthone, wherein procedure was limited to sleeve gastrectomy because of the complexity of the duodenal switch.[6] Gagner performed the first laparoscopic sleeve gastrectomy in high-BMI patient with subsequent Roux-en-Y gastric bypass.[7] Sleeve gastrectomy has been found to have a risk/benefit profile between laparoscopic adjustable gastric band (LAGB) procedure and Roux-en-Y gastric bypass (RYGB). American Society for Metabolic and Bariatric Surgery (ASMBS) recognizes SG as an acceptable primary bariatric procedure and as a first stage for a RYGB or a DS.[8]

Performing bariatric surgery can be technically demanding in many situations because of large patients, large livers, thick abdominal walls and substantial visceral fat making exposure, dissection and reconstruction difficult.[9] The super obese (SO) patients with a BMI greater than or equal to 50 kg/m^2 is a difficult to manage population because of limited working space, excessive torque, on instruments due to thick abdominal wall, comorbidities and high risk anesthesia.[10] The maneuvering of instruments while performing SG becomes challenging, especially while doing intracorporeal suturing. The surgeons have been looking for methods to improve the patient outcomes, surgical technique and decrease complications on one hand, and reducing the learning curve on the other hand.

Robotic surgery has provided the surgeons with the advantage of three-dimensional vision, increased dexterity and precision by downscaling surgeon's movements enabling a fine tissue dissection and filtering out physiological tremor.[11,12] It overcomes the restraint of torque on ports from thick abdominal wall and minimizes port site trauma by remote center technology.[13]

The main limitation with robotic surgery is the perceived higher cost and set-up time compared to laparoscopy. But with increased experience, it is seen that set-up times reduce and costs may also come down as material prices reduce.[14] As other players enter the market, the cost of robotic surgery is likely to come down.

SURGICAL PROCEDURE

Instrumentation

The following robotic instruments are used for a robotic sleeve gastrectomy (RSG) in a da Vinci Si system **(Fig. 5.1)**:

- Large needle driver
- Ultrasonic shears
- Atraumatic bowel grasper forceps
- Laparoscopic/Robotic staplers.

All three instrument arms of the robotic system are used with third arm coming from the left side of the patient (explained in docking).

Patient Positioning and Operating Setup (Fig. 5.2)

The patient is positioned in supine position with arms by the side under general anesthesia. The abdomen is cleaned and draped and orogastric tube/urinary catheter (optional) are placed. Footboard is properly secured and straps placed at level of upper thigh. The body warming blanket is placed. The master console is placed in a way that the surgeon is able to freely visualize the operative field while sitting on the console. Two video monitors are placed on either side of the patient to enable assistants easily watch and help at every step of procedure, with ergonomic comfort. The anesthesia machine is kept on right side of the head end as patient cart comes in from the left shoulder.

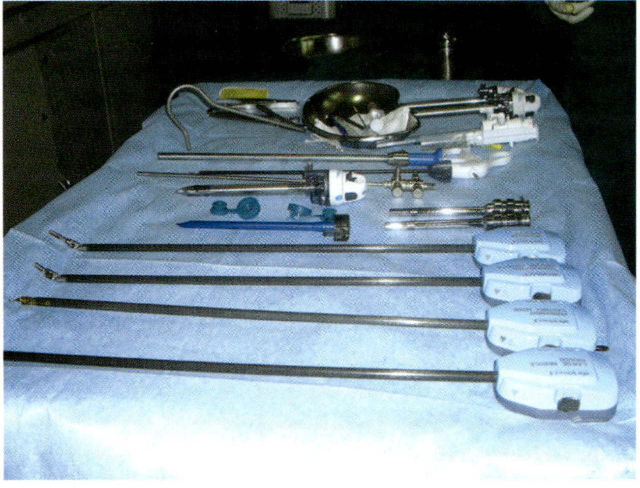

Fig. 5.1 : Instruments for robot-assisted sleeve gastrectomy

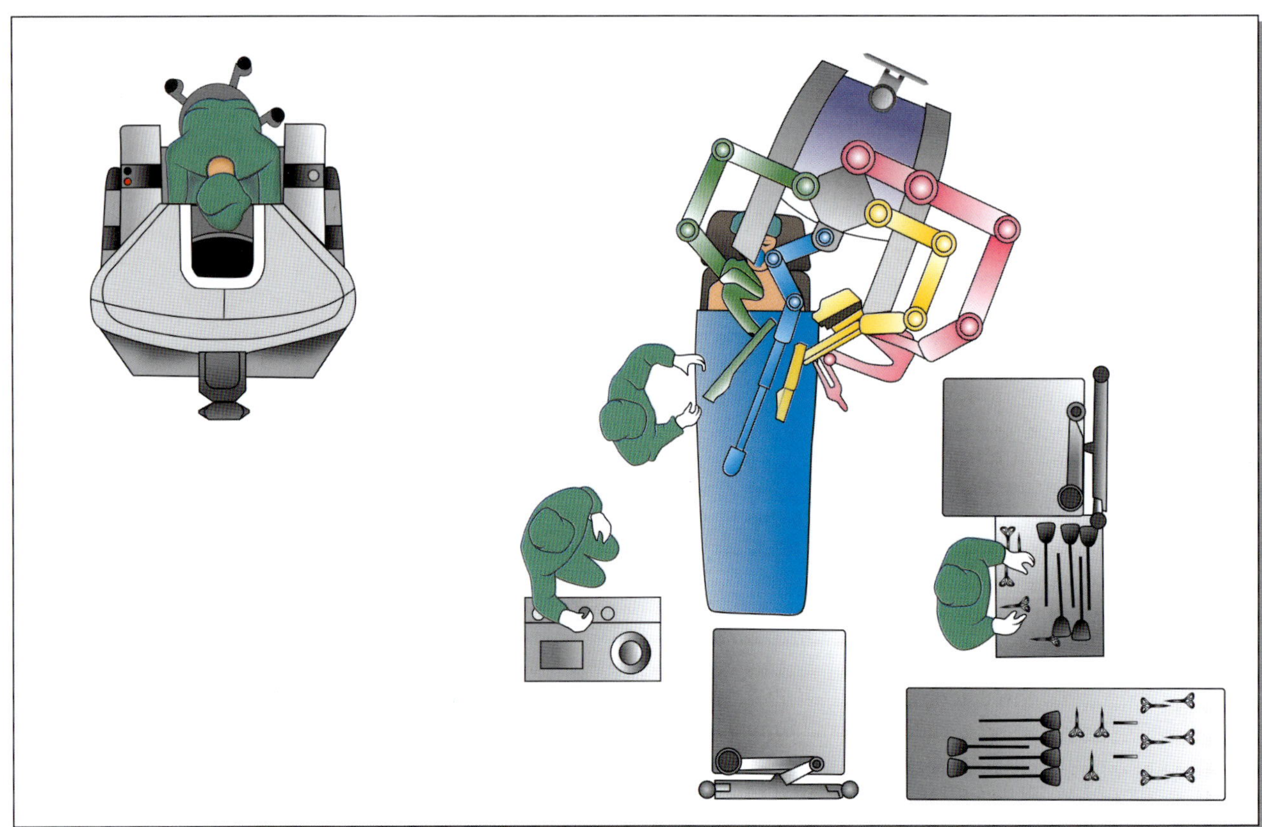

Fig. 5.2: Operating room set-up and patient cart positioning for robot-assisted sleeve gastrectomy (RASG)

Port Position and Docking

Pneumoperitoneum is achieved to 15 mm Hg using a Veress needle at Palmer's point (we prefer closed technique). All the distances are measured after insufflation of abdomen as they significantly change after pneumoperitoneum is created, especially in morbidly obese because of pendulous abdominal wall. The minimum intertrocar distance recommended in robotic surgery is 8-10 cm. But the actual distance intraperitoneally in morbidly obese individuals is significantly shorter than the distance measured on the skin. This factor has to be taken into account and trocars should be placed at maximum possible distance to avoid external arm

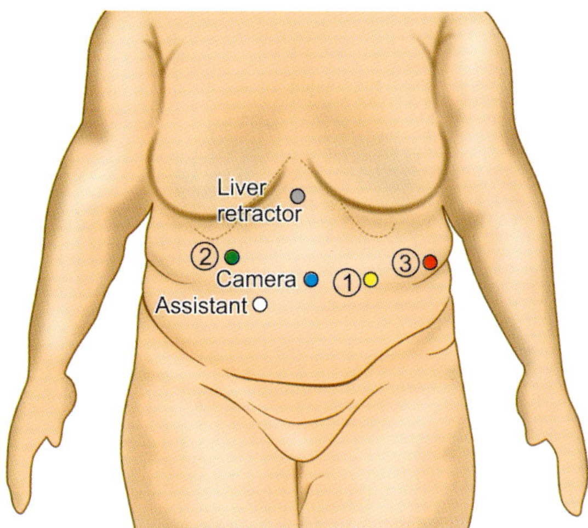

Fig. 5.3: Port position for robot-assisted sleeve gastrectomy

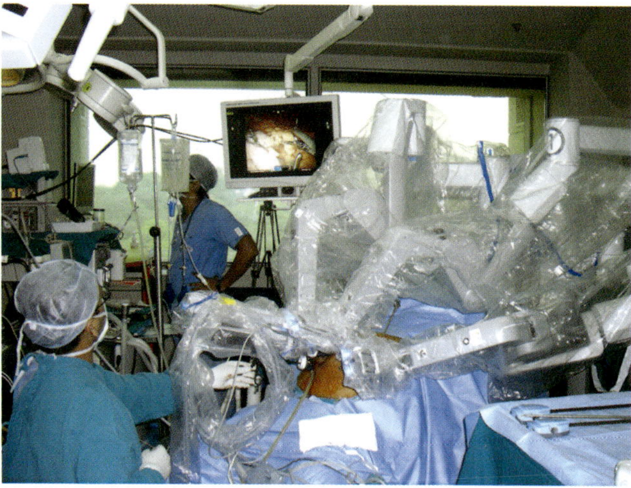

Fig. 5.4: Docking

clashing of robot. Pre-emptive 0.5% bupivacaine infiltration is done before incision at all port sites.

Camera port (12 mm diameter, 150 mm long trocar) is placed 20 cm below the xiphisternum slightly to left of midline under vision using a zero degree 10 mm scope to avoid any inadvertent visceral injury. Following this, one assistant and three da Vinci trocars are placed as follows **(Fig. 5.3)**:

R1 (8 mm da Vinci® cannula) is placed in left mid clavicular line approx. 20 cm from xiphisternum

R2 (8 mm da Vinci® cannula) is placed in right hypochondrium in midclavicular line taking care that the entry of port is below the margin of liver.

R3 (8 mm da Vinci® cannula) is placed in left flank at the level of camera port.

Assistant port (12 mm diameter) is placed in between camera port and R2 with a distance of at least 10 cm from both of them.

A 5 mm epigastric port is made and used for placing Nathanson liver retractor for retracting left lobe of liver.

The port placement needs to be adjusted based on the body habitus of the patient so as to prevent external arm collision and provide optimal exposure. A diagnostic laparoscopy is done to look for any adhesions/hernias/inadvertent injury during abdominal wall access.

The da Vinci® patient cart can either be brought from head end of the patient or from left shoulder (*parallel docking*) **(Fig. 5.4)**. Parallel docking gives more room to the anesthetist, as well as endoscopist for intraoperative gastroscopy. The third arm of the robot comes from left side of the patient. The assistant surgeon stands by the side for complimentary maneuvers (i.e. suction, stapling, retraction, etc.).

Surgical Technique

Operative Technique: RASG

The patient is placed in steep reverse Trendelenburg position. All three arms of da Vinci surgical system® (DVSS) are used.

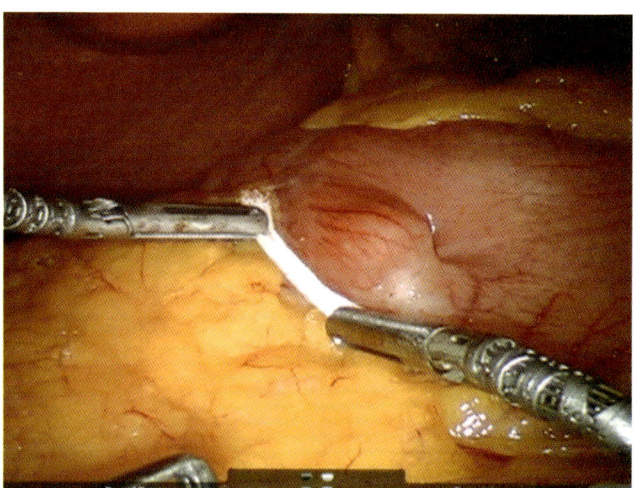

Fig. 5.5: Measuring proximal margin of gastrolysis using umbilical tape

A 38 Fr gastric calibration tube (GCT) is used after induction to empty out the gastric contents and kept in place to guide the sleeve formation. We place a nasogastric tube inside the GCT to be able to efficiently suck out the gastric secretions, which otherwise tend to pool in the wide end of GCT. Care is taken to empty out all the gastric secretions, especially from the fundus, so as to facilitate hiatal dissection. The GCT is then withdrawn into esophagus before starting the gastrolysis.

The first step is identification of pylorus. A 5 cm umbilical tape is taken to measure the distance from pylorus and gastrolysis is performed along the greater curvature of stomach using harmonic scalpel **(Fig. 5.5)**. Stomach is elevated using bowel grasper in R2, while bowel grasper in R3 is used to retract gastrocolic ligament laterally while harmonic scalpel in R1 is used for gastrolysis **(Fig. 5.6)**. Dissection is done close to the stomach in order to avoid injury to gastroepiploic vessels. The short gastric vessels from gastrosplenic ligament

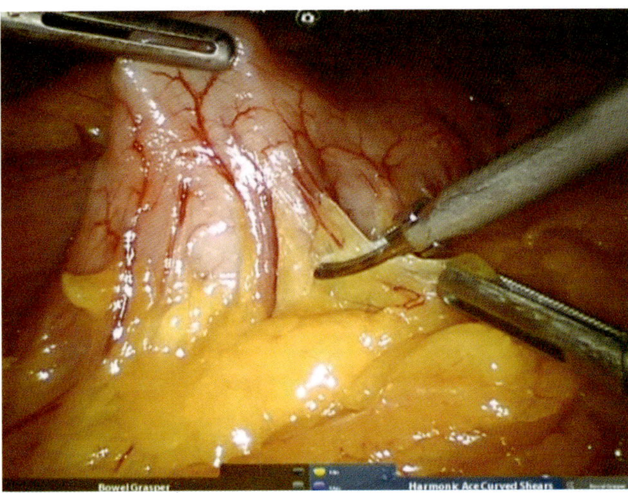

Fig. 5.6: Stomach is elevated using bowel grasper in R2, while bowel grasper in R3 is used to retract gastrocolic ligament laterally while harmonic scalpel in R1 is used for gastrolysis

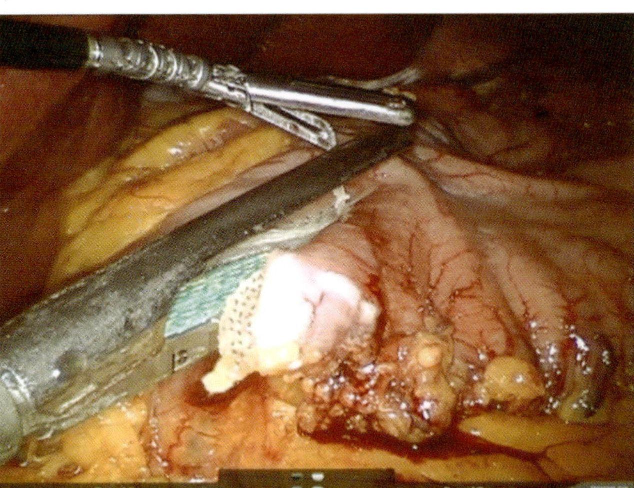

Fig. 5.7: Stapling started using green cartridge

and posterior gastric adhesions with pancreas are divided. *One can appreciate a bilaminar parchment like membrane if one remains close to stomach on the greater curvature.* This layer is relatively avascular and is the right plane for gastrolysis. Left crus is completely defined so that fundus is adequately mobilized. Care is taken that the bougie is withdrawn in the esophagus during this step; else it can lead to difficulty in dissection around the hiatus. If a hiatus hernia is identified, it should be repaired to avoid gastroesophageal reflux. Distal portion of gastrocolic ligament is divided until 4–5 cm from pylorus. Posterior adhesions of the stomach to the pancreas are taken down to fully mobilize the stomach.

Gastric calibration tube (GCT) is pushed forward by the anaesthetist and guided by the surgeon into first part of duodenum using bowel graspers. *Rotation of bougie by anesthetist and right traction by surgeon helps negotiate the pylorus. This leads to bougie nicely resting along the lesser curve of the stomach and helps in formation of an even sleeve.* Sleeve of stomach is created using articulating stapler from assistant port while the console surgeon applies traction on the stomach so that it lies in the right orientation. It is important to avoid any spiralling or uneven staple line. Sequential stapling with first green load and subsequent blue loads is performed while not being very snug to the bougie **(Fig. 5.7)**. Careful attention is given while stapling at incisura angularis to prevent narrowing. Transection is continued towards the angle of his along the lateral edge while maintaining lateral symmetrical traction. Staple line is not allowed to spiral either anteriorly or posteriorly to prevent a functional obstruction. Finally, transection is done at angle of HIS **(Fig. 5.8)**, avoiding an acute angle at gastroesophageal (GE) junction. Compression time of 30 seconds is allowed before and after every firing. The seven degrees of freedom help dissect in this area, especially around the left crus.

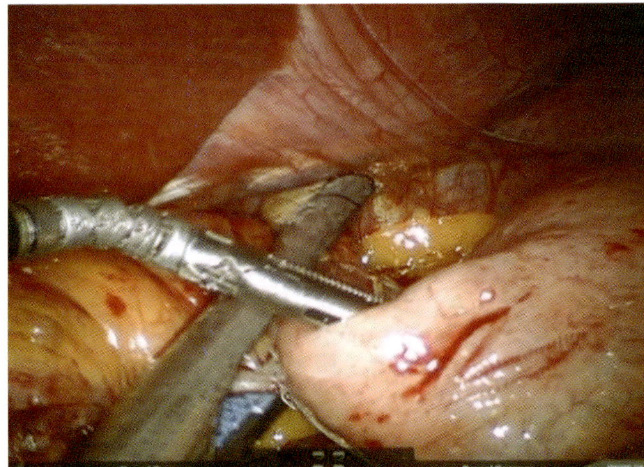

Fig. 5.8: Stapling at angle of HIS

Staple line reinforcements are used by some in the vertical firings at gastroesophageal junction. We imbricate the staple line keeping bougie in place using barbed 2-0 running suture **(Fig. 5.9)**. A check gastroscopy with saline immersion is done for all the cases so as to rule out any leak, bleed or obstruction.

Perioperative Care

The patients are given prophylaxis for deep venous thrombosis by mechanical (sequential compression devices, ambulation) and pharmacological (Low molecular weight heparin) methods. They are given a single shot of cephalosporin before induction for antimicrobial prophylaxis. Patients are encouraged to walk in the evening of surgery. All patients undergo an upper gastrointestinal series (gastrograffin study) the following day. If study shows no leak or stricture, patient is started on a clear liquid and discharged next day. The patients

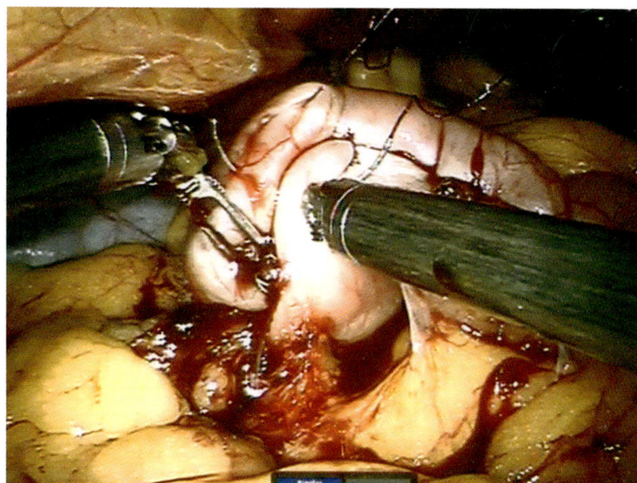

Fig. 5.9: Imbrication of staple line

are kept on liquid diet for two weeks followed by soft diet. Thereafter, they are progressed to normal diet intake.

REVIEW OF LITERATURE

Sleeve gastrectomy is increasingly becoming popular because of its low morbidity, excellent outcome and perceived technical simplicity. It is especially so in Indian subcontinent because of high prevalence of vegetarian population, who tend to choose a restrictive procedure rather than a malabsorptive one. But there are certain peculiarities in SG such as it has a long-stapled line with a potential to leak and a precise and safe dissection is required in the area of the left crus and hiatus to entirely mobilize the fundus. Compared to laparoscopic surgery, robotic surgery offers the possibility for endowrist, and this action facilitates the oversewing of the staple line.

Five studies have been published which focus on RSG.[15-19] Diamantis et al.[15] published a feasibility study that included 19 patients who underwent RSG. Their mean OR time was 95.5 minutes and reported complication rate was zero. Ayloo et al.[16] compared 30 robotic with 39 laparoscopic SG procedures and found no difference in length of hospital stay, complication rates or excess body weight loss at 1 year. They found a significantly longer OR time for RSG (135 vs 114 minutes), due to the fact that they had oversewn the staple line in the robotic arm and not in the laparoscopic arm.

Villalonga et al.[17] reported that the learning curve of performing RSG is over by 20 cases. He also published a large comparative series on SG including 100 patients each in robotic and laparoscopic arms.[18] They found that OR time was significantly longer in robotic group by 12 minutes. There was no significant difference in other perioperative parameters or complication rate. They did found that leaks occurred only in those patients in whom they did not oversewn the staple line, but used a buttress material. They concluded that RSG is a good stepping stone to robotic gastric bypass and revisional bariatric procedures. Romero et al.[19] published their experience of 134 RSG cases and compared it with descriptive results of a systematic review of laparoscopic SG (n = 3,148). The OR time was significantly higher by 12 minutes (p = 0.006), while the length of stay was lower by 1.1 days in robotic group (p =< 0.005). Leaks were found in 0 RSG versus 1.97% laparoscopic SG (p = 0.101); strictures in 0 versus 0.43% (p = 0.447); bleeding in 0.7 versus 1.21 % (p = 0.594); and mortality in 0 versus 0.1% (p = 0.714), respectively.

We conducted a study in patients who underwent RSG at our institution.[20] First 100 patients (41 females and 59 males) with a mean BMI of 48.17 ± 11.7 kg/m^2 were included. *The BMI ranged from 33 to 82.6 kg/m^2 with three patients above BMI of 80.* The super-obese group was compared to morbidly obese group based on patient demographics, BMI, comorbidities and perioperative outcomes, complications, weight loss. It revealed no significant difference in terms of operative time (p = 0.145), blood loss (p = 0.523) and length of hospital stay (p = 0.213). The operative time to BMI ratio was significantly lower for the SO group. There were no perioperative complications or mortality in either of the groups. The excess body weight loss at 6 month follow-up was also not significantly different among the two.

A steep decline in OT and DT was observed after initial 10 cases. We feel that the OR team got over the learning curve for robotic bariatric surgery by 10th case. The team was already well versed in laparoscopic bariatric procedures and could adjust to the new system pretty fast.

DISCUSSION

Robotic surgery is a team effort, and more so in bariatric surgery, where the role of an experienced bedside surgeon cannot be understated, as he is responsible for stapling (if robotic staplers are not used). The entire team learns with the surgeon and develops experience about patient safety precautions, operating room set-up, and type of instruments needed, thus leading to better OR times with better patient outcome.[21] As the main surgeon is separated from the patient while performing robotic surgery, the assistant surgeon has to be trained enough to help him perform difficult tasks and also to take care of any emergency situation arising during the procedure. The role of a trained scrub nurse and operating room technician is also very important in streamlining the conduct of the procedure and prevent any wastage of time and resources.

Another advantage which comes with use of robotic system is improved ergonomics and lesser operator fatigue. Ergonomics in laparoscopic surgery can be very challenging with big patients and uncomfortable postures, which lead to surgeon fatigue and work-related musculoskeletal symptoms.[22] Robotics provides the advantage of more degrees of freedom, which is advantageous in performing difficult dissection and sutured anastomosis.

There has been a concern about cost every time use of robotic system is considered, as the direct costs are generally higher for the robotic approach in bariatric procedures.

At the end of the day, the big question to be answered is whether the use of robotics is going to stay or will it perish with time like many fancy technologies. Looking at the basic concept of computer-assisted navigational surgery, robotics provide an enabling platform in between surgeon and the patient. It provides augmented and higher quality inputs from the patient to the surgeon and his output is refined to a superior quality before reaching back to the target. According to us, this should not be analyzed in terms of features of the present machine that is available for use, but in terms of the potential in the concept of using a digital interface to interact with patients and enhance the performance of the surgeon.[23] With the advent of newer technologies in robotics such as fluorescence, integration of images, virtual and augmented reality, telesurgery, single site platforms, natural orifice surgery and haptic feedback, we believe that digital platforms will provide an empowering tool to the surgeons which can potentially change the way surgery is practised today.

REFERENCES

1. Caballero. The Global Epidemic of Obesity. Epidemiol Rev. 2007;29(1):1-5.
2. Maggard MA, Shugarman LR, Suttorp M, Maglione M, Sugerman HJ, Livingston EH, et al. Meta-analysis: surgical treatment of obesity. Ann Intern Med. 2005;142(7):547-59.
3. Himpens J, Dapri D, Cadière GB. A prospective randomized study between laparoscopic gastric banding and laparoscopic isolated sleeve gastrectomy: results after 1 and 3 years. Obes Surg. 2006;16:1450-6.
4. D'Hondt M, Vanneste S, Pottel H, Devriendt D, Rooy FV. Laparoscopic sleeve gastrectomy as a single-stage procedure for the treatment of morbid obesity and the resulting quality of life, resolution of comorbidities, food tolerance, and 6-year weight loss. Surg Endosc. 2011;25:2498-504.
5. Hess DS, Hess DW. Billio pancreatic diversion with a duodenal switch. Obes Surg. 1998;8:267-82.
6. Hamoui H, Anthone GJ, Kaufman HS, Crookes PF. Sleeve gastrectomy in hig risk patient. Obes Surg. 2006;16:1445-9.
7. Regan JP, Inabnet WB, Gagner M. Early experience with two stage laparoscopic Roux-en-Y gastric bypass as an alternative in the super-super obese patient. Obese Surg. 2003;13:861-4.
8. ASMBS Clinical Issues Committee. Updated position statement on sleeve gastrectomy as a bariatric procedure. Surg Obes Relat Dis. 2012;8:21-6.
9. Wilson EB, Sudan R. The Evolution of Robotic Bariatric Surgery. World J Surg. 2013;37:2756-60.
10. Parikh MS, Shen R, Weiner M, Siegel N, Ren CJ. Laparoscopic bariatric surgery in super-obese patients (BMI>50) is safe and effective: a review of 332 patients. Obes Surg. 2005;15(6):858-63.
11. Talamini MA, Chapman S, Horgan S, Melvin WS. The Academic Robotic Group: a prospective analysis of 211 robotic-assisted procedures. Surg Endosc. 2003;17:1521-4.
12. Bindal V, Bhatia P, Kalhan S, Khetan M, John S, Ali A, et al. Robot-assisted excision of a large retroperitoneal schwannoma. JSLS. 2014;18(1):150-4.
13. Cadiere GB, Himpens J, Vertruyen M, Bruyns J, Germay O, Leman G, et al. Evaluation of telesurgical (robotic) Nissen Fundoplication. Surg Endosc. 2001;15(9):918-23.
14. Nakadi IE, Melot C, Closset J, DeMoor V, Betroune K, Feron P, et al. Evaluation of da Vinci Nissen Fundoplication Clinical Results and Cost Minimization. World J Surg. 2006;30(6):1050-4.
15. Diamantis T, Alexandrou A, Nikiteas N, Giannopoulos A, Papalambros E. Initial experience with robotic sleeve gastrectomy for morbid obesity. Obes Surg. 2011;21:1172-9.
16. Ayloo S, Buchs N, Addeo P, Bianco FM, Giulanotti PC. Robot-assisted sleeve gastrectomy for super-morbidly obese patients. J Laproendosc Advan Surg Tech. 2011;21:295-9.
17. Vilallonga R, Fort JM, Gonzalez O, Caubet E, Boleko A, Neff KJ, et al. The initial learning curve for robot-assisted sleeve gastrectomy: A surgeon's experience while introducing the robotic technology in a bariatric surgery department. Minimally Invasive Surgery. 2012;2012:347131. Epub 2012 Sep 17
18. Vilallonga R, Fort JM, Caubet E, Gonzalez O, Armengol M. Robotic Sleeve Gastrectomy Versus Laparoscopic Sleeve Gastrectomy: a Comparative Study with 200 Patients. Obes Surg. 2013;23:1501-7.
19. Romero RJ, Kosanovic R, Rabaza JR, Seetharamaiah R, Donkor C, Gallaset M, et al. Robotic Sleeve Gastrectomy: Experience of 134 Cases and Comparison with a Systematic Review of the Laparoscopic Approach. Obes Surg. 2013;23: 1743-52.
20. Bhatia P, Bindal V, Singh R, et al. Robot-assisted sleeve gastrectomy in morbidly obese versus super obese patients. JSLS. 2014;18(3).
21. Bindal V, Gonzalez-Heredia R, Masrur M, Elli EF. Technique Evolution, Learning Curve, and Outcomes of 200 Robot-Assisted Gastric Bypass Procedures: a 5-year experience. Obes Surg, 2014.
22. Esposito C, El Ghoneimi A, Yamataka A, Rothenberg S, Bailez M, Ferro M, et al. Work-related upper limb musculoskeletal disorders in paediatric laparoscopic surgery: A multicenter survey. J Pediatr Surg. 2013;48(8):1750-6.
23. Bindal V, Bhatia P, Dudeja U, et al. Review of contemporary role of robotics in Bariatric Surgery. J Min Access Surg. 2015;11:16-21.

CHAPTER

6

Robot-assisted Roux-en-Y Gastric Bypass

Parveen Bhatia, Vivek Bindal, Anand Kumar Yadav

INTRODUCTION

This chapter highlights the techniques and outcomes of Robot-assisted Roux-en-Y gastric bypass (RYGB). Robotic surgery is currently considered to be an attractive technology that could help perform RYGB, given its well-described advantages with the rise in obesity and bariatric procedures, surgeons are encountering patients with high body mass index (BMI) and revisional bariatric procedures. At present, the largest body of literature on application of the robotic platform in bariatric surgery is with RYGB. In this chapter we will describe the instrumentation, patient positioning, operating room set-up and surgical techniques of robotic RYGB.

Obesity is one of the greatest twenty first century public health challenge in both developed and developing regions of the world affecting 33% of world population.[1] Surgery currently represents the most successful long-term treatment of obesity and its associated comorbidities.[2]

Performing bariatric surgery can be technically demanding in many situations, as large patients having large livers, thick abdominal walls, and substantial visceral fat (more so in Asians) makes exposure, dissection, and reconstruction difficult.[3]

Super-obese (SO) patients with a BMI of 50 kg/m^2 or higher are difficult to manage because of thick abdominal walls, limited working space, excessive torque on instruments and high-risk anesthesia due to co-morbidities.[4] The maneuvering of instruments while performing LRYGB becomes challenging, especially while doing intracorporeal suturing.

Laparoscopic Roux-en-Y gastric bypass (LRYGB) as a bariatric procedure was described in the 1990s[5] and more than 100,000 procedures are being performed annually in United States alone.[6] Roux-en-Y gastric bypass (RYGB) constitutes 26.8% of total bariatric surgery volume according to an estimate published in July 2015 by the American Society for Metabolic and Bariatric Surgery (ASMBS).[7] The learning curve of LRYGB has been estimated to be about 75–100 cases.[8,9]

Because of adverse operating environment, surgeons encounter difficult ergonomic positions that can potentially shorten their careers, making them to look for methods that will improve surgical technique and patient outcomes, decrease complications, and also reduce the learning curve. Cadiere et al. reported the first use of robotics in bariatric surgery in 1999.[10]

Since then all of the commonly performed bariatric surgical procedures including RYGB, adjustable gastric banding, sleeve gastrectomy and biliopancreatic diversion with duodenal switch have been performed robotically and demonstrated to be feasible and safe. Robotic surgery has given surgeons the advantage of three-dimensional vision and has increased dexterity and precision by downscaling the surgeon's movements, enabling fine tissue dissection and filtering out physiological tremor.[11,12] It overcomes the restraint of torque on ports from the thick abdominal wall and minimizes port site trauma by remote center technology.[13] According to the consensus document on robotic surgery prepared by the Society of American Gastrointestinal and Endoscopic Surgeons (SAGES) and Minimally Invasive Robotic Association (MIRA), Robotic Surgery Consensus Group, robotic surgery holds particular value for gastric bypass amongst general surgical procedures.

Robotic surgery is facing challenges of higher cost and set-up time, compared with laparoscopy[14] but with increased experience, it is seen that set-up times are reduced, and as other companies enters the market, the cost of robotic surgery is likely to come down.

ADVANTAGES OF ROBOTIC ROUX-EN-Y GASTRIC BYPASS

Although sleeve gastrectomy has become the most common bariatric procedure being performed worldwide, many still consider RYGB to be the gold-standard surgical procedure for morbid obesity.[15,16] The overall results are good in terms of both weight loss and comorbidity resolution somewhere in between BPD and sleeve gastrectomy.[17] RYGB leads to 65.7%

excess weight loss and remission rates of 66.7% for type 2 diabetes mellitus and 60.4% for dyslipidemias.[18]

Roux-en-Y gastric bypass (RYGB) involves two anastomoses (gastrojejunostomy and jejunojejunostomy). A fundamental driver for the introduction of robotics to this procedure was the belief that a hand sutured gastrojejunal anastomosis would improve the quality of anastomosis when compared to stapled technique and that hand suturing would be greatly facilitated by the enhanced dexterity of the robotic system .

Robotic surgery is currently considered as an attractive technology that could help perform RYGB, given its well-described advantages.[19] It is also the most studied robotic bariatric procedure.[20,21]

SURGICAL TECHNIQUES

Various techniques of doing robotic RYGB are as mentioned below:

- Totally robotic RYGB (Single versus double docking)
- Hybrid technique
- Various techniques of doing gastrojejunostomy anastomosis [Hand-sewn or stapled (linear or circular stapler)].
- According to placement of Roux loop (antecolic or retrocolic).

The technique of choice at our center, IMAS (Institute of Minimal Access, Metabolic and Bariatric Surgery, Sir Ganga Ram Hospital, New Delhi) is to perform a Totally Robotic RYGB with a hand-sewn gastrojejunostomy. The instrumentation and technique are described below:

Instrumentation

Robotic Instruments (da Vinci® Si system (Intuitive Surgical, Sunnyvale, CA):

- R1—Ultrasonic shears—5 mm.
  Large needle driver—8 mm.
  Monopolar hook—8 mm.
- R2—Cadiere forceps—8 mm.
- R3—Double fenestrated grasper—8 mm.
- 12 mm camera—30° down
- Robotic port washers—3
- 4 arm robotic drapes—1 set

Laparoscopic Instruments

- Telescope 10-0°/10-30°
- Long ultrasonic probe—1
- Long hunter graspers—2
- Normal length hunter graspers—2
- Long Maryland dissector—1
- Long scissors—1
- Long needle driver 5 mm—1
- Nathanson's liver retractor—1
- Trumpet suction long—1
- Trocars:
  - 12 mm long trocar—2 (camera and assistant port).
  - 15 mm long trocar—1 (assistant port), if tristaples have to be used.
  - 8 mm robotic cannula with reducer—3 (R1, R2 and R3).
  - 5 mm long trocar (excel)—2.
- Clip applicator long—1.
- Laparoscopic staplers.

Technique

All patients receive subcutaneous low-molecular weight heparin 12 hours before along with below knee elastic stockings. Sequential compression devices are applied as prophylaxis against deep venous thrombosis on the operating table. Antibiotics (e.g. Cefuroxime 1.5 g) are administered within 30 minutes of incision.

Ideally, the room should be equipped with an operating table capable of holding 1,000 pounds and providing at least 30° of reverse Trendelenburg position. The table should also have the ability to be fitted with extenders for length and width. A footboard is essential to prevent patient movement during manipulation of the operating table.

Position

Position the patient supine position with left arm by the side and 20° of reverse Trendelenburg position with padding under both knees. Place a Foley catheter (optional) and secure the feet with tape and padding to the footboard. Place a safety strap just above the patient's knees. The abdomen is cleaned and draped, and an Gastric bougie of 38 Fr with an Ryle's tube inside placed in stomach. The assistant surgeon stands by the side of the patient with scrub nurse. The anesthesia machine is kept on one side of the head end, as the patient cart comes in from the head end.

Port Placement (Fig. 6.1)

- Pneumoperitoneum created at Palmer's point using Veress needle (closed technique).
- Using optical trocar, entry made at camera port. All other ports placed under vision to avoid any inadvertent injury.

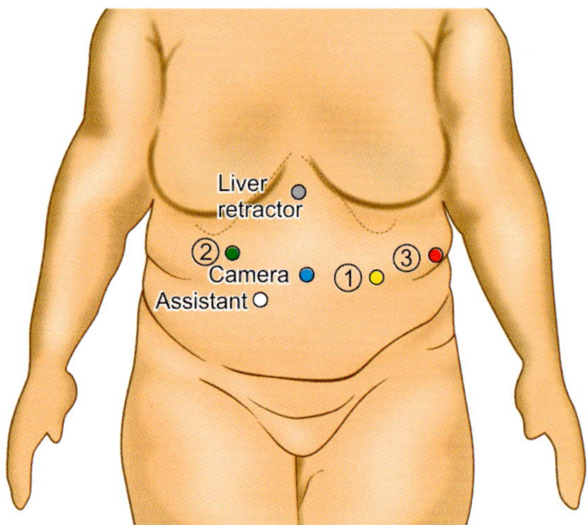

Fig. 6.1: Port positions for robot-assisted RYGB

- All the ports are marked after insufflation as port position shifts significantly after insufflation.
- C—Camera port, placed 20 cm from xiphisternum slightly to the left of midline.
- R2—In right midclavicular line, 20 cm from xiphisternum in arc like fashion.
- A (Assistant port)—between port C and port R2 at least 8 cm apart.
- R1—in left midclavicular line, 20 cm from xiphisternum.
- R3—in left anterior axillary line at the level of camera port.
- A 5-mm epigastric port is used to place a Nathanson liver retractor to retract the left lobe of the liver.
- The minimum intertrocar distance recommended in robotic surgery is 8–10 cm, but the actual distance intraperitoneally in morbidly obese individuals is significantly shorter than the distance measured on the skin.

Procedure

Gastrojejunostomy first technique

Diagnostic laparoscopy and bowel marking

- Diagnostic laparoscopy done. Nathanson's liver retractor placed.
- Assistant surgeon stands on the right side of patient.
- Omentum lifted upwards from left horizon and ligament of Trietz identified.
- Bowel walked 75 cm distal to ligament of Trietz, keeping proximal loop (biliopancreatic limb) on left side of patient, bowel hitched to stomach near lesser curvature at two sites using nonabsorbable suture.
- Bowel walking continued from 1st mark, 100 cm distally and marked using nonabsorbable suture at two sites 5 cm apart keeping proximal stitch small and distal stitch large.

Robot docking

- Robot docked in from head end.
- The master console is placed so that the surgeon can freely visualize the operative field while sitting on the console
- Patient cart brought in from head end. Patient's cart central column, target anatomy (stomach) and camera port, all lie in single straight line.
- Two video monitors are placed on either side of the patient to enable the assistants to easily watch and help at every step of procedure, with ergonomic comfort.

Operating room set-up: See **Figure 6.2**.

Gastric Pouch Formation

Taking following instruments in three arms, dissection is started:

- R1—Harmonic 5 mm long.
- R2—Cadiere forceps.
- R3—Double-fenestrated grasper.

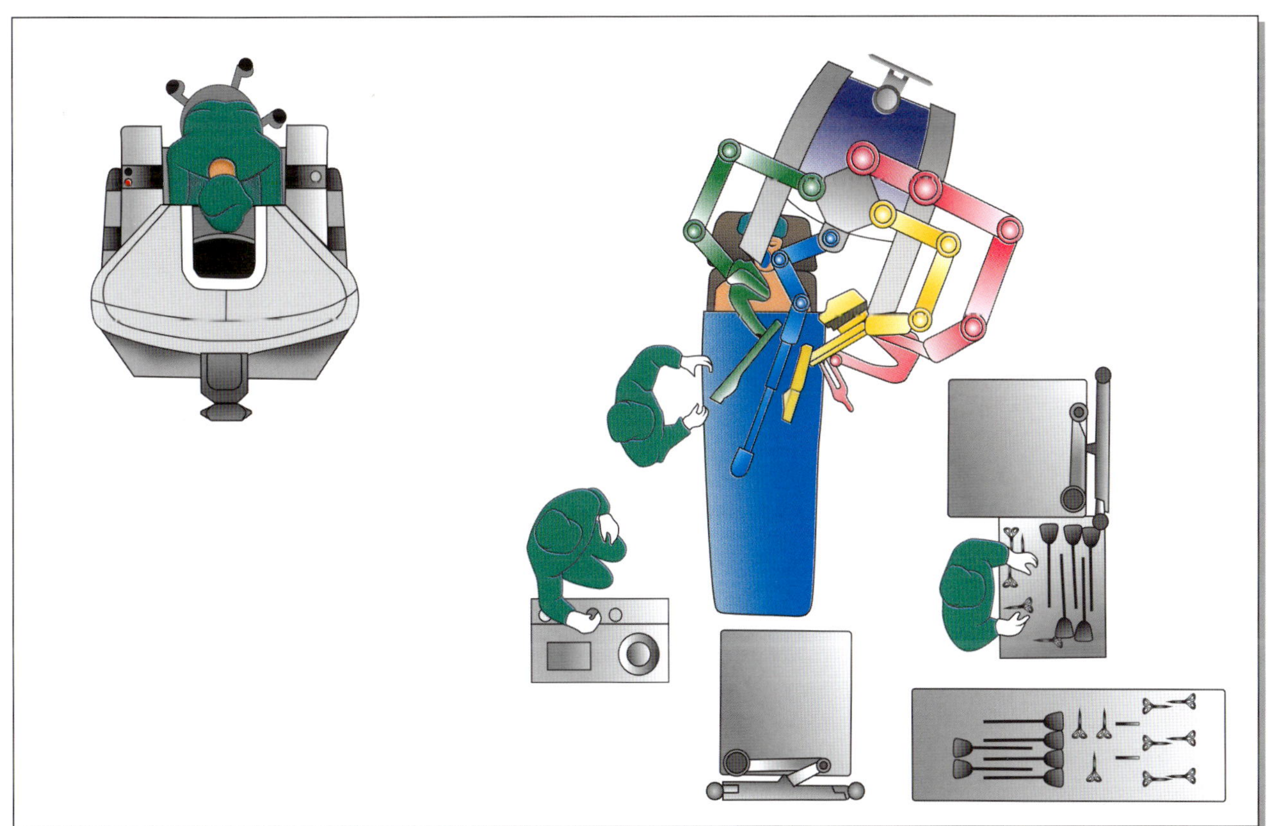

Fig. 6.2: Operating room set-up and patient cart positioning for robot-assisted Roux-en-Y gastric bypass (RYGB)

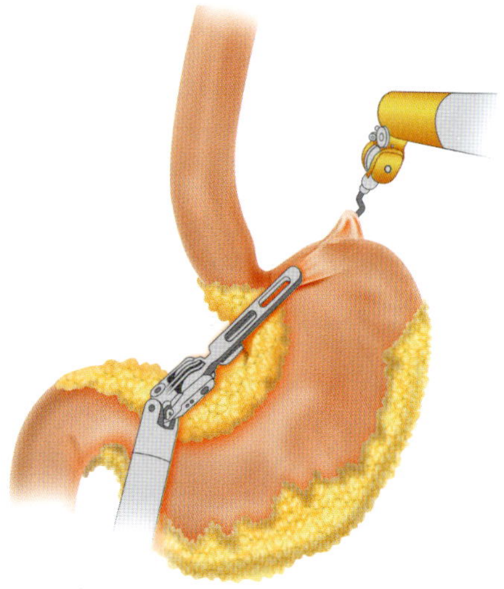

Fig. 6.3: Initial dissection around the left crus. The bowel grasper in the left hand retracts the fundus caudally while the monopolar hook divides the phrenoesophageal membrane, simplifying the final step of gastric pouch creation

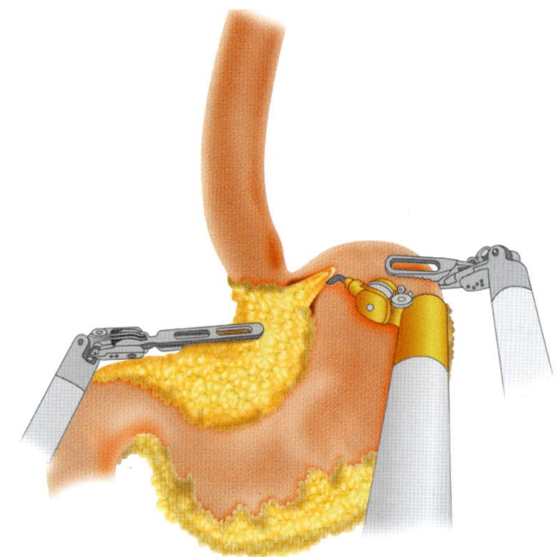

Fig. 6.4: Perigastric dissection is commenced at the level of second vessel from GE junction using the monopolar hook, avoiding injury to the vagus nerve. The third arm is used to retract the stomach anterolaterally, while fat is retracted medially by second arm

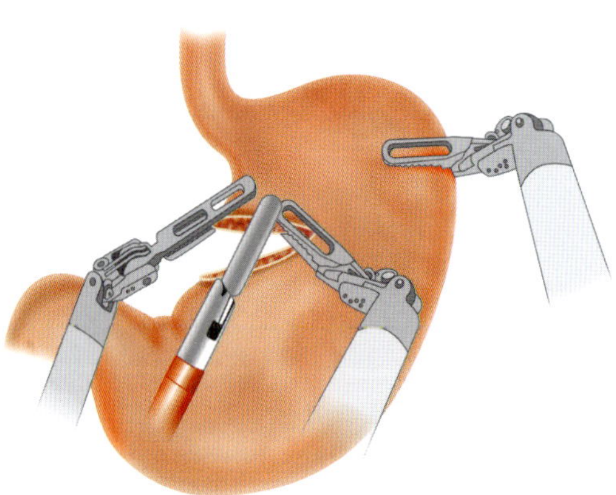

Fig. 6.5: A small gastric pouch is created by first horizontal fire followed by vertical firings using an endoscopic stapler with 60 mm cartridge

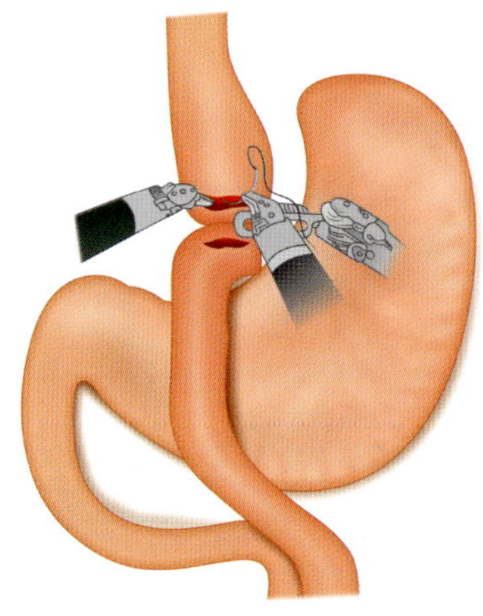

Fig. 6.6: Creation of the gastrojejunostomy (GJ). A hand-sewn GJ is being created . The third arm is holding the gastric pouch and Roux limb together

Dissection started by taking down the phrenoesophageal membrane, using energy source (monopolar hook or ultrasonic shears), after retracting the fundus of the stomach caudally **(Fig. 6.3)**.

Using perigastric dissection a small gastric pouch of capacity 20–30 mL is created starting between the first and second vessel from the gastroesophageal junction. R3 is used to retract the stomach laterally, while the harmonic scalpel in R1 is used to open up the gastrohepatic ligament. Perigastric dissection is commenced using the harmonic shears/hook, avoiding injury to the vagus nerve, and the lesser sac is reached **(Fig. 6.4)**. A horizontal fire of the stapler is done by the assistant using a 60 mm blue/tan cartridge. Dissection is continued superiorly to free the posterior adhesions of the stomach. Bougie is placed at this time to size the pouch. The vertical firing is done (60-mm blue/purple cartridge, two usually needed), and pouch creation is completed **(Fig. 6.5)**. Using barbed suture, staple line imbricated above downwards.

Gastrojejunal Anastomosis (Fig. 6.6)

- Barbed suture used for imbrication of vertical limb of gastric pouch is continued as fourth layer of Gastrojejunostomy.
- Gastrotomy and enterotomy made using monopolar hook/harmonic shears and stoma widened

using harmonic shears in R2 creating a stoma length of 2–2.5 cm approximately.
- Using a new barbed suture, third layer (posteriorly) started from left side, towards right side. Same suture reversed at opposite end (right) to form 2nd layer of anastomosis (anteriorly).
- Anterior—most layer completed using another barbed suture thus completing the anastomosis.

Jejunojejunal Anastomosis

- Window created in jejunum mesentery just proximal to gastrojejunostomy (towards left side) and jejunum transacted using white/tan- 60 mm cartridge thus creating a biliopancreatic limb of 75 cm.
- Roux limb measured for 100 cm from gastrojejunostomy till we reach the previously placed marking sutures.
- Enterotomies made at 100 cm mark and in the biliopancreatic limb.
- Jejunojejunostomy (side-to-side) made using blue/tan 60 mm cartridge).
- Enterotomy closed in single layer using nonabsorbable from below upwards in continuous fashion.

Closure of Mesenteric Defects

- Mesenteric defect (defect between small bowel mesenteries) closed using nonabsorbable suture 2-0 below upwards.
- Peterson defect (defect between the small bowel limb and transverse mesocolon) examined and closed using continuous nonabsorbable suture.

Intraoperative leak test done using upper GI endoscopy/methylene blue to rule out any intraluminal bleeding or leak.

Drain may be placed as per surgeon's preference and removed after 48 hours.

Jejunojejunostomy first technique

Creation of Gastric Pouch—as described above.

Creation of jejunojejunostomy: Focussing on the infracolic part, the transverse colon is lifted up, the ligament of Trietz is identified, and 75 cm of jejunum is measured and divided using the stapler. The third arm holds the biliopancreatic limb static while 100 cm of Roux limb is measured and the site for the jejunojejunostomy (JJ) is identified. The third arm holds the two bowel loops together while an enterotomy is created with the cautery hook **(Fig. 6.7)**.

A Jejunojejunostomy is created using a 60 mm white/blue/tan cartridge. The enterotomy is closed using delayed/nonabsorable running suture with large needle driver.

Then the omentum is divided using the Harmonic scalpel and the Roux limb is taken up to the gastric pouch for the gastrojejunostomy (GJ) **(Fig. 6.8)**.

Creation of Gastrojejunostomy

A totally hand-sewn GJ is done using delayed absorbable/barbed suture. While constructing the GJ, the third arm will hold the gastric pouch and small bowel together to release tension. Gastrojejunostomy is created as described above.

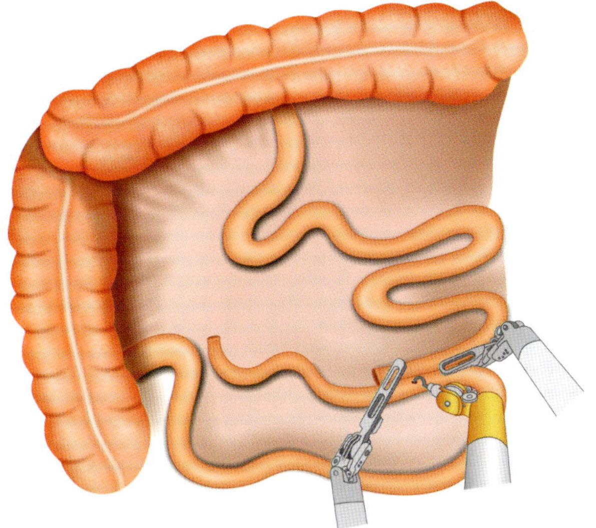

Fig. 6.7: Creation of the jejunojejunostomy. The second and third arms are holding both the loops of jejunum together. A monopolar hook is being used to create an enterotomy

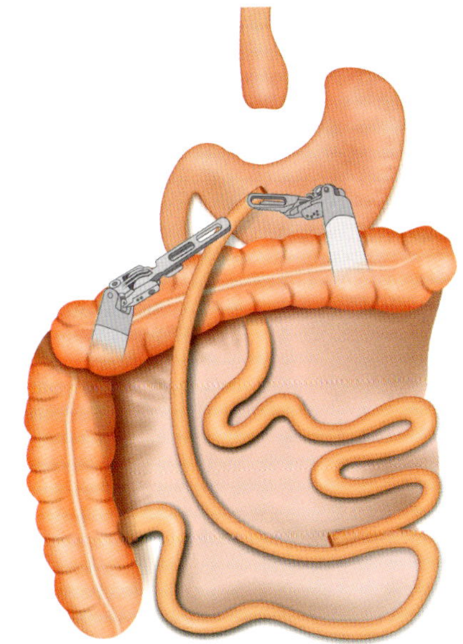

Fig. 6.8: The Roux limb is taken up to gastric pouch for gastrojejunostomy, using second and third arm

The jejunojejunostomy mesenteric defect is closed using nonabsorbable suture after gastrojejunostomy creation to avoid tension on the mesentery while the Roux limb is taken up to the gastric pouch.

PERIOPERATIVE CARE

Patients are given prophylaxis for deep venous thrombosis by mechanical (sequential compression devices, elastic stockings, ambulation) and pharmacological (LMWH—low molecular weight heparin) methods. LMWH started day before surgery and thereafter for 28 days. Patients are encouraged to walk in the evening of surgery and are started on a liquid diet. Upper GI gastrografin study is done on first postoperative day. Patient discharged on second day after ensuring adequate fluid intake. Drain removed. Patients are kept on a liquid diet for 1 week, followed by a week of a soft diet. Thereafter, they are progressed to a normal diet.

Follow-up: Patients are called on regular follow ups after 1 week, one month, 3 months, 6 months and every year thereafter.

ROBOTIC RYGB: CURRENT STATUS AND FUTURE

There are many significant published series comparing outcomes of robotic RYGB versus laparoscopic RYGB (LRYGB).[22-31]

Buchs et al.[30] found a significantly lower incidence of complications in the robotic group (11.6% vs 16.1%). The average leak rate across studies was 0.9% in RRYGB versus 1.6% in LRYGB, and the GJ stricture rate was 3.1% in the robotic arm and 3.2% in the laparoscopic arm. Snyder et al.[21] and Buchs et al.[30] found significantly lower leak rates in RRYGB. The overall mortality in both groups was 0.05%.

Bindal et al.[32] reviewed the published literature with a total of 3337 patients (1381 RRYGB and 1956 LRYGB). They found that mean OR time was 211.9 minutes in the robotic arm versus 185.1 minutes in the laparoscopic arm. This difference may be compounded by the fact that stapled GJ was done in the laparoscopic arm in six of nine studies whereas, a sutured GJ was done in the robotic arm in all studies. The average length of stay was 5 days for the robotic group as compared to 7.1 days for the laparoscopic group. The overall complication rate was 12.2% in the robotic group as compared to 13.3% in the laparoscopic group.

In our own patients, there has been no leak or stricture formation after RRYGB, a result that compares favorably with the published literature on LRYGB, and we believe that a hand-sewn GJ anastomosis done in a precise way decreases the anastomotic complication rate. Many large comparative studies and systematic reviews do offer some tendencies for robotic bariatric surgery.[33-35]

The learning curve has been studied for both LRYGB and RRYGB. The learning curve for LRYGB has been reported to be 75–100 cases,[8,36] whereas the learning curve for RRYGB is 14 cases shown by Buchs et al.[19]

Yu et al.[37] studied complications in the first 100 cases of RRYGB and found no leaks and one reoperation. The published literature is favorable to RRYGB than laparoscopic technique in terms of learning curve.

Robotic surgery is a team effort and entire team learns with the procedure and gets experienced in patient safety precautions, OR set-up, and instrumentation. As the main surgeon is away from the patient while performing robotic surgery, the assistant surgeon at the bedside must be trained enough for stapling (if robotic staplers are not used) and to deal with any emergency situation arising during the procedure. All the team members including scrub nurse and OR technician are also very important in streamlining the conduct of the procedure and getting a better patient outcome without any wastage of time and resources.

Improved ergonomics and reduced operator fatigue is an another advantage which comes with use of the robotic system as compared to laparoscopic surgery. Laparoscopic surgery can be very challenging in big patients and uncomfortable postures leading to surgeon's fatigue and work-related musculoskeletal symptoms.[38] Robotic surgery providing the advantage of more degrees of freedom, and a stable platform helps in performing difficult dissection and hand-sewn anastomosis.

There has been a concern about cost every time we talk of robotic surgery especially in developing countries like us. The direct costs are generally higher for the robotic approach in bariatric procedures like RYGB[39] but the overall cost of RRYGB was comparable than the cost of LRYGB when all the factors were accounted for as shown by Hagen et al.[27] A decrease in the number of laparoscopic staplers used in robotic procedures by doing a hand-sewn anastomosis also results in a saving.

With the advent of newer technologies in robotics, such as fluorescence imaging, virtual and augmented reality, integration of images telesurgery, natural orifice surgery, single-site platforms, and haptic feedback, we believe that digital platforms will provide an empowering tool to surgeons that potentially may change the way surgery is practiced today.

REFERENCES

1. World health organisation. *http://www.who.int/mediacentre/factsheets/fs311/en/*. Accessed 28 May 2013.
2. Gastrointestinal surgery for severe obesity. NIH consensus statement. 1991;9(1):1-20.
3. Wilson EB, Sudan R. The evolution of robotic bariatric surgery. World J Surg. 2013;37:2756-60.
4. Parikh MS, Shen R, Weiner M, Siegel N, Ren CJ. Laparoscopic bariatric surgery in super-obese patients (BMI >50) is safe and effective: a review of 332 patients. Obes Surg. 2005;15:858-63.
5. Wittgrove AC, Clark GW, Tremblay LJ. Laparoscopic gastric bypass, Roux-en-Y: preliminary report of five cases. Obes Surg. 1994;4:353-7.
6. Nguyen NT, Masoomi H, Magno CP, Nguyen XM, Laugenour K, Lane J. Trends in use of bariatric surgery, 2003–2008. J Am Coll Surg. 2011;213:261-6.
7. Ponce J, Nguyen NT, Hutter M, Sudan R, Morton JM. American Society for Metabolic and Bariatric Surgery estimation of bariatric surgery procedures in the United States, 2011-2014. Surg Obes Relat Dis. 2015;11(6):1199-200.
8. Schauer P, Ikramuddin S, Hamad G, Gourash W. The learning curve for laparoscopic Roux-en-Y gastric bypass is 100 cases. Surg Endosc. 2003;17:212-5.
9. Shikora SA, Kim JJ, Tarnoff ME, Raskin E, Shore R. Laparoscopic Roux-en-Y gastric bypass: results and learning curve of a high-volume academic program. Arch Surg. 2005;140:362-7.

10. Cadiere GB, Himpens J, Vertruyen M, MD, Favretti F. The world's first obesity surgery performed by a surgeon at a distance. Obes Surg. 1999;9:206-9.
11. Talamini MA, Chapman S, Horgan S, Melvin WS. The Academic Robotic Group. A prospective analysis of 211 robotic-assisted procedures. Surg Endosc. 2003;17:1521-4.
12. Bindal V, Bhatia P, Kalhan S, Khetan M, John S, Ali A, et al. Robot-assisted excision of a large retroperitoneal schwannoma. JSLS. 2014;18:150-4.
13. Cadiere GB, Himpens J, Vertruyen M, Bruyns J, Germay O, Leman G, et al. Evaluation of telesurgical (robotic) Nissen fundoplication. Surg Endosc. 2001;15:918-23.
14. Nakadi IE, Melot C, Closset J, DeMoor V, Betroune K, Feron P, et al. Evaluation of da Vinci Nissen fundoplication clinical results and cost minimization. World J Surg. 2006;30:1050-4.
15. Schauer PR, Ikramuddin S. Laparoscopic surgery for morbid obesity. Surg Clin North Am. 2001;81:1145-79.
16. Buchwald H, Williams SE. Bariatric surgery worldwide 2003. Obes Surg. 2004;14:1157-64.
17. Sjostrom L, Lindroos AK, Peltonen M, Torgerson J, Bouchard C, Carlsson B, et al. Lifestyle, diabetes, and cardiovascular risk factors 10 years after bariatric surgery. N Engl J Med. 2004;351:2683-93.
18. Puzziferri N, Roshek TB, Mayo HG, Gallagher R, Belle SH, Livingston EH. Long-term follow-up after bariatric surgery: a systematic review. JAMA. 2014;312:934-42.
19. Buchs NC, Pugin F, Bucher P, Hagen ME, Chassot G, Koutny-Fong P, et al. Learning curve for robot-assisted Roux-en-Y gastric bypass. Surg Endosc. 2012;26:1116-21.
20. Bindal V, Gonzalez-Heredia R, Masrur M, Elli EF. Technique evolution, learning curve, and outcomes of 200 robot-assisted gastric bypass procedures: a 5-year experience. Obes Surg. 2015;25:997-1002.
21. Bindal V, Gonzalez-Heredia R, Elli EF. Outcomes of robot-assisted Roux-en-Y gastric bypass as a reoperative bariatric procedure. Obes Surg. 2015;25:1810-5.
22. Sanchez BR, Mohr CJ, Morton JM, Safadi BY, Alami RS, Curet MJ. Comparison of totally robotic laparoscopic Roux-en-Y gastric bypass and traditional laparoscopic Roux-en-Y gastric bypass. Surg Obes Relat Dis. 2005;1:549-54.
23. Snyder BE, Wilson T, Leong BY, Klein C, Wilson EB. Robotic-assisted Roux-en-Y gastric bypass: minimizing morbidity and mortality. Obes Surg. 2010;20:265-70.
24. Ayloo SM, Addeo P, Buchs NC, Shah G, Giulianotti PC. Robot-assisted versus laparoscopic Roux-en-Y gastric bypass: is there a difference in outcomes? World J Surg. 2011;35:637-42.
25. Park CW, Lam ECF, Walsh TM, Karimoto M, Ma AT, Koo M, et al. Robotic-assisted Roux-en-Y gastric bypass performed in a community hospital setting: the future of bariatric surgery? Surg Endosc. 2011;25:3312-21.
26. Scozzari G, Rebecchi F, Millo P, Rocchietto S, Allieta R, Morino M. Robot-assisted gastrojejunal anastomosis does not improve the results of the laparoscopic Roux-en-Y gastric bypass. Surg Endosc. 2011;25:597-603.
27. Hagen ME, Pugin F, Chassot G, Huber O, Buchs N, Iranmanesh P, et al. Reducing cost of surgery by avoiding complications: the model of robotic Roux-en-Y gastric bypass. Obes Surg. 2012;22:52-61.
28. Benizri EI, Renaud M, Reibel N, Germain A, Ziegler O, Zarnegar R, et al. Perioperative outcomes after totally robotic gastric bypass: a prospective nonrandomized controlled study. Am J Surg. 2013;206:145-51.
29. Myers SR, McGuirl J, Wang J. Robot-assisted versus laparoscopic gastric bypass: comparison of short-term outcomes. Obes Surg. 2013;23:467-73.
30. Buchs NC, Morel P, Azagury DE, Jung M, Chassot G, Huber O, et al. Laparoscopic versus robotic Roux-en-Y gastric bypass: lessons and long-term follow-up learned from a large prospective monocentric study. Obes Surg. 2014;24:2031-9.
31. Markar S, Karthikesalingam A, Venkat-Ramen V, Kinross J, Ziprin P. Robotic vs. laparoscopic Roux-en-Y gastric bypass in morbidly obese patients: systematic review and pooled analysis. Int J Med Robot. 2011;7:393-400.
32. Bindal V, Bhatia P, Dudeja U, Kalhan S, Khetan M, John S, Wadhera S. Review of contemporary role of robotics in bariatric surgery. J Minim Access Surg. 2015;11:16-21.
33. Fourman MM, Saber AA. Robotic bariatric surgery: a systematic review. Surg Obes Relat Dis. 2012;8:483-8.
34. Kim K, Hagen ME, Buffington C. Robotics in advanced gastrointestinal surgery: the bariatric experience. Cancer J. 2013;19:177-82.
35. Toro JP, Lin E, Patel AD. Review of robotics in foregut and bariatric surgery. Surg Endosc. 2015;29:1-8.
36. Oliak D, Ballantyne GH, Weber P, Wasielewski A, Davies RJ, Schmidt HJ. Laparoscopic Roux-en-Y gastric bypass: defining the learning curve. Surg Endosc. 2003;17:405-8.
37. Yu CJ, Clapp BI, Lee MJ, Albrecht WC, Scarborough TK, Wilson EB. Robotic assistance provides excellent outcomes during the learning curve for laparoscopic Roux-en-Y gastric bypass: results from 100 robotic-assisted gastric bypasses. Am J Surg. 2006;192:746-9.
38. Esposito C, El Ghoneimi A, Yamataka A, Rothenberg S, Bailez M, Ferro M, et al. Work-related upper limb musculoskeletal disorders in paediatric laparoscopic surgery. A multicenter survey. J Pediatr Surg. 2013;48:1750-6.
39. Curet MJ, Curet M, Soloman H, Lui G, Morton JM. Comparison of hospital charges between robotic, laparoscopic stapled, and laparoscopic handsewn Roux-en-Y gastric bypass. J Robot Surg. 2009;3:75-8.

CHAPTER

7

Robotic Surgery for Benign Colorectal Diseases

Deepak Govil, Vivek Tandon, Vachan Hukkeri, Satyaprakash Jindal, Adithya GK

INTRODUCTION

The last decade has seen a progressive application of minimally invasive techniques in the surgical management of colorectal diseases, both benign and malignant. Simultaneously advances and increasing experience in robotic surgery has facilitated the increasing use of this modality in the field of colorectal surgery. The application of robotic surgery in rectal cancer is discussed in another chapter of this book. In the present chapter we will discuss the role of robotic surgery in the other colorectal diseases.

Minimal access laparoscopic surgery for colorectal disease has been shown to have several advantages over open surgery. Smaller incisions allow for a much less painful and a quicker postoperative recovery without any compromise in the quality and safety of the surgical procedure. With the increasing experience and wider availability, it is only natural that the use of robotics extend to the field of colorectal surgery. The use of robotic surgery to perform colectomies has been described since 2002.[1] In addition, procedures such as rectopexy for rectal prolapse, colectomies for benign diseases like diverticulitis and total proctocolectomy with pouch reconstruction for ulcerative colitis (UC) and familial adenomatous polyposis (FAP) are being increasingly done robotically. As in other areas of surgery, robotic surgery offers a definite advantage with respect to increased operative dexterity resulting from instruments with maneuverability greater even than the human wrist. Digital zoom allows for an enhanced vision aiding better tissue handling as compared to laparoscopic surgery. The deterrents of robotic surgery have been the long operative time and loss of tactile feedback as compared to open surgery. Additionally, certain surgeries like total proctocolectomy may require multiple dockings of the robot making the procedure time consuming and cumbersome. Inclusive of a docking time of about 30 minutes the operative time for most robotic colorectal surgeries has been in the range of 200–300 minutes.[2] We have found that with higher case load, increasing experience and familiarity of the staff with the robot, docking time can be substantially reduced. Also the enhanced range of instrument movement and the three-dimensional vision provided by the robotic operating system more than makes up for this operative delay. Of late a large number of publications are showing the feasibility of robotics in colorectal surgery. Robotic surgery has been compared to laparoscopic surgery in terms of operative time, blood loss and complications. No significant difference has been found between the two with respect to complications, mortality and rate of conversion to open surgery, though robotic surgery does significantly add to the total cost of the procedure.

In this chapter we will be detailing principles and technique of some common colorectal surgical procedures performed for benign colorectal diseases using the robotic system. We will discuss the procedures under the following headings:

- Colectomy (right, left, transverse and total)
- Rectopexy.

RIGHT HEMICOLECTOMY

Patient position: Supine with arms by the side of the patient. A 10°–15° reverse Trendelenburg position with a 10°–15° left side down position helps in better visualization of the target area **(Fig 7.1A)**.

Port placement: A 12 mm camera port in the left periumbilical region with a 10–20 cm distance from the target anatomy is initially placed. Three 8 mm operating arms as shown in the figure are used keeping an 8–10 cm distance between all robotic ports. An assistant port can be placed depending on the need of the surgeon and should be at least 5 cm from the robotic ports and avoid entering the area between the target anatomy and robotic ports **(Fig. 7.1B)**.

Docking: The robot can be brought in from either the right side of the patient or from the upper right abdomen depending on the surgeon's preference and the need for mobilization of the transverse colon. It is essential to maintain a straight line extending from the column of the robot to the target anatomy and the camera port.

Procedure: The three robotic arms allow for efficient traction and dissection. In case of requirement, an assistant port can be placed for suctioning and application of clips and staplers. The right hemicolectomy proceeds as in a

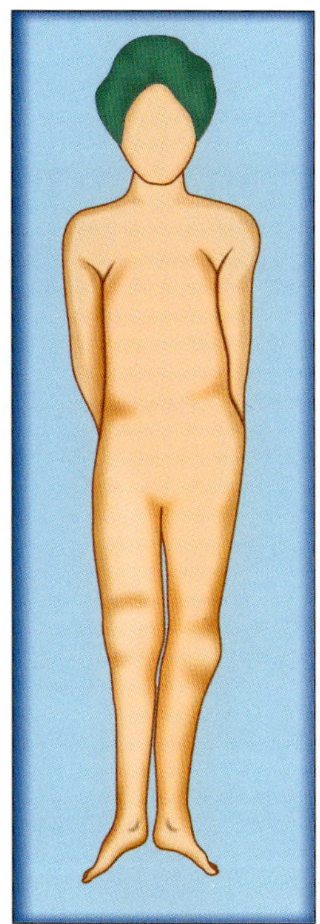

Fig. 7.1A

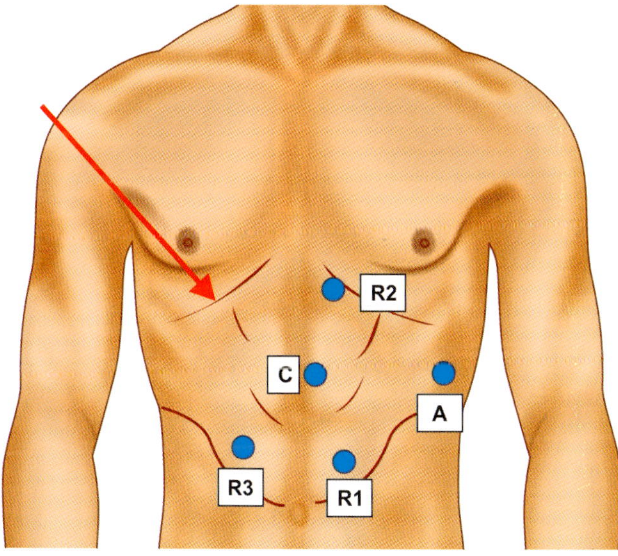

Fig. 7.1B

laparoscopic procedure. The ileocecal region is lifted and the ileocolic pedicle is skeletonized, clipped and cut. Then a medial to lateral mobilization of the ascending colon is done. The next vessel encountered is the right colic vein which is dealt with in a similar fashion. Next the hepatic flexure is mobilized and the dissection extended to or beyond the middle colic vessels depending on the extent of colonic resection planned. The need for division of the middle colic pedicle is also dependent on the same. The margin of resection of the bowel is then marked and divided. The ileocolic anastomosis can be performed either intracorporeally or extracorporeally using staplers. The three-dimensional vision available in the robotic system gives clear visualization of important structures like right ureter, duodenum and pancreatic head allowing them to be adequately protected despite the lack of tactile feedback.[3]

Robotic right hemicolectomy is considered by most surgeons as the initial learning platform before proceeding to complex colorectal surgery. In recent years multiple publications have highlighted the use of robotic system for performing a right hemicolectomy.

The results of robotic versus laparoscopic right colectomies have been compared in a recent meta-analysis by Huirong Xu et al. They included 7 studies, in their meta-analysis and compared 234 robotic with 415 laparoscopic right hemicolectomies. They found that the robotic procedures had longer operative times ($p < 0.00001$), lower estimated blood losses ($p = 0.0002$), lower postoperative overall complications ($p = 0.02$), and significantly faster bowel function recovery ($p < 0.00001$). There were no differences in the length of hospital stay ($p = 0.12$), conversion rates to open surgery ($p = 0.48$), postoperative ileus ($p = 0.08$), anastomosis leakage ($p = 0.28$), and bleeding ($p = 0.95$).[4] A similar meta-analysis by Niccolò Petrucciani et al. which included six studies, compared 168 patients undergoing robotic right hemicolectomy with 348 patients undergoing laparoscopic right hemicolectomy. They concluded that the only significant difference between the two groups was a longer operative time when the procedures were performed robotically.[5] The bowel anastomosis can be done either intracorporeally or extracorporeally. Intracorporeal anastomotic technique has been compared to the extracorporeal anastomotic technique and it has been found that the former technique results in a faster post operative recovery and lesser overall morbidity. Also a comparison between intracorporeal robotic and laparoscopic anastomosis has revealed no major difference in the functional outcome. Therefore, robotic right hemicolectomy should be considered as a safe and feasible procedure. Additionally, it is an ideal initial learning step before proceeding to complex pelvic bowel procedures.

TRANSVERSE COLECTOMY

Position: Supine with arms by the side of the patient **(Fig. 7.1A)**.

Port placement: A 12 mm camera port in the periumbilical region and three 8 mm operating arms as shown in the figure. An assistant port can be placed if required **(Fig. 7.1C)**.

Docking: The robot is brought in from the head end of the table.

Procedure: The transverse colon is lifted up with the omentum. This opens up the mesentry of transverse colon and the middle colic pedicle is clearly visualized and can be clipped and cut. The rest of the transverse mesocolon is then

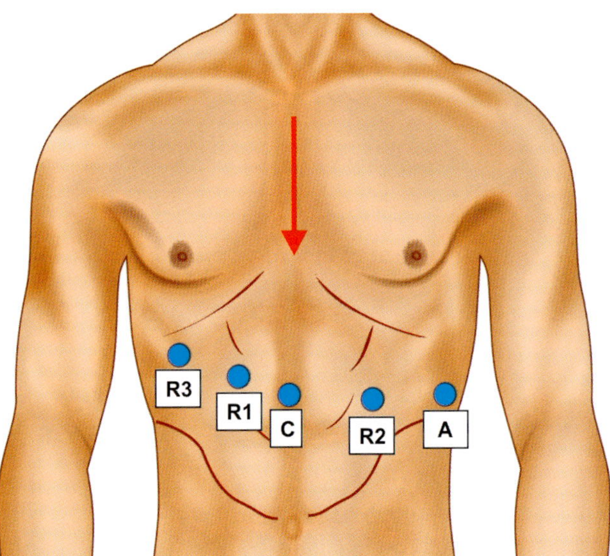

Fig. 7.1C

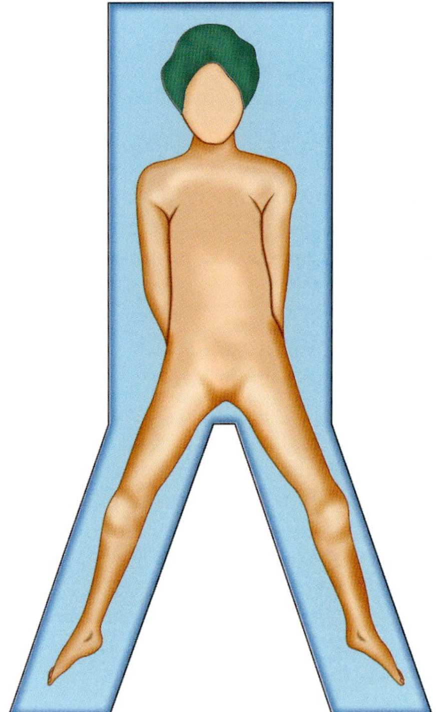

Fig. 7.1D

dissected separating it from the duodenum and pancreas. The enhanced three-dimensional vision of the robotic system helps avoid any injury to these structures. The splenic and hepatic flexure are then dissected and divided as per the extent of resection planned. The anastomoses between the two ends of the colon can then be done by the intracorporeal or extracorporeal technique using sutures or staplers as preferred by the surgeon. The ease of intracorporeal anastomosis using the robotic system usually does not warrant extensive mobilization of the hepatic and splenic flexures.

Kyung Uk Jung et al. in their series of 162 colectomies had three cases of transverse colectomy. The mean operative time for those cases was in the range of 300 minutes. They had no major complications and performed the anastomoses by the intracorporeal suturing technique.[6] There are limited indications for an isolated transverse colectomy but as the procedure can be performed with a single docking and operating in a single quadrant a robotic procedure is feasible and provides multiple advantages that are inherent to all robotic surgeries.

LEFT AND SIGMOID COLECTOMY

Position: Trendelenburg position, semilithotomy with the right side down with arms placed by the side of the patient **(Fig. 7.1D)**. If the splenic flexure needs to be mobilized then a lesser Trendelenburg position is preferred.

Port placement: A 12 mm camera port is placed in the right periumbilical region ensuring a 10–20 cm distance from the target anatomy. Three 8 mm operating arms are used as shown in the figure. Again it is important to adhere to the general principles of robotic port placement, i.e. keep at least an 8–10 cm distance between robotic ports and a 5 cm distance between an assistant port and any robotic port **(Fig. 7.1E)**.

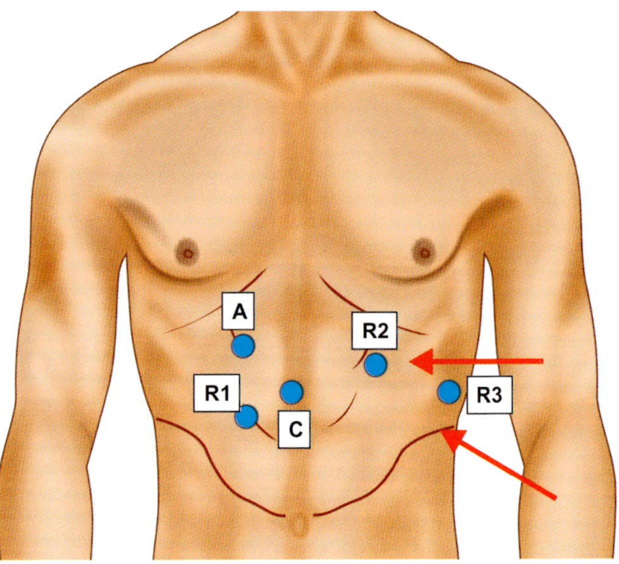

Fig. 7.1E

Docking: The robot is brought in from either the left of the abdomen or diagonally from the left thigh region again ensuring that the central column of the robot, the target anatomy and the camera port are in one straight line.

Procedure: Sigmoid colectomy is a relatively simpler procedure and the surgical technique is the same as when the procedure is performed laparoscopically. The sigmoid colon is lifted up exposing the mesentery with the inferior mesenteric vessels. The vein and artery are dissected, clipped and divided. The mesenteric fat is then divided gradually from the medial to the lateral aspect ensuring that the left ureter is protected. The superior and inferior dissection is performed similarly, the extent depending on the extent of colonic resection planned. Depending on the level of inferior dissection the anastomosis can either be with a linear stapler within or outside the abdomen (after giving a suprapubic incision). Alternatively, if the distal extent of colonic resection does not allow enough mobility to the residual colon for the same a circular stapler can be inserted through the anus to establish colo-colic continuity.

There are several reports of left and sigmoid colonic resections performed robotically. Also the single port technique has been applied to the procedure. Rami Makhoul et al. have reported 4 cases of robotic single-incision sigmoid colectomy performed for patients with diverticular disease of the colon. They used only two operating arms with a single incision port at the umbilicus. The mean operating time was 250 minutes with a mean blood loss of 75cc. They concluded that single-incision robotic colectomy (SIRC) was both safe and feasible in such cases.[7]

Robotic left hemicolectomy can be performed for both benign and malignant diseases of the left and sigmoid colon. The procedure is more cumbersome than the previously described procedures as there is a need to operate in more than one quadrant of the abdomen as the splenic flexure needs to be mobilized. This may warrant the need for more than one docking and different docking methods have been described, including:

- *Hybrid technique:* This technique involves initial laparoscopic mobilization of the splenic flexure followed by docking of the robot in the left lower quadrant to proceed with the left colonic mobilization.
- *Single-docking technique (described by Kim SH):* This technique involves single docking of the robot in the left lower quadrant with mobilization of the second and third robotic arm for the different parts of the procedure (splenic flexure mobilization and for the pelvic dissection).
- *Double-docking technique (described by KY Lee and BS Min):* This technique involves dual docking, once from the left hemi-abdomen for dissection of the splenic flexure and then changing the docking to the left lower quadrant for the pelvic dissection.[8]

A systematic review and meta-analysis conducted by Laura Lorenzon et al. evaluated a total of 400 left hemicolectomy, 143 robotic and 257 laparoscopic. The only significant difference noted was a lesser blood loss in robotic surgery as compared to the laparoscopic group. They concluded that robotic left hemicolectomy can be considered as a safe and feasible option for both benign and malignant diseases.[9]

TOTAL PROCTOCOLECTOMY WITH POUCH ILEO-ANAL ANASTOMOSES

Position: Supine or semilithomoty position with arms by the side of the patient. In case the multiple dockings technique is used the patients position would need to be adjusted depending on the part of the colon being dissected.

Port placement: A 12 mm camera port in the periumbilical region and three 8 mm operating arms as shown in the figure can be used. Again these would need to be modified depending on the type of docking being used and whether the hybrid technique is applied. Assistant ports can be placed depending on the need of the surgeon. Keeping in mind the general principles of robotic port placement, the distance between any robotic port and assistant port should be at least 5 cm.

Docking: The need to operate in multiple quadrants makes the procedure more cumbersome and time consuming as multiple docking is required. This docking can be a combination of the ones for both right and left colectomies. To overcome this problem, we have adopted the hybrid technique in which part of the procedure is done laparoscopically to avoid multiple dockings and part is done using the robot. This allows the surgeon to take advantage of the robot while performing the pelvic dissection without the drawback of multiple dockings.

Procedure: Total proctocolectomy entails excision of the complete colon and rectum. The reconstruction is done after constructing a pouch from the terminal ileum and anastomosing this to the anus. The pouch can either be hand sewn or stapled and it can be fashioned either within or outside the abdomen depending on surgeon. While many different types of pouch have been described, the most commonly used one is the 'J' shaped pouch. A covering ileostomy to protect this delicate pouch ileo anal anastomoses is usually made necessitating a second surgery for closure of the same.

Minimal access surgery has greatly helped in reducing the morbidity associated with this complex procedure. It is most commonly performed for diseases such as ulcerative colitis and familial adenomatous polyposis. Total proctocolectomy is plagued by the problem of multiple dockings being required to facilitate surgery in all quadrants of the abdomen. There are a few case reports in literature showing the feasibility of robotic total proctocolectomy.[10] Variants of the procedure include laparoscopic-assisted, totally robotic and single incision total proctocolectomy.[11-13] The procedure has also been shown to be useful in cases of ulcerative colitis with associated malignancy.[14] In our experience of laparoscopic assisted robotic total proctocolectomy with pouch ileo anal anastomoses we have found that increasing experience with robotic surgery in lower rectal cases rapidly brings down the docking and operating time. We have been able to reduce the average docking and operating time from 30 and 360 minutes to 10 and 240 minutes respectively.

RECTOPEXY

Rectal prolapse affects predominantly females and is associated with debilitating symptoms such as pain, rectal bleeding and tenesmus. Incarceration of the prolapse is a definite risk in some cases. Surgery is the treatment of choice

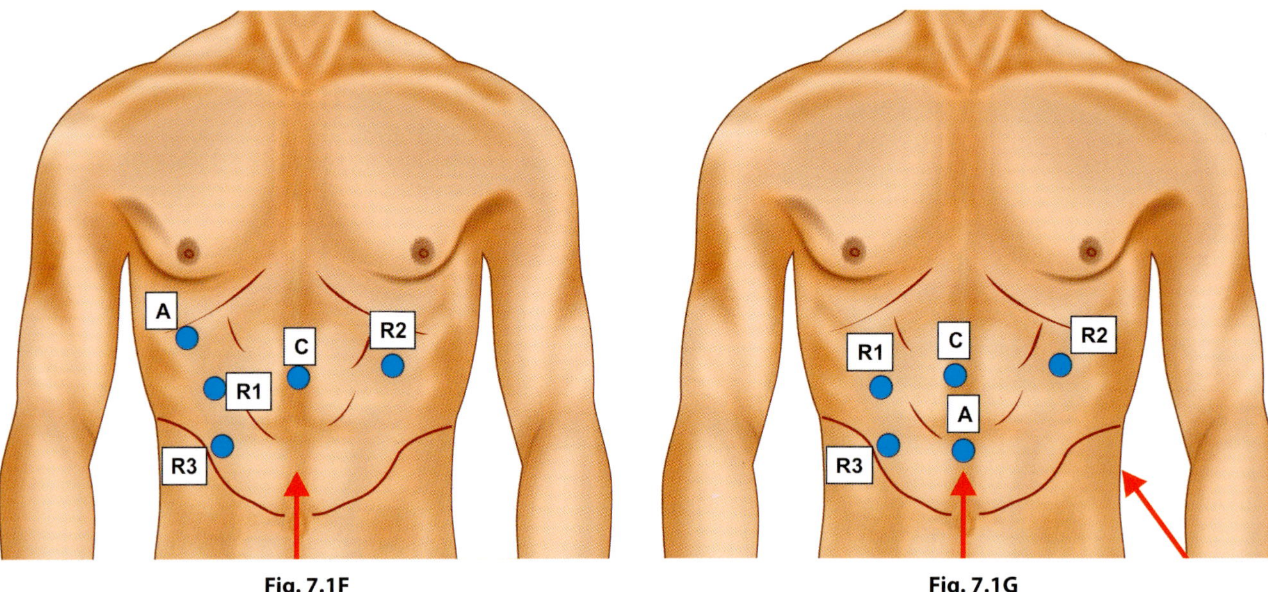

Fig. 7.1F

Fig. 7.1G

Figs 7.1A to G: The port sites are marked by dots, "C" denotes the 12 mm camera port, "R1" is the first robotic arm 8 mm, "R2" the second robotic arm 8 mm, "R3" the third robotic arm 8 mm, "A" 5 or 12 mm assistant port. The direction from which the robot is being wheeled in is shown by the red arrow

with a large variety of procedures being done to treat prolapse and this probably is testimony to the fact that no one surgical procedure is perfect. The surgical approach to correct the prolapse may be via the perineal or the abdominal route. The former is usually preferred in elderly patients, who have a high risk associated with the procedure due to multiple associated comorbid illnesses.[15-18] The abdominal route is preferred for the younger, fitter patients as the recurrence rates are lower.[19-21]

In last decade there has been, as in other surgeries, a significant shift to performing such procedures through the minimally invasive approach. Additionally, meshes are being used safely with limited complications.[22] The laparoscopic approach not only helps improve symptoms, it also has acceptably low recurrence rates and morbidity thus making it increasingly popular with both surgeons and patients.[23-26] However, it has its limitations and for most surgeons, it takes significant time to master. Laparoscopy in the pelvis is made difficult by the limitation of space restricting the freedom of instrument movement. This is further aggravated by a limited, two-dimensional vision and instrumentation which has limited mobility.

Robotic access to the peritoneal cavity allows for significantly better and three-dimensional visualization within the pelvic cavity. Additionally, robotic instruments have a greater degree of maneuverability allowing for enhanced dexterity which makes the dissection both easier and precise. It is therefore only logical that the advantages of robotic surgery be applied to surgical procedures for rectal prolapse done via the transabdominal route. However, limited availability and cost are two major limitations that will need to be overcome for this to happen on a wide scale.[27-29]

Position: The position may either be the Lloyd Davies (modified) with both arms by the side of the patient[30] or a steep Trendelenburg.[31] Both these positions allow for digital rectal or vaginal examination if required. The pneumoperitoneum may be created by using the Veress needle or by the open technique and is usually a matter of surgeon preference.

Port placement: The camera port (12 mm) is placed above the umbilicus. Three 8 mm ports are then placed as follows. The first is 2 cm above the midpoint of a line joining the camera port with the right anterior superior iliac spine (ASIS), the second is 2 cm medial to the right ASIS and a third 8 mm port is placed about 4 finger breaths lateral to the camera port. A final 12 mm assistant port is placed as per the surgeon's preference to help in mesh placement.[30] It must be emphasized again that as in all robotic procedures adequate distance (minimum 8–10 cm) between ports must be ensured to avoid collisions of the robotic arms **(Fig 7.1F)**.

Kaikkonen et al. prefer to place the camera port in the right paraumbilical region with three other 8 mm ports as is shown in **Figure 7.1G**. A 5 mm suprapubic port is placed to allow for fixation of the mesh to the sacral promontory using tackers.[32] While they place the robotic cart to the left of the patient it may be placed between the patient's legs with the camera port placed infraumbilically.[31]

Surgical Procedure

The procedure begins with retraction of the rectosigmoid junction to the left and a peritoneal incision made over the sacral promontory. Lifting up the uterus with stitch helps to improve the exposure in females and should be used if required. The peritoneal incision is extended along the rectum in an inverted "J" fashion, taking care to protect the right hypogastric nerve as one opens the Denonvillier's fascia in males or the rectovaginal septum in females. The plane between the mesorectum and retroperitoneum can be identified as the latter is whiter in color. The plane under the superior rectal artery is entered using a cautery or harmonic dissector and the left ureter and hypogastric nerves identified progressively carrying the dissection down in the presacral space. The lower extent of the dissection should be below the Waldeyer (retrosacral) facia. With an aim to protect rectal innervation, as much as possible lateral mobilization is done in a limited manner. Anteriorly the dissection is done in the rectovaginal plane to the upper limit of the vagina where, often, a hernia sac, if large, may need to be dissected and excised. In this area, it is important to preserve the left lateral ligament and the nervi erigentes.

If one opts for posterior placement of the mesh, this can now be assessed after pulling the rectum out of the pelvis. A small rectangular sheet of mesh is placed down up to the pelvic floor extending posterior to the mesorectum. Mesh fixation may be aided by placing a 5 mm suprapubic port. Fixation may be done using either a tacking device or suture. In either case it is important to take care not to injure the sacral plexus. It is suggested that the pexy be extended about 5 cm on either side and this requires about 3 tackers or sutures to be placed about a centimeter apart on the bony promontory. In the D'Hoore procedure once the anterior space is mobilized, polypropylene mesh is secured to the anterior aspect of the rectum and then secured to the sacral promontory using 0 Ethibond suture. This elevates the anterior wall without any traction on the rectum. The posterior vaginal fornix is lifted up and sutured to the mesh (anteriorly), aiding in the repair of rectocele, as well as prolapse.[33]

Results

Present data on results of robotic rectopexy is primarily from small nonrandomized reports. The primary question has been to try and assess any benefit over and above the laparoscopic approach to rectopexy.

Heemskerk et al. in 2007, reported their comparison of 14 patients who underwent robot-assisted rectopexy with 19 patients who underwent laparoscopic rectopexy in the same period. While their report suggested that robotic rectopexy was safe and effective with similar rates of complications compared to laparoscopic rectopexy, the operative time and costs were both significantly higher in the robotic group. With experience the time factor, as expected, is no longer a significant issue.[34] Kaikkonen et al. in 2013 reported their results of 20 patients who were operated for rectal prolapse compared to matched controls who underwent laparoscopic surgery for prolapse. They found robotic surgery to be as safe, effective and not more time consuming than laparoscopic rectopexy but suggested that routine use of robotic surgery for rectopexy did not have a strong argument.[35] Mehmood et al. in a nonrandomized study, compared 17 patients who underwent robotic rectopexy with 34 patients who underwent the procedure laparoscopically.[30] They assessed and compared the quality of life after surgery and reported that based on the SF-36 PCS (Physical Component Score) the robotic procedure may be superior and attributed this to the technical advantage of robotic surgery in the form of better visibility and enhanced dexterity due to superior instrumentation. However, definitive Level I evidence in this regard is still awaited.

Overall, robotic colorectal surgery is here to stay. There are specific advantages in the depth in pelvic surgery, specially in male patients with narrow pelvis and in difficult situations.

REFERENCES

1. Weber PA, Merola S, Wasielewski A, Ballantyne GH, Delaney CP, Telerobotic-assisted laparoscopic right and sigmoid colectomies for benign disease. Diseases of the Colon and Rectum. 2002;45(12):1689-96.
2. Tsoraides SS, Huettner F, Rawlings AL, Crawford DL. Robotic Surgery of the Colon. The Peoria Experience. Robot Surgery, Book edited by: Seung Hyuk Baik.
3. Witkiewicz W, Zawadzki M, Rząca M, Obuszko Z, Czarnecki R, Turek J, Marecik S. Robot-assisted right colectomy: surgical technique and review of the literature. Videosurgery Miniinv. 2013;8(3):253-7.
4. Huirong Xu, Jianning Li, Yanlai Sun, Zengjun Li, Yanan Zhen, Bin Wang, Zhongfa Xu. Robotic versus laparoscopic right colectomy: a meta-analysis. World Journal of Surgical Oncology. 2014;12:274.
5. Petrucciani N, Sirimarco D, Nigri GR, Magistri P, Torre MLa, Aurello P, D'Angelo F, Ramacciato G. Robotic right colectomy: A worthwhile procedure? Results of a meta-analysis of trials comparing robotic versus laparoscopic right colectomy. Journal of Minimal Access Surgery. 2015;11(1).
6. Jung KU, Park Y, Lee KY, Sohn SK. Robotic transverse colectomy for mid-transverse colon cancer: surgical techniques and oncologic outcome. J Robotic Surg. 2015;9(2):131-6.
7. Makhoul R, Obias V. Robotic single-incision sigmoid colectomy: initial case series. J Robotic Surg, DOI 10.1007/s11701-014-0449-0
8. Parra-Davila E, Diaz-Hernandez JJ. Totally robotic left colectomy. J Robotic Surg. 2011;5:57-64. DOI 10.1007/s11701-011-0254-y
9. Lorenzon L, Bini F, Balducci G, Ferri M, Salvi PF, Marinozzi F. Laparoscopic versus robotic-assisted colectomy and rectal resection: a systematic review and meta-analysis. Int J Colorectal Dis. DOI 10.1007/s00384-015-2394-4
10. Baca B, Aghayeva A, Ozben V, Bayraktar O, Atasoy D, Erguner I, Karahasanoglu T, Hamzaoglu I. Robotic total proctocolectomy for ulcerative colitis—a video vignette. Colorectal Dis. 2015;17(8): 736. doi: 10.1111/codi.13019.
11. Morelli L, Guadagni S, Mariniello MD, Furbetta N, Pisano R, D'Isidoro C, Caprili G, Marciano E, Di Candio G, Boggi U, Mosca F. Hand-assisted hybrid laparoscopic-robotic total proctocolectomy with ileal pouch-anal anastomosis. Langenbecks Arch Surg. 2015;400(6):741-8. doi: 10.1007/s00423-015-1331-x. Epub 2015 Aug 6.
12. Pedraza R, Patel CB, Diego I, Valdez RV, Haas EM. Robotic-assisted laparoscopic surgery for restorative proctocolectomy with ileal J pouch- anal anastomosis. DOI: 10.3109/13645706.2010.536355.
13. Roviello F, Piagnerelli R, Ferrara F, Scheiterle M, De Franco L, Marrelli D. Robotic single docking total colectomy for ulcerative colitis: First experience with a novel technique. Int J Surg. 2015;21:63-7.

14. Hanai T, Maeda K, Masumori K, Katsuno H, Matsuoka H. Technique of Robotic-assisted Total Proctocolectomy with Lymphadenectomy and Ileal Pouch-Anal Anastomosis for Transverse Colitic Cancer of Ulcerative Colitis, Using the Single Cart Position. Surg Technol Int. 2015;27:86-92.
15. Williams JG, Rothenberger DA, Madoff RD, Goldberg SM. Treatment of rectal prolapse in the elderly by perineal rectosigmoidectomy. Dis Colon Rectum. 1992;35:830-4.
16. Lasheen AE, Khalifa S, El Askry SM, Elzeftawy AA. Closed rectopexy with transanal resection for complete rectal prolapse in adults. J Gastrointest Surg. 2005;9:980-4.
17. Watkins BP, Landercasper J, Belzer GE, et al. Long-term follow-up of the modified Delorme procedure for rectal prolapse. Arch Surg. 2003;138:498-502.
18. Altemeier WA, Giuseffi J, Hoxworth P. Treatment of extensive prolapse of the rectum in aged or debilitated patients. AMA Arch Surg. 1952;65:72-80.
19. Chow PK, Ho YH. Abdominal resection rectopexy versus Delorme_s procedure for rectal prolapse: comparison of clinical and physiological outcomes. Int J Colorectal Dis. 1996;11:201-2.
20. Penninckx F, D_Hoore A, Sohier S, Kerremans R. Abdominal resection rectopexy versus Delorme_s procedure for rectal prolapse: a predictable outcome. Int J Colorectal Dis. 1997;12:49-50.
21. Steele SR, Goetz LH, Minami S, Madoff RD, Mellgren AF, Parker SC. Management of recurrent rectal prolapse: surgical approach influences outcome. Dis Colon Rectum. 2006;49:440-5.
22. Smart N, Pathak S, Boorman P, Daniels I. Synthetic or biological mesh use in laparoscopic ventral mesh rectopexy—a systematic review. Color Dis. 2013;15(6):650-4.
23. Solomon MJ, Young CJ, Eyers AA, Roberts RA. Randomized clinical trial of laparoscopic versus open abdominal rectopexy for rectal prolapse. Br J Surg. 2002;89:35-9.
24. Kairaluoma MV, Viljakka MT, Kellokumpu IH. Open vs. laparoscopic surgery for rectal prolapse: a case-controlled study assessing short-term outcome. Dis Colon Rectum. 2003;46:353-60.
25. Purkayastha S, Tekkis P, Athanasiou T, et al. A comparison of open vs. laparoscopic abdominal rectopexy for full-thickness rectal prolapse: a meta-analysis. Dis Colon Rectum. 2005;48:1930-40.
26. Kariv Y, Delaney CP, Casillas S, et al. Long-term outcome after laparoscopic and open surgery for rectal prolapse: a case-controlled study. Surg Endosc. 2006;20:35-42.
27. Munz Y, Moorthy K, Kudchadkar R, et al. Robotic assisted rectopexy. Am J Surg. 2004;187:88-92.
28. Wong MT, Meurette G, Rigaud J, Regenet N, Lehur PA. Robotic versus laparoscopic rectopexy for complex rectocele: a prospective comparison of short-term outcomes. Dis Colon Rectum. 2011;54:342-6.
29. Baik SH. Robotic colorectal surgery. Yonsei Med J. 2008;49:891-6.
30. Mehmood RK, Parker J, Bhuvimanian L, Qasem E, Mohammed AA, Zeeshan M, Grugel K, Carter P, Ahmed S. Short-term outcome of laparoscopic versus robotic ventral mesh rectopexy for full-thickness rectal prolapse. Is robotic superior? Int J Colorectal Dis. 2014;29:1113-8.
31. Haahr C, Jakobsen HL, Gögenur I. Robot-assisted rectopexy is a safe and feasible option for treatment of rectal prolapse. Dan Med J. 2014;61(5):A4842.
32. Mäkelä-Kaikkonen J, Rautio T, Klintrup K, Takala H, Vierimaa M, Ohtonen P, Mäkelaä J. Robotic-assisted and laparoscopic ventral rectopexy in the treatment of rectal prolapse: a matched-pairs study of operative details and complications. Tech Coloproctol. DOI 10.1007/s10151-013-1042-7
33. D'Hoore A, Cadoni R, Penninckx F. Long-term outcome of laparoscopic ventral rectopexy for total rectal prolapse. Br J Surg. 2004;91:1500-5.
34. Heemskerk J, Dominique E, de Hoog E, van Gemert W, Baeten C, Greve J, Bouvy N. Robot-assisted vs. conventional laparoscopic rectopexy for rectal prolapse: a comparative study on costs and time. Dis Colon Rectum. 2007;50:1825-30.
35. Kaikkonen J, Rautio T, Klintrup K, Takala H, Vierimaa M, Ohtonen P, Makela J. Robotic-assisted and laparoscopic ventral rectopexy in the treatment of rectal prolapse: a matched-pairs study of operative details and complications. Tech Coloproctol. DOI 10.1007/s10151- 013-1042-7.

CHAPTER

8

Carcinoma Rectum

Somashekhar SP

INTRODUCTION

Minimally invasive techniques have revolutionized surgical practice, especially surgery of the gastrointestinal tract. Benefits of such an approach include reduced postoperative pain, shorter hospital stay and an improved cosmetic outcome.

Mesorectal excision with autonomic nerve preservation, the gold standard procedure for rectal cancer was popularized by Heald. The underlying principle is the meticulous and precise dissection of an avascular plane between the presacral fascia and the fascia propria of the rectum. The complex anatomy of the pelvis, restricted space and visibility makes the surgery one of the technically demanding procedures. The pelvic size is regarded as a direct relating factor to the quality of the resected rectum.

Though slower to gain acceptance, laparoscopic rectal surgery has gained in popularity, and in experienced hands is now regarded as a safe and feasible alternative to open surgery. Nevertheless, the long learning curve, together with inherent difficulties such as two-dimensional imaging, limited dexterity and diminished tactile sense have meant that the application of laparoscopic surgery to technically demanding pelvic procedures continues to present a challenge, in particular for restorative resection of mid and low rectal cancers.

The use of the da Vinci robotic system has been postulated to compensate for these technical limitations. The benefits of robotic surgery as a minimally invasive surgical technique parallel those of traditional laparoscopy, with the added advantages of overcoming several barriers to the use of laparoscopy, such as limitations of the human hand (seven degrees of movement and elimination of hand tremors), elimination of the fulcrum effect of laparoscopy (the robotic arms imitate the movements of the surgeon's hand), improved visualization (three-dimensional stereoscopic imaging), and increased independence of the operating surgeon, thus enabling the surgeon to achieve a more complete mesorectal excision with better autonomic nerve preservation leading to superior bladder and sexual functions. Due to these advantages robotic-assisted management of rectal cancer has gained wide acceptance.

LAPAROSCOPIC SURGERY IN RECTAL CANCER

- Two trials, i.e. CLASICC trial, which recruited colon and rectal cancer patients, and the COREAN trial, which recruited rectal cancer patients only, showed feasibility and oncological safety
- There is strong concern about the higher rate of CRM involvement among rectal cancer patients in the laparoscopic arm (12.4%) of the CLASICC trial compared with the open arm (6.3%). This is especially in the mesorectal margin below rectrosacral ligament.
- In the CLASICC trial with 34% conversion rate, the morbidity and mortality rates were high among laparoscopic cases (colon and rectal cancer) converted to open surgery **(Table 8.1)**.

Laparoscopic rectal surgery could not achieve a high impact, mainly, because of the unstable video camera platform, 2-D imaging, limited dexterity of instrument, fixed tip of instrument, amplification of tremor leading to steep learning curve, high rate of conversion, and the technical challenge of work in a narrow pelvis with limited instruments maneuverability, especially in obese and in patients who were treated by preoperative chemoradiation **(Table 8.2)**.

Table 8.1: Findings of classical trials

	Classic, 2005	*Classic, 2010*
Conversion rate	82/242 (34%)	2/170 (1.2%)
Thirty-day morbidity in converted patients	48/82 (59%)	NA
CRM involvement	30/193 (16%)	5/170 (2.9%)
Mean procedures per surgeon (N)	20	75
Participating centers (N)	27	3
Mean BMI (kg/m^2)	25	24.1

Abbreviations: NA, not assessed; CRM, circumferential resection margin; BMI, body mass index

Table 8.2: Comparative features of robotic surgery versus laparoscopic surgery

	Robotic surgery	*Laparoscopic surgery*
Binocular stereoscopic vision with camera which is stable	Yes	No
Hi definition 3-D camera	Yes	No
12x magnification	Yes	No
Stability of camera	Yes	No
Endowrist technology	Yes	No
Degree of precision	Very high	Operator dependent
Ease of intracorporeal knotting	Very easy	Long learning curve
Multitasking instruments	Yes	No
Surgeon comfort	Very high	Fatigue
Elimination of tremors	Yes	No
Learning curve	Short	Long

PREOPERATIVE PREPARATION AND PRECAUTIONS

All patients who present with newly diagnosed rectal cancer undergo rigid sigmoidoscopy to identify the tumor location. Abdominal pelvic computerized tomography is performed to assess distant metastasis. According to our institution protocol all patients undergo pelvic MRI to assess local infiltration and nodal metastasis. Patients with local invasion (T3-T4) or node involvement are reviewed by the multidisciplinary team and recieve neo-adjuvant chemoradiotherapy. They receive 50.4 Gy dose of EBRT in 28 fractions over 5 and a half weeks, along with systemic 5-flurouracil based chemotherapy followed by surgery 6–8 weeks later.

Preoperatively patient is admitted 12 hours before surgery. He is advised to take clear liquids with an oral antibiotic (ciprofloxacin + tinidazole) for two days prior to surgery. Night before the surgery after admission proctoclysis enema and two dulcolax (bisacodyl) tablets are given per oral. We do not administer peglec at our institution because we observe that it causes dilatation of bowel.

ANESTHESIA

The procedure is performed under general anesthesia. The patient is placed in deep head down position with the legs placed in lithotomy position on the Allen stirups.

Port Placement and Instrumentation

The robotic surgery was performed using the four arm Da Vinci S surgical system (Intuitive Surgical Inc., Sunnyvale, CA, USA) **(Figs 8.1A to C)**. Rectal resection can be performed with a full robotic technique or using a hybrid procedure with some steps laparoscopically performed. We perform complete robotic approach. Total robotic colorectal mobilization and resection was performed in all. We used two types of port placements in our patients. Initially we used the port placement as depicted in **Figure 8.2**. For the subsequent cases we preferred the port placement as depicted in **Figure 8.3**. Both type involves dual docking but in fixed position of robotic cart.

Type 1: A 12 mm camera port is placed 3–4 cm above the umbilicus and 2–3 cm to the right side from the midline with optical trocar. Rest of the ports are placed after insufflating the abdomen with gas and marking the port measurements. Arm one (8 mm) port is placed on patient's right side, at crossing of mid-clavicular line (MCL) and spinoumbilical line. Arm two (8 mm) port is placed on patient's left side similar to the arm 1. Third arm (8 mm) is placed 3 cm below right costal margin and 2 cm medial to right MCL. Additional port (8 mm) is placed on the left 6–7 cm below left costal margin and 2 cm medial to MCL. Assistant port (12 mm) is placed on patient's right side, 8 = 10 cm lateral to the camera port **(Fig. 8.2)**.

Type 2: Here the camera is placed in the midline about 3 cm from the umbilicus. The R1 port is placed along the spinoumbilical line at level of midclavicular line. The R2 port is placed 2 cm to the right of the midline at the subcostal region. The R2I port is placed similarly to R1 at the left side along the spinoumbilical line at level of midclavicular line. The R3 is then placed 3 cm right of the midline just above the inguinal ligament. The R3I port is placed laterally **(Fig. 8.3)**. The advantage of using the second approach is less arm clashing and easier mobilization of left colon up to the splenic flexure. Further, it is easier to apply the linear stapler through the R3 port which is converted to assistant port during pelvic dissection.

Steps of Surgery

The low anterior resection is a technically demanding procedure in robotic assisted colorectal surgery because it needs not only the upper left quadrant approach for splenic flexure mobilization but also the lower left quadrant approach for total mesorectal excision in rectal cancer patients.

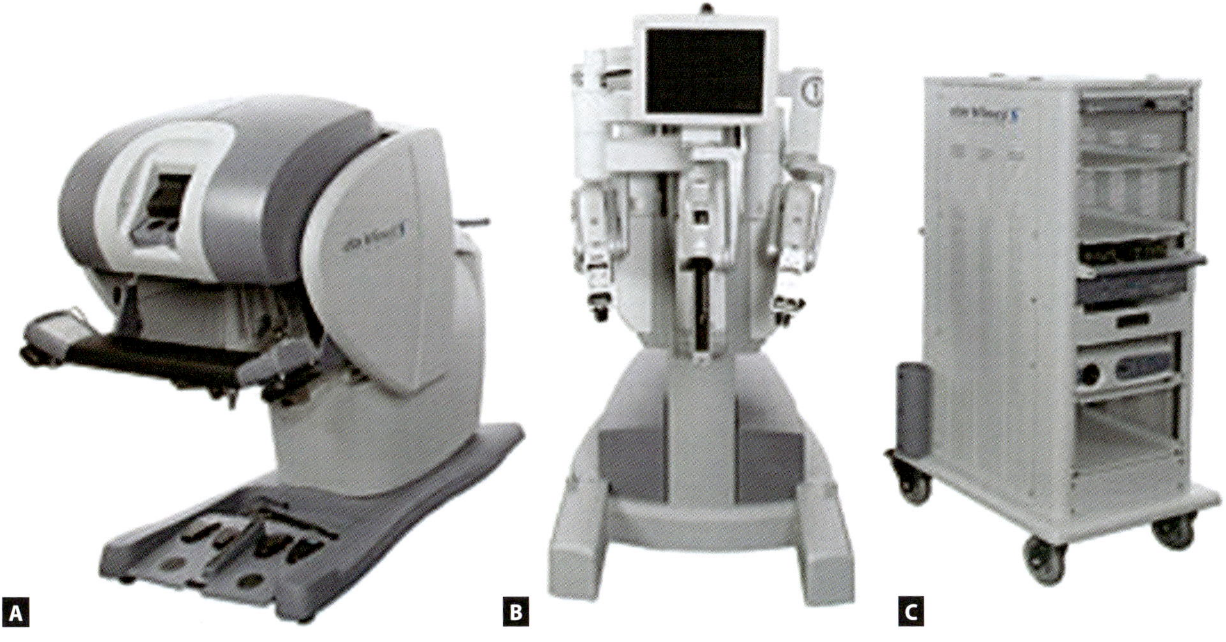

Figs 8.1A to C: The da Vinci robotic system. (A) Surgeon's console; (B) Patient cart; (C) Accessories shelf

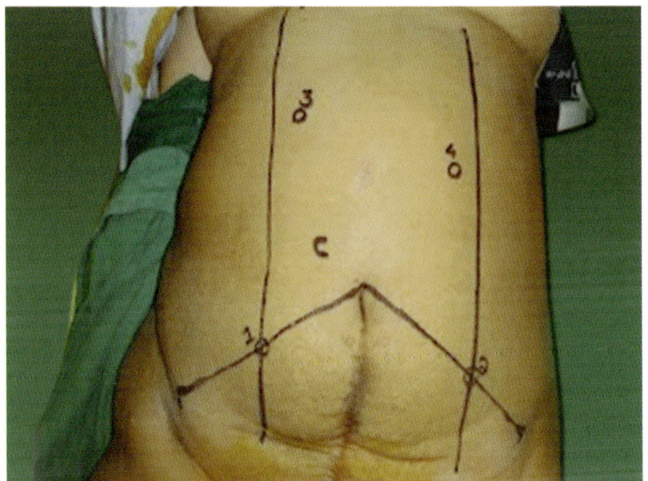

Fig. 8.2: Port placement in laparoscopic assisted robotic procedure

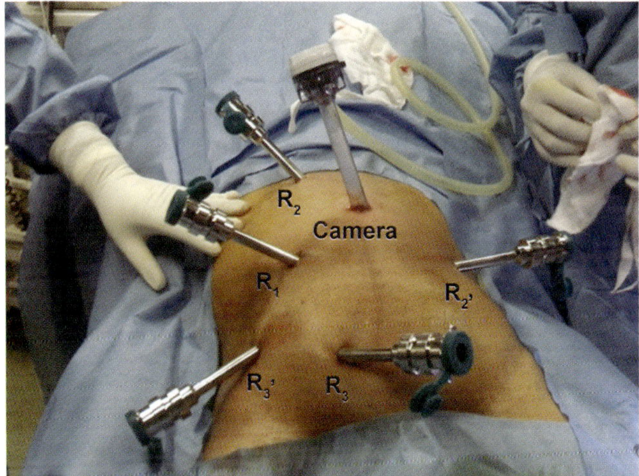

Fig. 8.3: Port placement in total robotic surgery

Patient positioning: The patient is placed supine on the operating table. After induction of general anesthesia and insertion of an oral gastric tube and Foley catheter the patient is rotated with the left side up and right side down, to approximately 20–30° tilt. The patient is then placed in the Trendelenburg position; this helps gravitational migration of the small bowel away from the operative field.

A 30° down facing camera is used. Hot shears is used in R_1, cadiere forceps in R_2 and double fenestrated grasper in R_3.

Robotic dissection is performed as follows:

- Initial metastatic survey of the abdomen
- Identification and clipping of IMA and IMV and division
- Safeguarding autonomic nerves followed by clipping and transection of IMA and IMV
- Medial to lateral dissection (identification of ureter and gonadal vessels)
- Left colon mobilization up to splenic flexure
- Pelvic dissection and total mesorectal excision
- Distal transection, exteriorization of specimen
- Anastomosis using circular stapler.

Postoperative Care

Patient is kept nil per oral with Ryles tube aspiration for 3–4 days. If the patient has a covering ileostomy the Ryles tube is removed in 24 hours. Patient is given IV fluids, and IV antibiotics and other supportive care. Low molecular weight heparin is started after 6 hours of surgery and is continued till patient is ambulating well. Serum electrolytes are monitored on alternate days. Urinary catheter clamping is started after 48 hours and catheter is removed once the patient gets bladder sensation. Majority of the patients are discharged on POD 5–6.

Complications and Their Management

The major complication that we have faced is anastomotic leak especially in patients who have received preoperative chemoradiation. Now as a protocol, we do a covering loop ileostomy in patients with ultralow anterior resection or those who have received preoperative chemoradiation. A few patients who received preoperative chemoradiation developed prolonged ileus and they were treated conservatively.

ROBOTICS IN RECTAL CANCER

Initial published studies are small, not randomized, single center series. Most of the published studies are mainly retrospective or prospective single center series, comparing mainly robotic rectal resection to laparoscopy. Five meta-analyses have already been published on this technique, indicating the marked interest in robotic surgery for rectal cancer.

The operative approaches were evaluated in terms of:
- Operative time
- Estimated blood loss
- Conversion to open procedure
- Length of hospital stay
- Number of lymph nodes harvested
- Margin status
- Time to return of bowel function
- Perioperative complications.

Conversion Rate

In comparison with standard laparoscopy, the most important finding for robotic rectal surgery is the lower rate of conversion to open surgery. Conversion to open surgery is an important indicator of proficiency, generally being ~10–15% in laparoscopic rectal surgery, except for the COREAN trial, where the conversion rate was 1.1%. A preliminary publication of the COLOR II trial reported a 17% conversion rate to open surgery. An RCT [robotic versus laparoscopic resection for rectal cancer (ROLARR)]—comparing laparoscopic with robotic rectal resection for cancer—is ongoing, and its first end-point is the conversion rate to open surgery **(Fig. 8.4)**.

In a meta-analysis, robotic rectal resection was associated with a significant reduction of conversion rate in comparison with laparoscopy **(Table 8.3)**. In another meta-analysis, conversion rates and estimated blood loss were significantly lower in robotic rectal cancer patients than in rectal cancer patient undergoing conventional laparoscopic resection.

Learning Curve

Learning curve for minimally invasive surgery is a crucial issue, because laparoscopic colorectal surgery has a steep learning curve, particularly for rectal cancer, and robotic surgery seems to reduce the learning curve to 15/20 cases **(Fig. 8.5)**. This is an important benefit as the conversion is directly related to a higher rate of postoperative complications and mortality as shown by CLASICC trial.

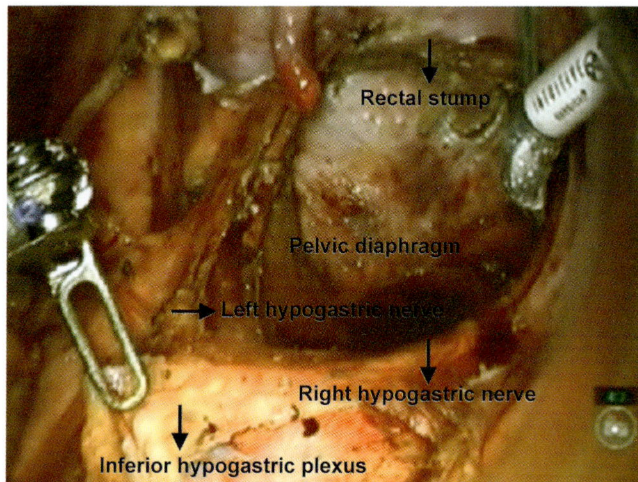

Fig. 8.4: Relation of nerves to rectum

Table 8.3: A meta-analysis of conversion rate

	Conversion rate		*p value*
	R	*L*	
Park, 2010	0/41 (0%)	0/82 (0%)	1.0
Kim, 2010	2/100 (2%)	3/100 (3%)	1.0
Kwak, 2011	0/59 (0%)	2/59 (3.4%)	0.496
Baek, 2011	3/41 (7.3%)	9/41 (22%)	0.116
Bianchi, 2010	0/25 (0%)	1/25 (4%)	1.0
Baik, 2009	0/56 (0%)	6/57 (10.5%)	0.013
Patriti, 2009	0/29 (0%)	7/37 (19%)	<0.05

SHORT-TERM CLINICAL OUTCOMES

In comparison with open surgery, robot-assisted surgery maintains all the advantages of minimally invasive procedures. The clinical outcomes of robotic surgery did not show any significant difference from laparoscopic technique. Overall complications rate and length of hospital stay are similar for both techniques **(Table 8.4)**.

Sexual and Urinary Functions

Laparoscopy did not add any advantage in term of sexual/urinary dysfunction preservation. In fact MRC CLASICC trial raised a concern that laparoscopic TME may be associated with increased rates of male sexual dysfunction. Only three studies evaluating genitourinary function after robotic rectal surgery have been published **(Table 8.5)**. A similar trend for sexual function has been observed, with a decrease at one

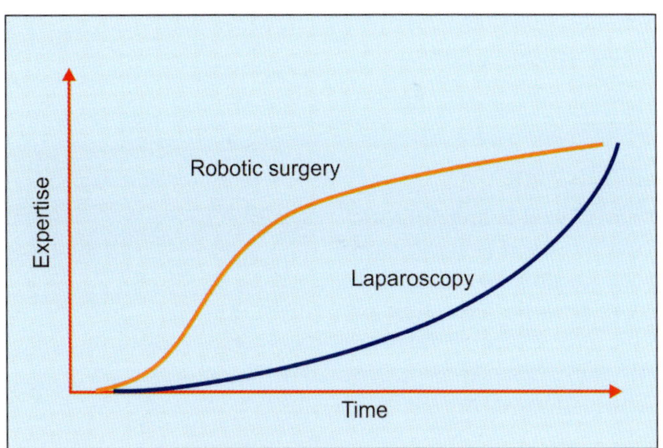

Fig. 8.5: The learning curve

Table 8.4: Various study comapring hospital stay and postoperative complications in robotic procedure and laparoscopic surgery						
	Hospital stay (days)			*Postoperative complications (%)*		
	ROB	*LAP*	*p*	*ROB*	*LAP*	*p*
Park, 2010	9.9	9.4	0.5	29.3	23.2	0.4
Kim, 2010	11.7	14.4	0.006	20	27	0.4
Kwak, 2011	NA	NA		32	27	NS
Baek, 2011	6.5	6.6	0.8	22	27	1
Bianchi, 2010	6.5	6	0.4	16	24	0.5
Baik, 2009	5.7	8.6	0.001	10.7	19.3	0.025
Patriti, 2009	11.9	9.6	>0.05	30.6	18.9	>0.55

Table 8.5: A comparison of urinary and sexual function following robotic versus laparoscopic surgery		
Reference	*Study*	*Results*
Kim, 2012	39 LAP versus 30 ROB (urinary) 20 LAP versus 18 ROB (sexual male only)	Earlier recover of normal voiding and sexual function
D'Annibate, 2013	30 LAP versus 30 ROB (*male only*)	Erectile function was restored completely in the ROB group and partially in the LAP group
Luca, 2013	74 ROB (38 *males* and 36 *females*)	Sexual function and general sexual satisfaction were restored completely. Urinary function unchanged after surgery

Abbreviations: LAP, laparoscopic rectal surgery; ROB, robotic rectal surgery

month after surgery and subsequent progressive recovery. Surgeons agree that an easier identification of the nerves and of the planes of dissection is provided by the robotic system.

Oncological Outcomes

A multivariate analysis that included potent parameters, i.e. SSO types, preoperative CRT, T-category, and growth pattern, showed that patients with distal resection margin ≥2 cm were significantly more likely to be in the robotic than in the open group (OR, 2.415; 95% CI, 1.233–4.73; P = 0.01). The mean number of harvested lymph nodes and lymphovascular or perineural invasion was similar in the two groups.

Concern about the CRM involvement was reported in CLASICC trial. Studies so far available demonstrate comparable oncologic results with laparoscopy **(Table 8.6)**.

Cost

Robotic surgery is expensive, due to the cost of robot purchase, maintenance, and instruments. Therefore, a careful analysis of costs and of cost effectiveness is mandatory, even if it is difficult to perform because of the lack of available data about the potential benefits of robotic surgery. A recent costs analysis demonstrates that robotic surgery is more expensive.

Table 8.6: Oncological outcomes (robotic vs open procedure)

	LNs (mean)			*Distal margin (mean, cm)*			*Positive CRM (%)*		
	ROB	*Open*	*p*	*ROB*	*Open*	*p*	*ROB*	*Open*	*p*
De Souza, 2011	15	16.8	0.26	NA	NA		0	3	0.25
Kim, 2011	20	19.6	0.7	2.7	1.9	0.001	1	1	1
Pakr, 2011	19.4	18.5	0.06	2.8	2.3	0.002	1	2	0.9

Abbreviations: LNs, lymph nodes; CRM, circumferential resection margin; NA, not assessed; ROB, robotic procedure

Table 8.7: Oncological outcomes (robotic vs laparoscopic procedure)

	LNs (mean)			*Distal margin (mean, cm)*			*Positive CRM (%)*		
	ROB	*LAP*	*p*	*ROB*	*LAP*	*p*	*ROB*	*LAP*	*p*
Park, 2010	17.3	14.2	0.06	2.1	2.3	NS	4.9	3.7	0.5
Kim, 2010	14.7	16.6	NS	2.7	2.6	0.09	3	2	NS
Kwak, 2011	20	21	0.7	2.2	2.0	0.8	1.7	0	>0.9
Baek, 2011	13	16	0.07	3.6	3.8	0.6	2.4	4.9	1
Bianchi, 2010	18	17	0.7	2	2	1.0	0	4	0.9
Baik, 2009	18.4	18.7	0.8	4	3.6	0.4	7	8	0.7
Patriti, 2009	10.3	11.2	>0.05	2.1	4.5	>0.05	0	0	NS

Abbreviations: LNs, lymph nodes; CRM, circumferential resection margin; NS, not significant; ROB, robotic procedure; LAP, laparoscopic procedure

INDIAN EXPERIENCE

A prospective randomized comparative study was undertaken from August 2011 to December 2012 at Manipal comprehensive cancer centre, Bengaluru.

Majority of the patients had the growth in the mid or lower rectum with only 14% having upper rectal cancer. Thirteen patients in the RA had lower rectal cancer out of which 3 patients underwent abdominoperineal resection (APR), while 5 out of 12 patients in the OA with low rectal cancer required APR. Temporary diverting loop ileostomy was performed in patients who underwent ultra-low anterior resection or in low anterior resection patients who had received preoperative chemoradiotherapy. In our study 20 patients underwent ileostomies (9 in RA and 11 in OA). The conversion rate was nil.

The mean total operative time was significantly longer in patients who underwent robotic surgery than open surgery (310 vs 246 minutes $p < 0.001$). However, in the RA the operative time which was initially high reduced significantly in the subsequent cases. Estimated blood loss was significantly less with robotic-assisted surgery (165.14 mL) compared to open method (406.04 mL).

Circular stapled anastomosis was performed in all patients who underwent LAR and the donuts were sent for frozen section analysis. The distal and proximal margins were negative for tumor in all the patients. The mean distal resection margin was significantly longer in the RA than OA (3.6 vs 2.4 cm, $p < 0.001$). The circumferential resection margins (CRM) were inked to assess the completeness and subjected to pathological analysis. The CRM was negative in all patients. Besides the CRM status, the quality of mesorectum was scored by the pathologist using three grades (complete, near complete and incomplete) as defined by the Dutch TME trial. None of the patients in RA had incomplete mesorectum while 1 patient in OA had an incomplete mesorectal excision. Number of lymph nodes removed by robotic method (16.88) was equal or slightly higher than the open method (15.20) but with no significant difference **(Tables 8.7 and 8.8)**.

All patients were assessed for urinary and sexual function disorders. As a part of the trial all patients underwent urinary catheter removal on the second postoperative day. Five patients in OA and two patients in RA developed urinary retention and required recatheterization and had catheter removal after 7 days following catheter clamping exercises. Post void residual volume was assessed at end of 1 month in all patients with the help of ultrasound, 3 in OA and one patient in RA had significant residual urine **(Tables 8.9 and 8.10)**. Erectile dysfunction and retrograde ejaculation was assessed in all male patients during follow-up using the European Organization for Research and Treatment of Cancer (EORTC) questionnaire QLQ-C38. 18% of male patients in RA and 25% in OA group had sexual dysfunction features.

ONGOING TRIALS

ROLARR trial: RObotic versus LAparoscopic Resection for Rectal cancer. This trial is a randomized two-arm control

Table 8.8: Nerve preservation

Total mesorectal excision + autonomic nerve preservation	n = 50
Robotic	25
Open	25

Table 8.9: Mean results of a prospective study at Mount Carmel College, Bengaluru

Characteristics	*Robotic n = 25*	*Open n = 25*
Male : Female	17 : 8	15 : 10
Age (years)	56.36 ± 8.21	59.56 ± 5.75
Mean BMI (kg/m^2)	28.19 ± 3.02	26.84 ± 2.75
Site: Upper third	2	5
Mid third	10	8
Lower third	13	12
Preoperative CTRT	7	9
Operation type		
Low anterior resections	22	20
Abdominoperineal resections	3	5
Mean blood loss (mL)	165.14 ± 11.25	406.04 ± 111.32
Mean operative time, minutes	310.32 ± 47.62	246.32 ± 17.45
Margins		
Proximal/Distal	Negative	Negative
Circumferential/Radial	Negative	Negative
Mean total lymph nodes	16.88 ± 2.18	15.20 ± 1.65
Mean hospital stay (days)	7.52 ± 1.38	13.24 ± 2.43
Intraoperative complications	1	0
Postoperative complications		
Minor	0	4
Major	0	1

Table 8.10: Results of a prospective study at Mount Carmel College, Bengaluru

Variable	*Robotic n = 25*	*Open n = 25*	*P value*
Age, years	56.36	59.56	0.117
BMI (kg/m^2)	31.19	28.84	0.105
Operating time (minute)	398 in first 5 cases	240	<0.001
	288 in next 20 cases	247	<0.001
Estimated blood loss (mL)	165.14	406.04	<0.001
Number of lymph nodes removed	16.88	15.20	0.055
Hospital stay (days)	7.52	13.24	<0.001

trial; worldwide study involving 28 centers in the United States, Europe, Asia, and Australia. The primary endpoint is the rate of conversions to open surgery, secondary endpoints are circumferential resection margin positivity and local recurrence, safety of the technique, functional results, quality of life, and economics considerations.

COLRAR trial: Trial to assess robot-assisted surgery and laparoscopy-assisted surgery in patients with mid or low rectal cancer. This study is designed to assess whether robotic surgical system improves the quality of rectal cancer surgery, especially in total mesorectal excision and a circumferential margin positivity rate. Secondary endpoints are to compare 3- and 5-year disease-free survival and overall survival after robot and laparoscopic resection of distal rectal cancer. This study will also assess the pelvic autonomic nerve preservation, short-term morbidity, pathological quality (i.e. number of harvested lymph node), local recurrence, and blood loss during surgery.

Advantages of Robot-assisted TME for Rectal Cancer

- Precise pelvic dissection especially for the narrow male pelvis
- Preservation of bladder and sexual function
- Low conversion rate
- Rectal transection under robotic setting
- Transanal specimen extraction and single stapling anastomosis
- Lateral pelvic LN dissection.

BIBLIOGRAPHY

1. Baik SH, Kim NK, Lee KY, Sohn SK, Cho CH, Kim MJ, et al. Factors influencing pathologic results after total mesorectal excision for rectal cancer: analysis of consecutive 100 cases. Ann Surg Oncol. 2008;15:721-8.
2. Berguer R, Rab GT, Abu-Ghaida H, et al. A comparison of surgeon's posture during laparoscopic and open surgical procedures. Surg Endosc. 1997;11:2139.
3. Bianchi PP, et al. Robotic versus laparoscopic total mesorectal excision for rectal cancer: a comparative analysis of oncological safety and short-term outcomes. Surg Endosc. 2010;24(11):2888-94. DOI: 10.1007/s00464-010-1134-7
4. Bokhari MB, Patel CB, Ramos-Valadez DI, et al. Learning curve for robotic-assisted laparoscopic colorectal surgery. Surg Endosc. 2011;25:855-60.
5. Brown G, Daniels IR. Preoperative staging of rectal cancer: The MERCURY research project. Recent Results Cancer Res. 2005;165:58-74.
6. Buunen M, et al. COLOR II A randomized clinical trial comparing laparoscopic and open surgery for rectal cancer. Dan Med Bull. 2009;56(2):89-91.
7. Cadiere GB, Himpens J, Germay O, Izizaw R, Degueldre M, Vandromme J, et al. Feasibility of robotic laparoscopic surgery: 146 cases. World J Surg. 2001;25:1467-77.
8. Collinson FJ, et al. An international, multicentre, prospective, randomised, controlled, unblinded, parallel-group trial of robotic-assisted versus standard laparoscopic surgery for the curative treatment of rectal cancer. Int J Colorectal Dis. 2012;27:233-41.
9. Current status of robotic rectal cancer surgery Jose Reinan Ramos J. Coloproctol. (Rio J.) Rio de Janeiro. 2014;34(3).

10. Ficarra V, et al. Systematic review and meta-analysis of studies reporting potency rates after robot-assisted radical prostatectomy. Eur Urol. 2012;62(3):418-30. DOI: 10.1016/j.eururo.2012.05.046
11. Guillou PJ, et al. Short-term endpoints of conventional versus laparoscopic assisted surgery in patients with colorectal cancer (MRC CLASICC trial): multicentre, randomised controlled trial Lancet. 2005;365:1718-26.
12. Heald RJ. A new approach to rectal cancer. Br J Hosp Med. 1979;22:277-81.
13. Jiménez-Rodríguez RM, Díaz-Pavón JM, de la Portilla de Juan F, Prendes-Sillero E, Dussort HC, Padillo J. Learning curve for robotic-assisted laparoscopic rectal cancer surgery. Int J Colorectal Dis. 2013;28:815-21.
14. Kim JC, et al. Open versus robot-assisted sphincter-saving operations in rectal cancer patients: techniques and comparison of outcomes between groups of 100 matched patients. Int J Med Robotics Comput Assist Surg. 2012;8(4):468-75.
15. Luca F, et al. Full robotic left colon and rectal cancer resection: technique and early outcome. Ann Surg Oncol. 2009;16:1274-8. DOI: 10.1245/s10434-009-0366-z
16. Martel G, Boushey RP. Laparoscopic colon surgery: past, present and future. Surg Clin N Am. 2006;86:867-97.
17. Memon S, et al. Robotic versus laparoscopic proctectomy for rectal cancer: a meta-analysis. Ann Surg Oncol. 2012;19:2095-101.
18. Morino M, et al. Male sexual and urinary function after laparoscopic total mesorectal excision. Surg Endosc. 2009;23:1233-40.
19. Park JS, et al. S052: a comparison of robot assisted, laparoscopic, and open surgery in the treatment of rectal cancer. Surg Endosc. 2011;25:240-8.
20. Se-Jin Baek, et al. Robotic versus conventional laparoscopic surgery for rectal cancer: a cost analysis from a single institute in Korea. World J Surg. 2012;36(11):2722-9.
21. Somashekhar SP, Ashwin KR. Prospective randomized study comparing robotic-assisted surgery with traditional laparotomy for rectal cancer—Indian Study Indian Journal of Surgery, 2013,1.
22. Spinoglio G, et al. Robotic laparoscopic surgery with the da Vinci® system: an early experience. Surg Technol Int. 2009;18:70-4.
23. Sung-Bum Kang, et al. Open versus laparoscopic surgery for mid or low rectal cancer after neoadjuvant chemoradiotherapy (COREAN trial): short-term outcomes of an open-label randomised controlled trial. Lancet Oncol. 2010;11:637-45.
24. Taylor GW, Jayne DG. Robotic applications in abdominal surgery: their limitations and future developments. Int J Med Robot. 2007;3:3-9 Review DOI: 10.1002/rcs.115
25. Trastulli S, Farinella E, Cirocchi R, Cavaliere D, Avenia N, Sciannameo F, Gullà N, Noya G, Boselli C. Robotic resection compared with laparoscopic rectal resection for cancer: systematic review and meta-analysis of short-term outcome. Colorectal Dis. 2012;14: e134-e156.
26. Yang Y, et al. Robot-assisted versus conventional laparoscopic surgery for colorectal disease, focusing on rectal cancer: a meta-analysis. Ann Surg Oncol. 2012;19(12):3727-36.

CHAPTER

9

Robotic Surgery for Bile Duct Tumors

Vivek Bindal, Anand Kumar Yadav

INTRODUCTION

Cholangiocarcinoma (CCA) may originate from any part of biliary tree as a primary cancer.[1] It is typically classified into hilar tumors which are intrahepatic, extrahepatic in nature and distal bile duct tumors which can be extrahepatic, corresponding to the anatomical relation to the biliary tree structure.[2] Histopathologically adenocarcinoma type of tumors accounts for over and above 95% of cholangiocarcinoma, whether it is anatomically extrahepatic or intrahepatic in origin. There were some other histological varieties of cholangiocarcinoma had been identified which included carcinoma of squamous or mucoepidermoid type, papillary carcinoma, leiomyosarcoma, rhabdomyosarcoma, cystadenocarcinoma, carcinoid tumor, etc.

As per the anatomical sites of origin in the biliary tree, cholangiocarcinoma can be classified into mainly intrahepatic and extrahepatic types. The intrahepatic type of tumors are again classified macroscopic four growth types: (1) Mass forming tumors; (2) Periductal infiltrating tumors; (3) Mass forming plus periductal infiltrating tumors; and (4) Intraductal tumors.[3]

The extrahepatic tumors are further divided into: (1) Hilar or Klatskin; (2) Middle; and (3) Distal tumors. Klatskin tumors represent approximately 60% of all extrahepatic tumors.

Macroscopically, extrahepatic cholangiocarcinoma presents as sclerosing, nodular, or papillary phenotypes.[3] The sclerosing type is the most common; it is characterized by annular thickening of the bile duct wall due to infiltration of the periductal connective tissue.

Benign tumors of the biliary tract are exceedingly rare, but can cause symptoms not dissimilar from those resulting from malignant causes. The most common benign biliary tumors are papillomas and adenomas.

Risk factors for bile duct cancer:

- Primary sclerosing cholangitis[4]
- Liver flukes infestation (Opisthorchisviverrini and clonorchissinensis)[5,6]
- Choledochal cysts (Caroli's disease)[7]
- Hepatolithiasis[8,9]
- Chemicals (e.g. thorotrast and dioxin)[10-13]
- Hepatitis C[14]
- Lynch syndrome II
- Bile duct adenoma and multiple biliary papillomatosis.

SURGICAL TREATMENT

Preoperative Assessment

Removal of cancer tissues surgically by complete resection or R0 resection to achieve histologically negative resection margins is the one and only hope for cure in the cases of cholangiocarcinoma. On the other hand, only a few of the patients are considered suitable for surgical resection procedures. Hence, preoperative evaluation and assessment of patients for resectability is considered mandatory and ideally to be carried out by a team of specialist surgeons. Both cancer patient and the tumor factors need preoperative consideration.

Initially the evaluations should begin with the assessments of general systemic medical condition of the cancer patient in terms of cardiac, respiratory and kidney function before the surgical procedure. Assessment of the patients has to be done for their performance status and fitness for a major surgical procedure which may involve partial hepatectomy. Additionally in cases of obstructive jaundice patients, the irregularity in pathophysiology related to the conditions such as changes in liver, pancreas and immunological function, the hemostatic mechanisms, the gastrointestinal barrier, and healing of wound needs to be taken into consideration.[15]

At the time of preoperative assessments, nearly one-third of patients may be regarded as unresectable disease condition. Additionally, at the time of laparoscopic procedure, 25–30% of cases who were considered to be suitable for radical surgical procedure will be identified to have unresectable condition.

Medical conditions like chronic liver disease (CLD) or presence of portal hypertension usually makes the patient unfit for surgery. In case there is any proof about cholangitis, it is to be treated with appropriate drainage and systemic antibiotics prior to surgery.[6]

The main aim of the operation is R0 resection procedure with free proximal margin and distal margin, tumor bed resection (involving caudate lobe and vascular components) and appropriate lymphadenectomy. In cases of cholangiocarcinoma to have longer term of survival complete resection with margins being negative histologically is considered a critical criterion.

In cases of Klatskin tumor, which makes the majority of patients, which may require extended hepatectomy, along with complete surgical resection of structures like extra-hepatic bile duct and also radical lymphadenectomy.[16] This kind of aggressive surgical strategy has increased the rate of curative resections and longer duration of survival for the patients having this type of disease.[17]

There are number of challenges and various technical complex issues in this surgical approach like control of inflow, caudate lobe of liver inclusion and reconstructive surgical procedure involving many separate ducts of small caliber size. The feasibleness and surgical safety of laparoscopic techniques in hepatic resections had been reported, specifically for anterior segment and lateral segment of liver. But, the acceptance of laparoscopy procedure for biliary tumors is limited due to technical challenges and cancer-related concerns.[18]

Robotic surgical procedure might help to overcome certain challenges of laparoscopic procedure and offer the minimal invasive surgical advantages to the patients, who would instead usually undergo the extensive open method of surgery. The major limitations observed during these surgical procedures are mobilization of the right hepatic lobe, dissection of the hepatic hilum, control of hemorrhage during transaction of hepatic parenchyma, and complicated biliary reconstruction. Already many advantages offered by robotic platform had been described well. Robotic surgery helps the operating surgeon by increasing the precision of surgical dissection while facilitating the suturing procedure in many difficult situations. It also gives the surgeon comfort ergonomically during this longer duration of challenging surgical procedures so that the operating surgeon can work to the full potential and abilities. In all these highly advanced surgical methods, it is quite important to learn that with the use of minimally invasive surgical procedure, the major indications and selection of patients for the procedure do not usually change. The basic principles of any safe R0 type of surgical resection procedure and appropriate lymphadenectomy would not be compromised. A lower threshold of option for convert to an open surgical method may be kept if the major aim of the operation cannot be achieved safely by adopting the minimal invasive techniques.

The situations for unresectable conditions are:[19]

- Presence of major comorbidities which excludes safe surgery
- Metastasis of the disease
- Invasion of cancer to the main portal vein or involvement of hepatic artery vessel proximal to the bifurcation site
- Bilateral cancer invasion of vessels like portal veins or hepatic arteries and their vascular branches
- Cancer involvement of hepatic ducts bilaterally up to secondary radicles, and
- Unilateral cancer involvement of hepatic duct and/or blood vessel with contralateral hepatic lobe atrophy.

Many of those restrictions could be overcome by applying surgical techniques like embolization of portal vein, which may induce contralateral hepatic hypertrophy to expand the remnant part of liver volume in future.

Patient Positioning and Docking

Under the influence of general anesthesia, the selected patient is kept in supine position for surgery with parted legs involving reverse—Trendelenburg tilt of approximate 20°. Cleaning and draping of the abdomen is done and the orogastric tube or urinary catheter is also placed. During surgery the assistant has to stand in between the parted legs. Pneumoperitoneum can be achieved to the level of 15 mm Hg by using a Veress needle inserted at palmer's point.

Placement of a 10/12 mm size of trocar at supraumbilical position is usually done (which may be used like an assistant port during the surgical procedure). Placement of one optical trocar and insertion of three da Vinci trocars are done as described in **Figure 9.1**.

Optical trocar of 12 mm size: In the region of mid-clavicular line towards right side, nearly 10 cm away from the assistant trocar, superior to the umbilicus level.

R1: In the region of mid-clavicular line towards left, around 10 cm distant from the assistant trocar, superior umbilicus level.

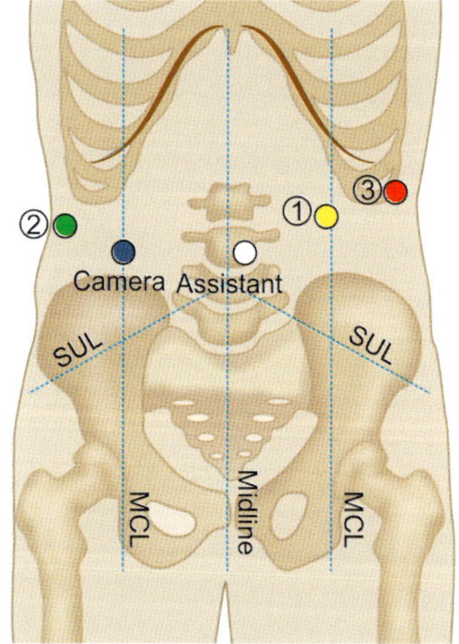

Fig. 9.1: Port position

Abbreviations: SUL, spinoumbilical line; MCL, midclavicular line; 1, 2, 3, represent positions for robotic arms 1, 2 and 3, respectively

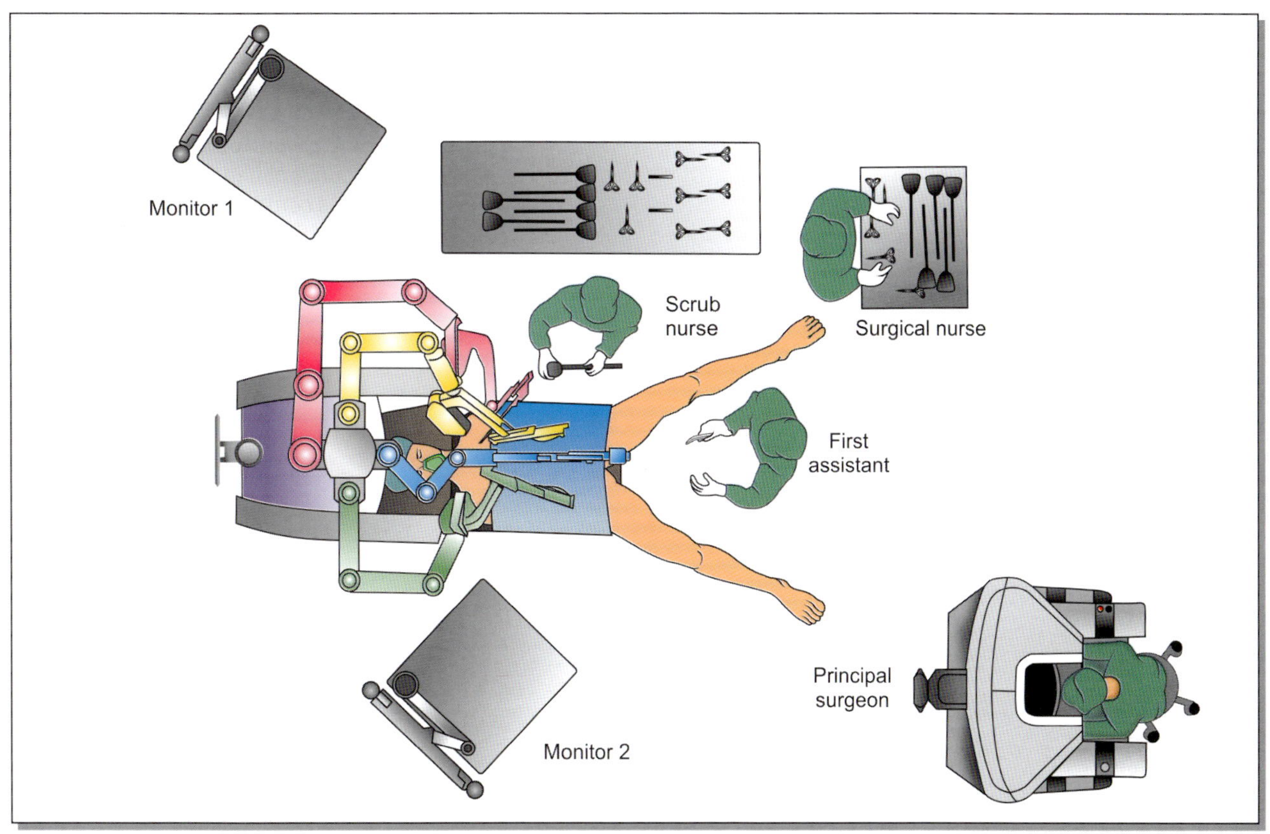

Fig. 9.2: Operating room setup for robot-assisted right extended hepatectomy

R2: In the region of anterior axillary line on right side, minimum 10 cm distant from the optical trocar insertion site.

R3: In the region of anterior axillary line towards left side, mostly used for the purpose of retraction procedure.

The placement of these ports may require adjustment based on the body shape and physique of the selected patient for prevention of collision of the external arm and to offer optimum exposure for surgery.

Usually a laparoscopy procedure for diagnostic purpose is carried out to check for any metastatic deposits identification or presence of free fluid. In case any deposit of suspicion is detected, to rule out metastasis it is to be biopsied and sent for examination in frozen condition. In case any free fluid is identified, it is then sent for cytology to check for presence of cells of malignant origin. During the operation an ultrasonogram can be done to exclude any unidentified metastatic deposits present in liver.

The patient cart of da Vinci® surgical system is positioned by bring it from the direction of patient's head end, and then the robotic arms are docked to the ports placed. The robotic third arm comes from the direction of left side of patient. To begin the surgical procedure, a monopolar hook, bipolar forceps and grasping forceps are taken in R1, R2 and R3 respectively. The supporting assistant surgeon has to stand in between the parted legs for the required complementary manipulative movements (i.e., suctioning, staple, retraction, and laparoscopic ultrasonogram). A sample of OR setup for extended right hepatectomy for cholangiocarcinoma is shown in **Figure 9.2**.

Bile Duct Resection

Mobilization of the hepatic flexure portion of the colon is done towards medial side and caudally along with a partial Kocher maneuver. Using R3 for retraction dissection is started at the hepatic hilum. Gallbladder is usually taken down while keeping the cystic duct which remains attached to common bile duct (CBD) as such. Indocyanine green (ICG) fluorescence helps in the identification of common bile duct and any aberrant structures in biliary anatomy. Common bile duct is dissected clearly and it is transected distally near the upper border of pancreas, and then the oversewing of the distal stump is done. A frozen section biopsy of the distal margin is sent to check for malignant cells, if found positive, there is a need for pancreaticoduodenectomy with or without hepatic resection, depending on site of cancer, metastasis and performance status of the cancer patient. The hepatoduodenal ligament is dissected and proximal part of bile duct is pulled up and separated from hepatic artery and portal vein. Lymphadenectomy operation is done alongside the common hepatic artery. Exposure of gastroduodenal artery at its origin is performed. Usually, the dissection of lymph nodes in hepatoduodenal ligament is considered appropriate. Resection of the fat tissue and lymph nodes is performed en bloc along with the bile duct. Near the hilum, hepatic ducts on both right and left side are dissected and then circled with vessel loops to help in traction. If a surgeon can reach near proximal to the site of tumor, division of bile ducts is performed and to check spread of malignant cells a frozen section biopsy of margin is sent to know about the R0 resection procedure.

In presence of Bismuth type III tumor, there is a requirement of extended hepatectomy either right or left side alongside bile duct resection for R0 resection. Details of technique of the surgical procedure are explained below in another section.

Resection of vascular areas and reconstructive surgeries are considered in the cases of portal veins or hepatic arteries are involved. This should be performed only by surgeons with higher experience and hospitals or institutions showing better perioperative reports in these high risk surgical procedures.

Reconstruction: Roux-en-Y Hepaticojejunostomy

For procedures like Roux-en-Y hepaticojejunostomy, infracolic area has to be reached for the preparation of the loop for reconstructive surgical procedure. The division of proximal jejunal loop is performed with the help of a stapler, and to make a roux loop jejunojejunostomy is done by laparoscopic stapler. The distal loop is later brought into the supracolic area in a transmesocolic approach. At that moment, a surgical anastomosis in between bile duct and the loop is performed in end-to-side method, by using 4-0, 5-0 or 6-0 PDS (Ethicon, Somerville NJ) based on the diameter size of bile duct. A ductoplasty could be considered if the bile duct diameter is of smaller size. Generally a single layer anastomosis with half running layers of suture is performed, one for the posterior wall and another for the anterior wall. Small number of interrupted stitches could be placed to provide adequate reinforcement to the anastomosis. Occasionally, the anterior layer is to be created with the help of interrupted stitches, in case of smaller diameter size or thinner walled ducts. The possibility of performing interrupted stitches microsurgical way is one of the significant benefits of using robot. For reducing the tension of the anastomosis, jejunal loop is fixed to hilum using two surgical stitches of Prolene 3-0 (Ethicon, Somerville, NJ, USA). Using fibrin glue might be considered towards the end of anastomosis. Mostly at the end of the surgical procedure, a drain may be inserted near the biliary anastomosis.

Extended Left Hepatectomy with Caudate Lobe Resection

The placement of ports and trocars has already been described. A detailed laparoscopy for diagnostic purpose is performed along with ultrasonogram of hepatic area to exclude metastasis of disease. The patient cart of robotic surgical system is docked and procedure begins by taking down the gallbladder, mostly keeping the attachment of cystic duct intact. Indocyanine green (ICG) fluorescence is mostly used to detect the biliary structures and look for any anatomical variations. Complete dissection of common bile duct is performed which is later tied and transected. The tissues from distal margin area of CBD are sent for evaluation of frozen section biopsy and oversewing of the stump is done with help of PDS sutures. Lymphadenectomy procedure is performed alongside the hepatoduodenal ligament. Dissection of the left hepatic artery is done, but before its transaction by a stapler, it is evaluated and confirmed by clamping test which will show a color change in liver parenchyma towards the left side. Dissection of the left side branch of portal vein is done following which the ligation and division is performed. Parenchymal transection is performed alongside the line of ischemia usually with the help of ultrasonic shears. To perform parenchymal transaction procedure a bipolar radiofrequency device known as Habib™ or Cavitational Ultrasonic Surgical Aspirator (CUSA) might be used.

Dissection of the anterior branch and posterior branch of right hepatic duct is done after which it is transected and the margins tissues are sent for frozen section biopsy. The caudate lobe of liver is usually dissected from the structures like inferior vena cava (IVC). The parenchymal tissue transection is performed and the hemostasis secured. The reconstructive surgery is performed in a Roux-en-Y method. The roux limb is made by stapling jejunojejunostomy and it is moved cranial direction in a transmesocolic (occasionally retrogastric) method. With help of 5-0 PDS, the two right sided ducts are connected. One opening is created in the roux limb and then a posterior layer of anastomosis is done with the help of continuous 5-0 suturing procedure. One interrupted anterior layer is usually thrown and small numbers of stitches are performed between liver and roux limb so as to prevent unnecessary tension on the anastomosis. The fibrin glue may be used over the anastomotic site and the raw surface area of transected hepatic parenchyma. The biological specimen can be retrieved in an endobag generally performing a pfannenstiel incision.

Extended Right Hepatectomy

At the beginning, the hepatic flexure portion of the colon gets mobilized, and a partial Kocher maneuver is conducted. Beginning at the upper border of the pancreas head, the lymphadenectomy procedure near the common hepatic artery is completed, with the help of monopolar hook and bipolar forceps, the site of origin of the gastroduodenal artery is exposed. The lower aspect of segment IV is pulled upward with the help of the fourth robotic arm, and dissection of the common bile duct (CBD) is completed and it is sectioned at the upper border of the pancreas head. The distal portion of stump of the common bile duct is sutured, and a frozen section biopsy specimen is sent to exclude cancer invasion. Dissection of the right hepatic artery is performed and then it is divided at its place of origin from the main hepatic artery. Transaction of the left hepatic duct is done near the left umbilical fissure and then a frozen section biopsy specimen is sent at this level also. After this, dissection of the right portal vein is completed and it is divided between the ligatures. Mobilization of the right hepatic lobe is performed from the peritoneal attachments. It is usually done by falciform ligament sectioning and the anterior half of the coronary ligament, until the frontal region of the inferior vena cava and the right hepatic vein is secured. Division of the hepatorenal ligament and the right triangular ligament are done with the help of a monopolar hook. The fourth arm of robot is used to pull the lower part of the right hepatic lobe upwards. By this method, the right side of the inferior vena cava gets exposed.

The ligation of the accessory hepatic vein is done by a suture and then the dissection procedure advances until the lower part of the right hepatic vein is reachable. Following the sectioning of the bridge of liver parenchyma in between the segments IV and III, the transection of parenchymal tissue is performed alongside the right side of the falciform ligament by help of harmonic scalpel, beginning at the anterior border of liver. With the help of staplers the division of the recurrent blood vessels from the umbilical fissure to segment IV, middle hepatic vein and right hepatic vein are performed. The reconstructive surgical procedures are performed as per the already explained method. Retrieval of the biological specimen is done in an endobag.

PALLIATIVE SURGERY

A greater number of patients with cholangiocarcinoma usually have tumors which are surgically unresectable during diagnosis. The aim in these cases is palliative treatment of symptoms using surgical interventions with lower morbidity and maximum efficacy.[20,21] For distal cholangiocarcinoma, generally endoscopic stent placement is the preferred procedure while for proximal cholangiocarcinoma, percutaneous stenting methods with or without endoscopic interventions are useful. In few difficult cases, a biliary and/or digestive surgical bypass could be required, but it may involve higher morbidity and fatal outcomes when performed by open surgical approach.[22] With the help of robotic surgery, the provision of minimally invasive surgical method will be significantly beneficial to these cases with a lower morbidity.[23]

LIVER TRANSPLANTATION

Liver transplantation of orthotopic type, in addition to multimodality treatment management, is rarely considered as an option in advanced stages of tumors like cancer invading portal veins, bilateral hepatic ducts involvement and atrophy of liver lobes. But, there are very few studies on transplantation of liver as a modality for managing cholangiocarcinoma. There is shortage of donor organs and poor therapeutic outcomes, the treatment indications of liver transplant are very few and it is not adopted as a standard treatment. In smaller number of cases when transplant is required, the use of robotic surgery may be an option for hepatectomy in a living donor.[24]

POSTOPERATIVE OUTCOMES

Surgical procedures of bile duct tumors are accompanied with substantial postoperative morbidity and fatality. The major complications observed perioperatively with the surgical procedure are biliary leakage, hemorrhage, cholangitis, abscess of liver, failure of liver, organ space or surgical site infections superficially and respiratory system complications. The factors which mostly increase the chances of complications after a minimal invasive bilioenteric anastomosis procedure are iatrogenically made bile duct injury and size of duct diameter ≤5 mm. These reports are better placed than many of the clinical studies with open method and laparoscopic hepaticojejunostomy operations.

As per published literatures, less than 50% of cases of cholangiocarcinoma are able to have a resection of curative nature. The survival rate for five years found to be highly variable, it may range from 8 to more than 50%.[25] The attributes which indicate a better patient outcome are negative margins detected on histopathology, no lymph nodes affected, concomitant hepatic resection, tumors which are well differentiated, papillary type of tumors and lack of any perineural invasion.[26] Generally, the best patient outcomes are in cases where R0 resection is performed and it is considered as a best predictor for five year survival.

REFERENCES

1. Jarnagin W, Winston C. Hilar cholangiocarcinoma: diagnosis and staging. HPB. 2005;7:244-51.
2. Joo I, Lee JM. Imaging bile duct tumors: pathologic concepts, classification, and early tumor detection. Abdominal Imaging. 2013;38:1334-50.
3. Hirohashi K, Uenishi T, Kubo S, Yamamoto T, Tanaka H, Shuto T, Kinoshita H. Macroscopic types of intrahepatic cholangiocarcinoma: clinicopathological features and surgical outcomes. Hepatogastroenterology. 2002;49:326-9.
4. Shaib YH, E1-Serag HB. The epidemiology of cholangiocarcinoma. Semin Liver Dis. 2004;24:115-25.
5. Taylor-Robison SD, Toledano MB, Arora S, Keegan TJ, Har- greaves S, Beck A, Khan SA, Elliott P, Thomas HC. Increase in mortality rates from intrahepatic cholangiocarcinoma in England and Wales 1968-1998. Gut. 2001;48:816-20.
6. Lazaridis KN, Gores GJ. Cholangiocarcinoma. Gastroenterology. 2005;128:1655.
7. Lipsett PA, Pitt HA, Colombani PM, Boitnott JK, Cameron JL. Choledochal cyst disease: A changing pattern of presentation. Ann Surg. 1994;220:644-52.
8. Pitt HA, Dooley WC, Yeo CJ, Cameron JL. Malignancies of the biliary tree. Curr Probl Surg. 1995;32:36-75.
9. Longmire WP, McArthur MS, Bastounis EA, et al. Carcinoma of the extrahepatic biliary tract. Ann Surg. 1973;178:333-40.
10. Liu D, Momoi H, Li L, Ishikawa Y, Fukumoto M. Microsatellite instability in thorotrast-induced human intrahepatic cholangiocarcinoma. Int J Cancer. 2002;102:366-71.

11. Hardell L, Bengtsson NO, Jonsson U, Eriksson S, Larsson LG. Aetiological aspects on primary liver cancer with special regard to alcohol, organic solvents and acute intermittent porphyria; an epidemiological investigation. Br J Cancer. 1984;50:389-97.
12. Szendroi M, Nemeth L, Vajta G. Asbestos bodies in a bile duct cancer after occupational exposure. Environ Res. 1983;30:270-7.
13. Brown DP. Mortality of workers exposed to polychlorinated biphenyls: an update. Environ Health. 1987;42:33-40.
14. Kobayashi M, Ikeda K, Saitoh S, et al. Incidence of primary cholangiocellular carcinoma of the liver in Japanese patients with hepatitis C virus-related cirrhosis. Cancer. 2000;88:2471-7.
15. Thompson JN, Cohen J, Moore RH, et al. Endotoxemia in obstructive jaundice: observations on cause and clinical significance. Am J Surg. 1988;155:314-21.
16. Giulianotti PC, Sbrana F, Fransesco BM, Addeo P. Robot-assisted laparoscopic extended right hepatectomy with biliary reconstruction. J Laparoendosc Adv Surg Tech. 2010;20(2): 159-63.
17. Ito F, Agni R, Rettammell RJ, et al. Resection of hilar cholangiocarcinoma: concomitant liver resection decreases hepatic recurrence. Ann Surg. 2008;248:273-9.
18. Simillis C, Constantinides VA, Tekkis PP, et al. Laparoscopic versus open hepatic resections for benign and malignant neoplasms—a meta analysis. Surgery. 2007;141:203-11.
19. Whang EE, Duxbury M, Rocha FG; Zinner MJ. Cancer of the gallbladder and bile ducts. In: Maingot R, Zinner M, Ashley SW (Eds). Maingot's abdominal operations. 12th edition. New York: McGraw-Hill Medical; 2013.
20. Date RS, Siriwardena AK. Current status of laparoscopic biliary bypass in the management of non-resectable periampullary cancer. Pancreatology. 2005;5:325-9.
21. Smith AC, Dowsett JF, Russell RC, et al. Randomised trial of endoscopic stenting versus surgical bypass in malignant low bile duct obstruction. Lancet. 1994;344:1655-60.
22. Lesurtel M, Dehni N, Tiret E, et al. Palliative surgery for unresectable pancreatic and periampullary cancer: a reappraisal. J Gastrointest Surg. 2006;10:286-91.
23. Buchs NC, Addeo P, Bianco FM, Elli FM, Ayloo S, Giulainotti PC. Robotic palliation for unresectable pancreatic cancer and distal cholangiocarcinoma. Int J Med Robotics Comput Assist Surg. 2011;7:60-5.
24. Giulianotti PC, Tzvetanov I, Jeon H, et al. Robot assisted right lobe donor hepatectomy. Transp Int. 2012;25(1):e5-e9.
25. Ito H, Matros E, Brooks DC, et al. Treatment outcomes associated with surgery for gallbladder cancer: a 20-year experience. J Gastrointest Surg. 2004;8:183.
26. Santibanes ED, Ardiles V. High malignant biliary tract obstruction. In: Fischer JE (Ed). Fischer's Mastery of Surgery, 6th edition. Lippincott Williams & Wilkins; 2012.

SECTION 3

Thoracic and Vascular Surgery

- **Thymus**
  Arvind Kumar, Belal Bin Asaf
- **Lung Resection**
  Belal Bin Asaf, Arvind Kumar
- **Esophagectomy**
  Arvind Kumar, Belal Bin Asaf
- **Vascular Surgery**
  Arvind Kumar, Belal Bin Asaf

CHAPTER

10

Thymus

Arvind Kumar, Belal Bin Asaf

ROBOTIC SURGERY FOR THYMUS AND ANTERIOR MEDIASTINUM

There have been many reports on the efficacy of robotic surgery for mediastinal diseases.[1-8] The robotic system appears to be ideally suited for the surgery on anterior mediastinal lesions. The robotic approach saves the patient from the morbidity of sternotomy. We will briefly discuss the use of the surgical robot in diseases of the mediastinum with emphasis on thymic disorders, which comprise the majority of the surgical indications in anterior mediastinum.

Myasthenia gravis (MG) is an autoimmune neuromuscular disease leading to fluctuating weakness and fatigue of different muscle groups. Fifteen percent of MG patients have thymoma.[9] The thymus gland is located in the anterior mediastinum between right and left phrenic nerves. Ectopic thymic tissue can be located at various locations throughout the anterior mediastinum.[10] The radical excision of thymus and pericardial fat therefore, is crucial both for tumor resection and achieving complete stable remission (CSR) of MG.[11] Robotic approach allows for a radical thymectomy, thereby improving the complete remission rate for MG when compared with the conventional thoracoscopic technique.[12] For patients with thymoma, the oncologic outcome in terms of overall survival and thymoma-related survival is promising, but a longer follow-up is needed to consider robotic thymectomy a standard approach.[13]

PREOPERATIVE PREPARATION AND PRECAUTIONS FOR PATIENTS UNDERGOING THYMECTOMY

- All patients who are to undergo a thymectomy should be evaluated thoroughly by a neurologist—ideally one with special training and interest in the diagnosis and management of MG.
- Confirmatory tests to diagnose MG and other potential diseases should be reviewed. Acetylcholinesterase receptor antibody (ACh-Ab) antibody test seems to be most specific.
- All patients should undergo a contrast-enhanced high-resolution computed tomography (CT) scan with 5–8 mm slices because thymoma or thymic carcinoma may be present.
- Pulmonary function tests, including vital capacity, forced expiratory volume, maximal expiratory force, arterial blood gas, and a flow-volume loop, should be performed.
- A thorough assessment for cardiac dysfunction, including echocardiography or a formal cardiology evaluation, may be beneficial.
- In view of the autoimmune etiology for MG, preoperative blood tests should include thyroid function testing, antinuclear antibody, and rheumatoid factor in addition to routine preoperative studies.
- Plasmapheresis or intravenous immunoglobulin should be considered for patients with advanced disease, bulbar symptoms, or poor pulmonary function.

A careful selection of candidates for surgery should optimize the long-term results for patients with MG. Special consideration should be given to patients with thymoma. About 10–15% of MG patients have thymoma and conversely 40–50% of patients with thymoma may eventually develop MG. Utmost care is therefore, required in evaluating thymoma patients preoperatively to rule out MG. Some of these patients may develop myasthenia in the post-operative period.

Patients referred for thymectomy for thymoma should have a latest imaging study with either CT scan or magnetic resonance imaging (MRI). Radiographic characteristics that must be assessed include size, heterogeneity, and presence of infiltration of adjacent structures. Though there is no size limit for performing minimally invasive thymic resection, but in our experience tumors greater than 4 cm should be approached only by experienced robotic surgeons. Moreover, while invasion of adjacent structures, such as the pericardium or lung does not preclude a robotic approach, careful selection of these cases should be done to adhere to the principles of oncological resection.

- Surgical resection of thymoma should be attempted only by trained thoracic surgeons or surgical oncologist with significant experience in treating thymic tumors.

- Surgical biopsy should be avoided if clinical and radiological features raise a strong possibility of resectable thymoma.
- Adequate neurological evaluation should be done to exclude MG and those with MG should be well controlled.
- The aim of resection is complete removal of the thymoma with intact capsule along with all thymic tissues, pericardial and anterior mediastinal fat between the two phrenic nerves and from both thyrothymic ligaments cranially to bilateral pericardiophrenic recesses caudally.
- Robotic resection of thymoma should only be attempted by surgeons with significant expertise in minimal invasive resection of thymoma.

ANESTHESIA AND POSITION

The procedure is done under general anesthesia. All patients should have invasive blood pressure monitoring using arterial line. Urinary catheterization should be considered judiciously keeping in mind the age of the patient and expected duration of procedure. All minimally invasive chest surgery including those done with robotic assistance requires lung isolation using double lumen endotracheal tube **(Fig. 10.1)**. For mediastinal robotic surgery including thymus a left sided double lumen tube is used and selective lung deflation is used depending on the side from which the thymus gland is approached.

The patient is positioned supine at the left edge of the operating table with the left chest elevated by 30°. Left upper limb is lowered below the table level with flexion at elbow (to allow unhindered access of robotic arms to left chest) being supported on a bean bag as shown in the **Figure 10.2**. For a right side approach, the position is same except that the right side is elevated and the right upper limb is positioned off the edge of the table instead of left **(Fig. 10.3)**.

Thymectomy can be done from either the right side or left side or bilaterally. The robotic system allows us to do a radical thymectomy from one side only. The choice of the side of approach is controversial topic. Proponent of left-sided approach site the following reasons for choosing the left side:

- Thymic tissue may extend lateral to or under the left phrenic nerve.[14]
- Occasionally the thymic gland descends totally or partially posterior rather than anterior to the innominate vein.
- The left thymic portion is usually larger and extends up to the cardiophrenic area thereby needing more dissection on left side.
- The aortopulmonary window is a frequent site of ectopic thymic tissue and can be accessed better or exclusively from the left side.[15]

On the other hand, points in favor of a right-sided approach include better visualization of both the brachiocephalic veins from the right side by following the superior vena cava, the visualization and dissection of the aortocaval groove is easier and better ergonomic position to accomplish dissection in caudal to cephalad direction from the right side. Cerfolio and

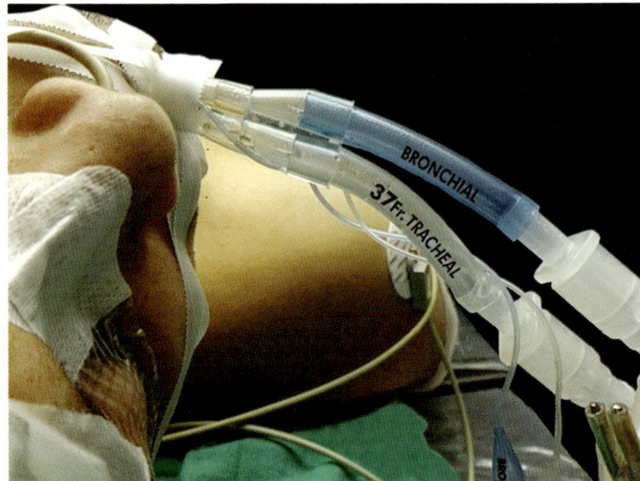

Fig. 10.1: Double-lumen endotracheal tube with bronchial lumen clamped for a left-sided robotic thymectomy

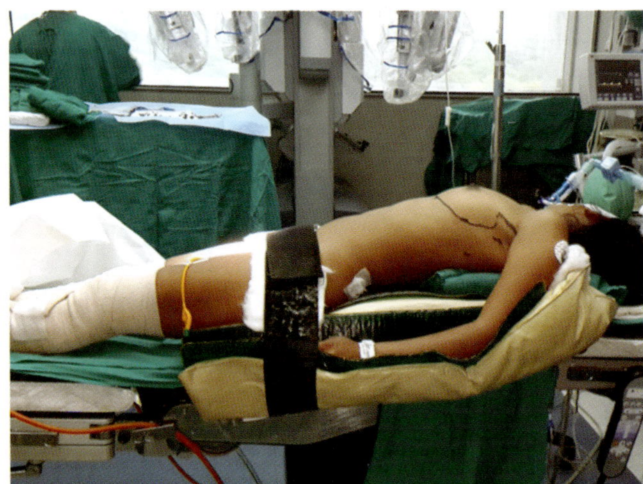
Fig. 10.2: Position for left side approach to thymectomy

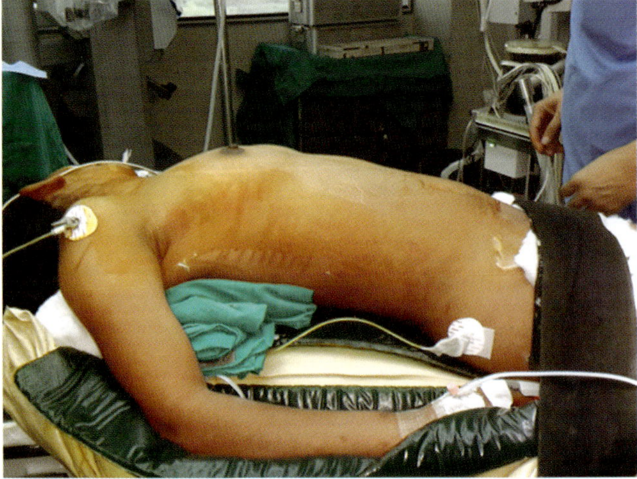
Fig. 10.3: Position for a right side approach to thymectomy

colleagues also suggested that a right-sided approach may be easier and safer during the early part of the surgeon's learning curve.[16]

Regardless of the preference, it is important to use a tailor-made approach for each patient. Our approach is from the left side for all patients undergoing thymectomy for MG without thymoma also for patients with thymoma with the tumor in the midline or towards the left side. We use the right side approach only for patients with thymoma who have the bulk of the tumor lying on the right of midline.

PORT PLACEMENT

We use a three port thoracoscopic approach for thymectomy. Occasionally a 5 or 12 mm port is placed additionally for assistance in cases of thymoma or in those patients with excessive pericardial fat **(Fig. 10.4)**. CO_2 insufflation is used at a pressure of 8 cm H_2O.

Three standard robotic ports are placed as follows:

- 5 mm port for initial thoracoscopic exploration in the 5th ICS just anterior to the midaxillary line which is later converted to 12 mm for the robotic camera. (**C**)
- 8 mm robotic port in 3rd intercostal space (ICS) anterior axillary line. (**R1**)
- 8 mm port in the 5th or 6th ICS in the midclavicular line. (**R2**)
- It is important to maintain a minimum of 8–10 cm distance between the ports to avoid external arm collisions.
- Accessory port wherever required can be a 5 or 12 mm port between camera and the caudal port at least two spaces at the apex of an imaginary triangle formed by the camera (C), the caudal port (R2) and the assistant port (A).

DOCKING

The patient cart is brought from over the right shoulder in such a way that the central column of the patient cart, the target anatomy and the camera port should be in one straight line. It is absolutely essential to arrange the robotic arms with regard to the sweet point before the docking is initiated **(Fig. 10.5)**.

Steps of Surgery

Important landmarks:

- The phrenic nerves (right and left)
- Pericardium
- Aorta
- Subclavian artery
- Superior vena cava
- Internal mammary vessels.

Steps

- The dissection is started caudally in the middle of the pericardium just adjacent and parallel to the left phrenic nerve. Mobilization of the thymus gland is then continued cranially along the left phrenic nerve.
- The dissection of the tissue in the aortopulmonary window is performed and further dissection is performed cranially along the phrenic nerve until the entrance of left brachiocephalic vein is reached at which point the cervical pleura is opened. The opening is then extended to mediastinal pleura up to to the median retrosternal line. The dissection is continued to the right side until the subxiphoid pleural fold is reached. With blunt gentle dissection, the right lung is made visible covered only by the right parietal pleura. At this stage, all attempt should

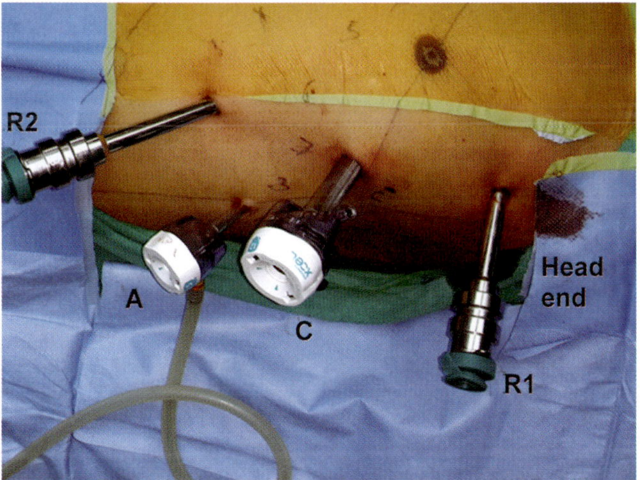

Fig. 10.4: Port placement for robotic thymectomy—Left sided 3 + 1 port approach

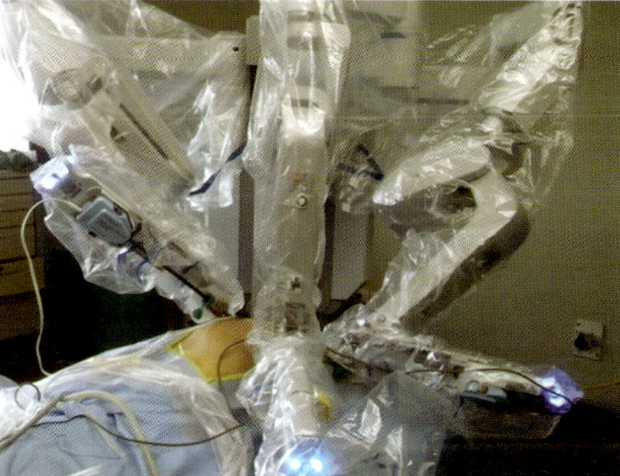

Fig. 10.5: Patient cart docked from over the opposite shoulder

be made to prevent opening the right pleura to avoid insufflation of CO_2 into the right thoracic cavity.

- Careful mobilization of the thymic tissue is then done from over the left brachiocephalic vein. Usually there are 2–4 thymic veins that drain into the brachiocephalic vein. These veins have to be very carefully dissected avoiding any undue tension keeping in view that any undue traction can lead to torrential bleed from the brachiocephalic vein due to avulsion tear of these fragile vessels. These veins are therefore, dissected with either bipolar forceps or ultrasonic scalpel. Relatively larger vessels should be divided between clips.
- Mobilization of the upper poles up to the thyrothymic ligament is the next step. The upper poles are gently pulled down after careful dissection revealing the thyrothymic ligaments. After complete exposure of the upper thymic pole, this ligament is severed.
- At this stage after the right mediastinal pleura has been swept off the right lobe of thymus gland, we open the right mediastinal pleura and all tissues medial to the right phrenic nerve are mobilized off the pericardium. We insist on visualization of the right phrenic nerve and removal of all fibrofatty tissue medial to it.
- If the visualization of the right phrenic nerve is difficult due to excessive pericardial fat, we use thoracoscopic guidance using a 5 mm 30° thoracoscope through a 5 mm port on the right side.
- In the end a complete mobilization of all thymic tissue, pericardial and mediastinal fat between the two phrenic nerves is achieved.
- The specimen is then placed in a specimen bag and retrieved through the camera port after undocking using conventional video-assisted thoracoscopic surgery (VATS) camera and instruments.
- The cavity is washed with normal saline and extrasaline is sucked out. Hemostasis is secured.
- An intercostal nerve block is performed from 3rd to 10th ICS.
- A single 28 Fr chest tube is placed on the left side and the port incisions are closed in layers using subcuticular closure for the skin.

Postoperative Care

Every attempt is made to extubate the patient immediately after the surgery in the operating room. All patients particularly with myasthenia gravis should be observed in a high dependency or intensive care unit. The chest drain is removed if a postoperative chest radiograph shows normal findings during the first 24 hours postoperatively.

Patients are usually discharged on the second and fourth postoperative day. It is mandatory to get the patient evaluated by a neurologist for the first few postoperative days.

Complications and their Management

The potential complications associated with robotic thymectomy are no different from those faced with conventional VATS. Some of the commonly reported complications include:

Phrenic Nerve Injury

Utmost care should be taken to avoid phrenic nerve injury in myasthenic patients. Apart from direct nerve injury, one should be mindful of the lateral damage caused by monopolar diathermy. Avoidance of monopolar current (use bipolar forceps instead) in close proximity to the nerve goes a long way in preventing this dangerous complication.

Excessive Bleeding due to Injury to Great Vessels

In the event of a bleed, the first response should be to apply pressure using a rolled gauze piece (already placed inside the pleural cavity). If the bleeding is a major one, immediate undocking followed by conversion to open approach and control of bleeding should be done. Minor bleeding not from major vessels usually responds to packing with gauze piece and patient waiting.

Cardiac Arrhythmias

Careful monitoring of the ECG during dissection over the pericardium is required. Minor arrhythmias are common and controlled awareness of the situation usually suffices. Sterile defibrillating pads must be available along with a defibrillator machine inside the operating room at all times, but are rarely required.

Exacerbation of Myasthenia Gravis and Myasthenic Crisis

Meticulous preoperative preparation and adequate control of MG prevent this complication which is a cause of major morbidity after thymectomy. Such patients may require prolonged ventilator support till the crisis tides over. Some patients may require intravenous immunoglobulin (IVIG) or plasmapheresis for achieving a rapid control.

REFERENCES

1. DeRose JJ, Jr, Swistel DG, Safavi A, Connery CP, Ashton RJ, Jr Mediastinal mass evaluation using advanced robotic techniques. Ann Thorac Surg. 2003;75:571-3.
2. Morgan JA, Kohmoto T, Smith CR, Oz MC, Argenziano M. Endoscopic computer-enhanced mediastinal mass resection using robotic technology. Heart Surg Forum. 2003;6:E164-6.
3. Bacchetta MD, Korst RJ, Altorki NK, Port JL, Isom OW, Mack CA. Resection of a symptomatic pericardial cyst using the computer-enhanced da Vinci Surgical System. Ann Thorac Surg. 2003;75:1953-5.
4. Bodner J, Wykypiel H, Greiner A, Kirchmayr W, Freund MC, Margreiter R, et al. Early experience with robot-assisted surgery for mediastinal masses. Ann Thorac Surg. 2004;78:259-65.
5. Savitt MA, Gao G, Furnary AP, Swanson J, Gately HL, Handy JR. Application of robotic-assisted techniques to the surgical evaluation and treatment of the anterior mediastinum. Ann Thorac Surg. 2005;79:450-5.

6. Augustin F, Schmid T, Bodner J. The robotic approach for mediastinal lesions. Int J Med Robot. 2006;2:262-70.
7. Rea F, Schiavon M, Di Chiara F, Marulli G. Single-institution experience on robot-assisted thoracoscopic operations for mediastinal diseases. Innovations Phila. 2011;6:316-22.
8. Melfi F, Fanucchi O, Davini F, Viti A, Lucchi M, Ambrogi MC, et al. Ten-year experience of mediastinal robotic surgery in a single referral centre. Eur J Cardiovasc Surg. 2012;41:847-51.
9. Papatestas AE, Genkins G, Kornfeld P, Eisenkraft JB, Fagerstrom RP, Pozner J, et al. Effects of thymectomy in myasthenia gravis. Ann Surg. 1987;206:79-88.
10. Ashour M. Prevalence of ectopic thymic tissue in myasthenia gravis and its clinical significance. J Thorac Cardiovasc Surg. 1995;109:632-5.
11. Jaretzki A. 3rd Thymectomy for myasthenia gravis. Ann Thorac Surg. 1990;49:688.
12. Ruckert JC, Swierzy M, Ismail M. Comparison of robotic and nonrobotic thoracoscopic thymectomy: A cohort study. J Thorac Cardiovasc Surg. 2011;141:673-7.
13. Marulli G, Schiavon M, Perissinotto E, Bugana A, Di Chiara F, Rebusso A, et al. Surgical and neurologic outcomes after robotic thymectomy in 100 consecutive patients with myasthenia gravis. J Thorac Cardiovasc Surg. 2013;145:730-5.
14. Ismail M, Swierzy M, Rückert RI, Rückert JC. Robotic thymectomy for myasthenia gravis. Thorac Surg Clin. 2014;24:189-95.
15. Mineo TC, Pompeo E, Ambrogi V. Video-assisted thoracoscopic thymectomy: From the right or from the left? J Thorac Cardiovasc Surg. 1997;114:516-7.
16. Augustin F, Schmid T, Sieb M, Lucciarini P, Bodner J. Video-assisted thoracoscopic surgery versus robotic-assisted thoracoscopic surgery thymectomy. Ann Thorac Surg. 2008;85:S768-71.

CHAPTER

11

Lung Resection

Belal Bin Asaf, Arvind Kumar

INTRODUCTION

The first report of the use of Robotic System for primary lung cancer came from Melfi et al.[1] in 2002. Due to safety concerns, the surgery was converted to thoracotomy in two of five patients. Nevertheless, the report demonstrated the feasibility of the procedure. Since then numerous reports have been published. Most of the authors have reported the use of three robotic arms with the four-arm technique being reported only by Veronesi et al. Cerfolio et al. and Park et al.[2-4] We believe that the completely portal four port approach (CPRL-4) is much simpler and more standardized and can be adapted for all the lobes.

It also allows for a relatively more efficient use of assistant port by the bedside surgeon. Reported complications range from 10.5 to 43.5% across various case series. The most commonly reported complications were prolonged air leak and arrhythmia. None of the reports have attributed any complication specific to the use of robotic system. The operative time shortens along the learning curve, and this shortening is evident after doing 20–30 cases in many reports.[5,6] The mortality is 0–3%, which is similar to that after conventional lung cancer surgery. Park et al.[4] recently reported a multicenter study involving 325 patients, in which the 5-year survival rate in all patients was 80% (Stage IA, 91%, Stage IB 88%, Stage II 49%), showing a favorable outcome.

INDICATIONS

- Early stage (Stage I and IIa) peripheral lung cancers
- Small peripheral aspergillomas
- Localized bronchiectasis.

PREOPERATIVE PREPARATION AND PRECAUTIONS

All patients undergoing resectional lung surgery should be thoroughly evaluated for fitness to undergo the resection. Therefore, pulmonary function evaluation by spirometry, lung volumes, diffusion capacity, arterial blood gas analysis, radionuclear lung scanning, cardiopulmonary exercise testing with forced expiratory volume 1 (FEV1) and DLCO is recommended.

All cases of lung cancers should be staged adequately by imaging (PET Scan and MRI brain wherever indicated). It is mandatory to have the histological nodal status staging using endobronchial ultrasound (EBUS) or mediastinoscopy to rule out N2 disease before surgery.

All patients should receive perioperative DVT prophylaxis to reduce the chances of pulmonary embolism.

ANESTHESIA AND POSITIONING

The patient is given general anesthesia with lung isolation achieved by appropriate double lumen endotracheal tube. We prefer invasive blood pressure monitoring through arterial line for all patients. Foley's catheterization should be used depending on the expected duration of surgery. Deep venous thrombosis (DVT) prophylaxis using compression devices are used routinely before induction. The position of the double lumen endotracheal tube is confirmed by bronchoscopy and patient is positioned for surgery.

The patient is placed in a typical lateral position with table breaks as shown in the **Figure 11.1** to achieve maximum opening of the intercostal spaces and moving the hip away to prevent interaction with the robotic camera and telescope. The position of the double lumen endotracheal tube is rechecked after final position.

PORT PLACEMENT

We prefer the CPRL-4 method as popularized by Cerfolio et al.[7] A total of five ports are used without any utility incision as described ahead **(Fig. 11.2)**. The pleural cavity is first explored via a 5 mm port placed over the seventh rib in the mid-axillary line or as anteriorly as possible. A 5-mm VATS camera is used to ensure entry into the pleural space and an initial exploration is done to assess the feasibility of resection and to detect any evidence of metastatic disease. Warm CO_2 insufflation is used to push the diaphragm inferiorly and aid in lung collapse. The port is eventually enlarged to allow 8–12 mm port for robotic arm 1 (for right-sided operations)

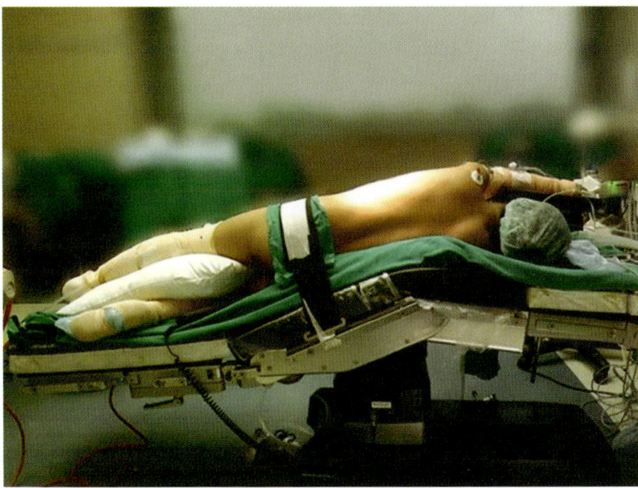

Fig. 11.1: Position for lobectomy

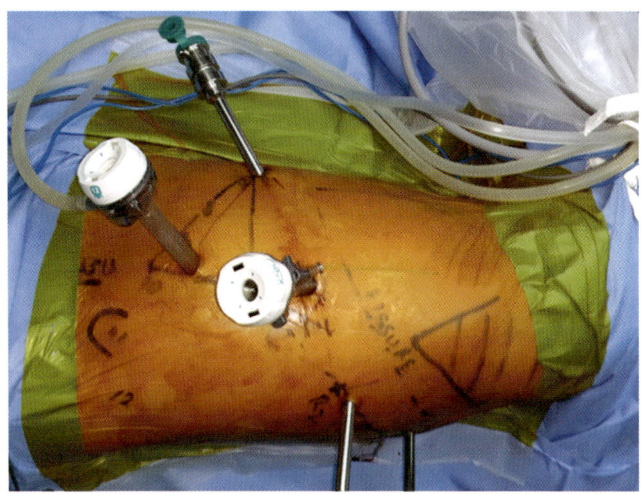

Fig. 11.2: Ports for completely portal robotic lobectomy

and also allow the passage of staplers when required. A paravertebral block is performed posteriorly using a local anesthetic and a 21-gauge needle from ribs 3 to 11. The needle is used to seek the ideal position for the second incision, which is 2 ribs below the major fissure and as far posterior in the chest as possible about 2–3 cm away from the lateral edge of vertebral column. A 5-mm incision is made and a 5-mm reusable metal da Vinci trocar is placed. This serves as the port for robotic arm 3 (R3). The remaining incisions are carefully planned and marked on the skin before actual incision. Ten centimeters anterior to R3 and along the same intercostal space mostly 8th ICS third incision is planned for an 8-mm port through which 8-mm metal reusable da Vinci trocar will be introduced. This serves as the port for robotic arm 2 (R2). The camera port (C) is then marked 9 cm anterior to this R2 in the same ICS **(Fig. 11.3)**. A 12-mm plastic disposable port will be used for the 12-mm robotic camera. Before making these 2 incisions a 21-gauge needle is used to identify the most anterior and inferior aspect of the chest that is just above the diaphragm. This will be the site for a 15-mm port which serves as the access port (A). This incision is carefully planned. It is made just above the diaphragm as anterior and inferior as possible in order to be between the ports used for robotic arm 1 and the camera. The access port can alternatively be placed more posteriorly if anatomy dictates; between the camera and robotic arm 2. It should be at least 2 or 3 ribs lower than these two ports. This position affords room for the bedside assistant to work. Once these incisions are carefully planned and their location is confirmed, they are made and the appropriate trocars are placed. In addition, the initial 5-mm anterior port that was made first is converted to a 8 or 12-mm double cannulated port for robotic arm 1.

DOCKING

The robot is driven over the patient's shoulder on a 15° angle and attached to the 4 ports. We use only 4 robotic instruments for all of these operations. These include the Cadiere grasper,

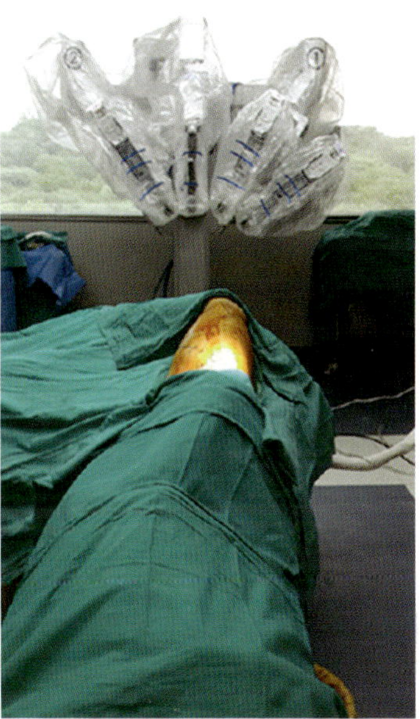

Fig. 11.3: The robot is brought from the head end at an angle of 15° anteriorly

a 5-mm bowel grasper (used exclusively through R3 and serves as a lung retractor), the Maryland forceps or the Curved bipolar forceps, and a monopolar cautery hook or spatula.

STEPS OF SURGERY

The standard anatomical lobectomy is then performed with individual division of the lobar vein, artery and bronchus. In cases with very well defined fissures we go through the fissure to identify the lobar branches of pulmonary artery which are dissected, looped and divided using staplers with vascular cartridge. The vein is similarly divided next followed by the bronchus. This sequence of division is not fixed and is changed as per the need of the individual case. A thorough three-dimensional orientation of the vascular and bronchial anatomy is mandatory for performing a safe lobectomy. For patients with thick fissures we use the fissure-less technique wherever possible to avoid prolonged postoperative air leaks. The steps for lobectomy can be summarized as follows:

- *Routine thoracoscopic exploration* using a 30° videoscope to evaluate the feasibility of a minimally invasive procedure and look for unsuspected findings.
- *Port placement and docking.*
- *Robotic pulmonary vein preparation:* The main superior or inferior pulmonary vein depending upon the lobe to be resected is isolated, encircled with a vascular loop and divided.
- *Dissection of the fissures.*
- *Hilum dissection:* The main trunk of the pulmonary artery is isolated and the interlobar nodes are removed. Transection of the arterial branches to the lobe is then completed using vascular staplers or division between Hem-o-lok clips.
- *Division of the bronchus:* Once the division of arterial branches and lobar vein have been completed, the lobar bronchus is isolated and all peribronchial nodes are removed. The lobar bronchus is then divided with a green load endostapler.
- *Completion of lymphadenectomy:* For cases with lung cancer, a systematic mediastinal lymph node dissection is then performed.
- *Specimen retrieval* specimen is retrieved in an endobag through the assistant port by increasing it to 4 cm in length. A 28 F chest tube the camera port.

POSTOPERATIVE CARE

The postoperative care is no different from the care of regular lobectomy patients. The chest tube is removed after cessation of air leak and when drainage is less than 3 mL/kg. Adequate analgesia is given, though in our experience we have found the requirement to be lower than after an open procedure. An aggressive postoperative respiratory physiotherapy is required to ensure rapid lung expansion and prevention of pulmonary complications.

COMPLICATIONS AND THEIR MANAGEMENT

The complications encountered after or during a robotic lobectomy do not differ much from those after VATS lobectomy. One of the most dreaded complications of lobectomy is pulmonary artery injury and torrential bleeding which can be potentially fatal. Lack of tactile feedback makes dissection of these fragile vessels tricky. The lack of tactile feedback is compensated by the magnified 3D vision. But it requires significant experience with robotic procedures to be able to do lobectomy safely. *We do not recommend starting the robotic thoracic program with lobectomy. Lung resection should be last procedure during the learning curve of robotic thoracic surgery.*

Two rolled gauze pieces should be inside the cavity before attempting to dissect the pulmonary artery. Special care is required while engaging staplers for division of the vessels. In the event of any injury the first response should be to apply pressure with a gauze piece to stop the bleeding and immediate undocking followed by conversion to open surgery and control of the bleed. *The emergency protocol of undocking and conversion should have been simulated and discussed with the team before initiation of surgery.*

Robotic lobectomy is an extension of the minimally invasive lobectomy spectrum and is therefore, naturally expected to have all the advantages of VATS lobectomy when compared with conventional open technique. But whether it is better than VATS lobectomy remains to be seen. There are very few reports comparing robotic lobectomy with conventional VATS lobectomy.[8-11] At present, only data on short-term results can be compared. Paul et al.[12] compared in-hospital mortality, complications, length of stay, and cost for patients undergoing robotic-assisted lobectomy and those undergoing thoracoscopic lobectomy. 2498 robotic-assisted and 37,595 thoracoscopic lobectomies performed from 2008 to 2011 were analyzed. In this early experience with robotic surgery, robotic-assisted lobectomy was found to be associated with a higher rate of intraoperative injury and bleeding than thoracoscopic lobectomy at a significantly higher cost. Swanson et al.[13] compared hospital costs and clinical outcomes for VATS lobectomies and wedge resections versus robotic-assisted thoracoscopic surgery using the Premier hospital database. The association between VATS or robotic approach and adverse events, hospital costs, surgery time, and length of stay was examined. Robotic lobectomy and wedge resection were found to have higher hospital costs and longer operating times, without any differences in adverse events. Jang et al.[8] compared 40 patients treated with robot-assisted lobectomy for lung cancer and 40 treated with thoracoscopic surgery. Postoperative complications occurred in 4 (10%) and 13 (32.5%) patients, respectively, the intraoperative blood losses were 219 and 374 mL, respectively, and the postoperative length of hospital stay were 6 and 9 days, respectively. They showed that the outcome of robot-assisted surgery was significantly more favorable than that of thoracoscopic surgery. In a case-controlled analysis by Louie et al.[9] patients treated with robot-assisted surgery used fewer analgesics and returned to daily activities earlier when compared with VATS, although there was no marked difference in the perioperative results between the surgical procedures. On the other hand, Augustin et al.[10] reported that the operative time, postoperative hemoglobin level, and cost of surgery were superior in thoracoscopic surgery. Veronesi et al.[14] summarized that the curability and safety of robot-assisted surgery for lung cancer are equivalent and the operability and length of the learning curve are superior to thoracoscopic surgery, but a high cost, limited devices, and a long operative time are disadvantageous. Therefore, at present, the merits of robot-assisted surgery have not been verified.

In conclusion, robotic surgery for pulmonary resections is safe and efficient and has similar survival rates compared with the open and VATS approaches. Based on our experience, we believe that the robotic platform helps in achieving, with far more finesse, an outstanding lymph node dissection. The other advantages offered by robotics in lung resectional surgery is debatable, but there is more or less a consensus on some of its obvious disadvantages so very rightly pointed out by Cerfolio, namely, the cost, lack of consistent platform availability, and lack of tactile feedback.[7,15]

REFERENCES

1. Melfi FM, Menconi GF, Mariani AM, Angeletti CA. Early experience with robotic technology for thoracoscopic surgery. Eur J Cardiothorac Surg. 2002;21:864-8.
2. Veronesi G, Galetta D, Maisonneuve P, Melfi F, Schmid RA, Borri A, et al. Four-arm robotic lobectomy for the treatment of early stage lung cancer. J Thorac Cardiovasc Surg. 2010;140:19-25.
3. Cerfolio RJ, Bryant AS, Skylizard L, Minnich DJ. Initial consecutive experience of completely portal robotic pulmonary resection with 4 arms. J Thorac Cardiovasc Surg. 2011;142:740-6. [PubMed]
4. Park BJ, Melfi F, Mussi A, Maisonneuve P, Spaggiari L, Da Silva RK, et al. Robotic lobectomy for non-small cell lung cancer (NSCLC): Long-term oncologic results. J Thorac Cardiovasc Surg. 2012;143:383-9.
5. Cerfolio RJ, Bryant AS, Minnich DJ. Starting a robotic program in general thoracic surgery: Why, how, and lessons learned. Ann Thorac Surg. 2011;91:1729-37.
6. Melfi FM, Mussi A. Robotically assisted lobectomy: Learning curve and complications. Thorac Surg Clin. 2008;18:289-95.
7. Cerfolio RJ. Total port approach for robotic lobectomy. Thorac Surg Clin. 2014;24(2):151-6.
8. Jang HJ, Lee HS, Park SY, Zo JI. Comparison of the early robot-assisted lobectomy experience to video assisted thoracic surgery lobectomy for lung cancer: A single-institution case series matching study. Innovations (Phila) 2011;6:305-10.
9. Louie BE, Farivar AS, Aye RW, Vallières E. Early experience with robotic lung resection results in similar operative outcomes and morbidity when compared with matched video-assisted thoracoscopic surgery cases. Ann Thorac Surg. 2012;93: 1598-604.
10. Augustin F, Bodner J, Maier H, Schwinghammer C, Pichler B, Lucciarini P, et al. Robotic-assisted minimally invasive vs. thoracoscopic lung lobectomy: Comparison of perioperative results in a learning curve setting. Langenbecks Arch Surg. 2013; 398:895-901.
11. Kent M, Wang T, Whyte R, Curran T, Flores R, Gangadharan S. Open, video-assisted thoracic surgery, and robotic lobectomy: Review of a national database. Ann Thorac Surg. 2014;97:236-44.
12. Paul S, Jalbert J, Isaacs AJ, Altorki NK, Isom OW, Sedrakyan A. Comparative effectiveness of robotic-assisted vs thoracoscopic lobectomy. Chest. 2014;146(6):1505-12. doi: 10.1378/chest. 13-3032.
13. Swanson SJ, Miller DL, McKenna RJ, Jr, Howington J, Marshall MB, Yoo AC, et al. Comparing robot-assisted thoracic surgical lobectomy with conventional video-assisted thoracic surgical lobectomy and wedge resection: Results from a multihospital database (Premier). J Thorac Cardiovasc Surg. 2014;147:929-37.
14. Veronesi G. Robotic surgery for the treatment of early-stage lung cancer. Curr Opin Oncol. 2013;25:107-14.
15. Cerfolio RJ. Pulmonary resection in the 21st century: The role of robotics. Tex Heart Inst J. 2012;39:848-9.

CHAPTER

12

Esophagectomy

Arvind Kumar, Belal Bin Asaf

INTRODUCTION

The first robotic-assisted esophagectomy was reported in 2003. The esophagus was resected using the transhiatal route with the da Vinci robot. Foregut continuity was re-established by a gastric pull-up with cervical anastomosis. Most reports have described transthoracic esophagectomy and have demonstrated the feasibility and safety of esophagectomy using the surgical robot.

PREOPERATIVE PREPARATION AND PRECAUTIONS

A detailed preoperative work up aimed at assessment of the stage of esophageal cancer, its resectability and patient's fitness for surgery, should be undertaken. The ability to tolerate single lung ventilation is mandatory. Although robotic surgery can be performed in patients with history of prior thoracic surgery, extensive pleural adhesions may preclude a safe dissection. Pulmonary function testing and preoperative cardiac testing will determine if the patient is physiologically fit to undergo esophagectomy. Due consideration should be given to perioperative DVT prophylaxis.

Indications and Prerequisites for Surgery

- Performance status ECOG 0, 1
- Adequate cardiopulmonary reserve assessed by PFT + DLCO, echocardiography
- Potentially resectable lesion on available investigations like CT chest
- Localized disease as evidenced by PET scan (Early stage disease T1/T2, N0)
- Locally advanced disease T3/T4a, N+ following neo-adjuvant treatment.

ANESTHESIA AND POSITIONING

The patient is induced with general anesthesia. We prefer to use lung isolation for esophagectomy cases and therefore use a double lumen endotracheal tube. A central venous access along with invasive blood pressure monitoring is routinely used. All patients are catheterized for monitoring the urine output.

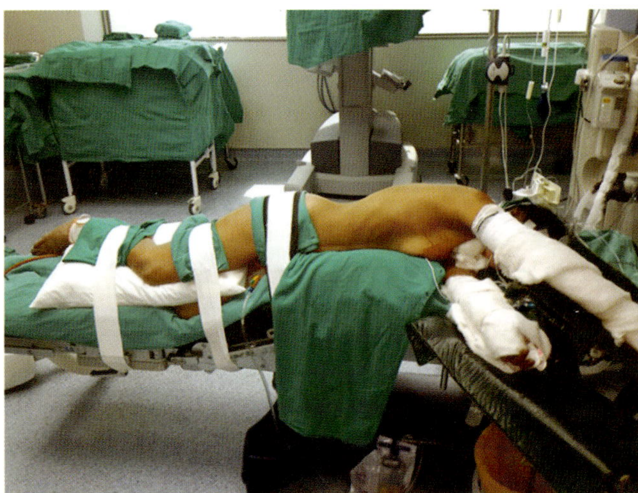

Fig. 12.1: Positioning for robotic esophagectomy

The patient is placed in a left lateral position and allowed to tilt anteriorly by 30° to achieve a somewhat semi prone position **(Fig. 12.1)**. All pressure points are adequately padded, and the patient must have sequential compression anti-DVT device applied to the lower extremities. The shoulder of the right arm is externally rotated, and the arm is put at near full extension (near 160°). The table is tilted as far anteriorly as required to achieve a semi-prone position. The robot is positioned to the right of the patient.

We have found this position to be more convenient and less time consuming with advantages similar to full prone position including:

- Lungs fall anteriorly away from area of dissection
- Ports are placed anteriorly where the intercostal spaces are wider
- Docking is also similar to that in prone position
- In the event a conversion is required, it can be done without any problem.

PORT PLACEMENT

We use a 4 port technique with 3 ports for the robotic system (1 camera and 2 working ports) and 1 assistant port. They are placed anterior to the lateral edge of scapula just anterior to posterior axillary line as shown in the figure. An assistant port is placed in between the camera port and R2 **(Fig. 12.2)**.

- 5 mm port—in 8th ICS just anterior to the postaxillary line. This is later converted to 12 mm port for robotic camera after initial exploration (C)
- 8 mm metallic daVinci canula for robotic arm 1 (R1) 8–10 cm cranial to the camera port.
- 8 mm metallic daVinci canula for robotic arm 2 (R2) 8–10 cm caudal to the camera port
- 12 mm disposable plastic port in between C and R2 about 2 rib spaces away. This will be the assistant port (A).

Carbon dioxide at a pressure of 8–10 mm Hg is used to insufflate the thoracic cavity; this improves visibility, pushes the lung and diaphragm away from the operative field. After the placement of 5 mm port for initial thoracoscopic exploration a posterior intercostal block is performed with a local anesthetic on the 3rd to 11th intercostal nerve. A 30° telescope in down orientation is used. The 12 mm assistant port is used for suctioning and assistance.

Important Landmarks

- Esophagus
- Azygous vein
- Intercostal neurovascular bundle
- Trachea, carina and right main bronchus
- Subclavian artery
- Recurrent nerves.

STEPS OF SURGERY

Intrathoracic Esophageal Mobilization

The mediastinal pleura is opened and esophageal mobilization is started from the mid part in the region of azygous vein and continued downward to the hiatus till the crural fibers are visualized. The azygous vein is then divided and further mobilization of the esophagus is continued upwards with enbloc removal of all subcarinal and periesophageal lymph nodes which often requires mobilization of the inferior pulmonary ligament and adherent lung. A combination of hook cautery, bipolar forceps and cadiere forceps is what we use for the entire procedure. The left pleura, hiatus, and pericardium are completely cleaned. The dissection continues into the neck by resecting the supra-azygos esophagus and periesophageal tissue. We routinely doubly clip the thoracic duct near the hiatus in all our patients. A single 28 F drain is inserted in a posteroapical position with extra holes in it. The drain is inserted through the assistant port. The robot is undocked and after ensuring hemostasis the port incisions are closed and dressed with sterile dressings.

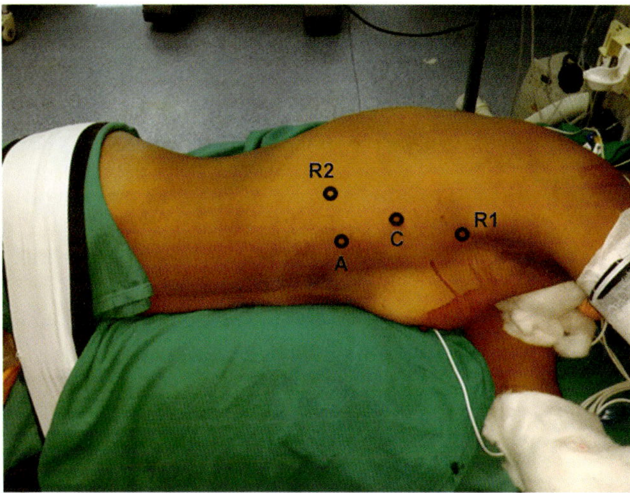

Fig. 12.2: Ports for robotic esophagectomy

The abdominal phase of the operation is then carried out by placing the patient in supine position with neck extended and turned towards right. The gastric mobilization and conduit creation is carried out laparoscopically. The neck exploration is started simultaneously and esophagus is divided in the neck. The specimen is delivered through the abdomen. An esophagogastric conduit anastomosis is then carried out by conventional hand sewn technique.

POSTOPERATIVE CARE

We keep all our patients in a high dependency unit after the surgery. They usually do not require ICU stay. The nasogastric tube is left in place for 3–4 days. We start the enteral feeding through feeding jejunostomy (FJ) on the second postoperative day. On postoperative day 7, a gastrografin swallow is performed. Patients with a normal study are allowed small frequent soft and liquid meal while they are continued on FJ. Patients with evidence of leak are kept on nil by mouth, and an esophagram is repeated after 10 days. The chest tubes and the neck drain are removed after there is no longer a concern for a leak.

Current Status

The first robotic-assisted esophagectomy was reported in 2003.[1] The distal esophagus was resected using the transhiatal route with the da Vinci robot. Foregut continuity was re-established by a gastric pull-up with cervical esophagogastrostomy. Till date there are 26 articles in the literature on this topic reporting experience with approximately 295 robotic esophagectomies in the management of malignant and benign esophageal diseases including transthoracic esophagectomy with lymphadenectomy and transhiatal esophagectomy. Most reports have described transthoracic esophagectomy and have demonstrated the feasibility and safety of esophagectomy using the surgical robot. Few of the largest reported series are described below.

The first report of completely robotic esophagectomy was by Kirnstine KH et al.[2] in 2007 who reported the use of surgical robot in 14 patients undergoing esophagectomy. Eight of the 14 patients underwent completely robotic esophagectomy with operating room time of 11.1 +/- 0.8 hours and estimated blood loss was 400 +/- 300 mL.

Boon J et al.[3] reported their experience of 47 transthoracic robotic esophagectomy (TRE). They reported a 14.9% conversion rate. The median operating time was 450 minutes and median blood loss of 625 mL with a mean hospital stay of 18 days. Twenty-one of 47 patients had pulmonary complications with three in-patient mortalities. A median of 29 (range 8–68) lymph nodes were dissected and R0 resection was achieved in 76.6 % patients.

From India, Puntambekar SP et al.[4] have reported a series of 32 cases. The mean total operative time was 210 minutes with average blood loss of 80 mL. They reported no conversions and conclude that TRE is a better alternative than thoracoscopic esophagectomy in view of the reduced stress to surgeon. Certfolio RJ et al.[5] reported successful robotic ivor lewis with chest anastomosis in 22 patients. Dunn DH et al.[6] presented their 3 year single center experience with transhiatal robotic esophagectomy (THRE) for dissection of thoracic esophagus and its associated morbidity. 40 patients with resectable esophageal carcinoma underwent THRE at their institute. Five patients were converted from robotic to open. Median operative time and estimated blood loss were 311 minutes and 97.2 mL, respectively. Postoperative complications frequently observed were anastomotic stricture, recurrent laryngeal nerve paresis, anastomotic leak, pneumonia and pleural effusion. Incidence of laryngeal nerve paresis (35%) and leak rate (25%) were somewhat higher in comparison with that reported in literature. They reported no in-hospital mortality with a 30-day mortality of 2.5% (1/40). R0 resection was achieved in 94.7% of patients.

Sarkaria IS[7] reported an early, single-institution experience of combined thoracoscopic and laparoscopic robotic-assisted minimally invasive esophagectomy using a four-arm robotic platform, with special attention given to the pitfalls and complications during procedure development. A total of 21 patients underwent the procedure with a four-arm robotic platform (17 by Ivor Lewis and 4 by McKeown). Of the patients, 17 (81%) had a complete (R0) resection, and 16 (76%) received induction treatment, the majority (14/21 [67%]) with combined chemoradiation. The median operative time was 556 minutes, which decreased to 414 minutes for the last 5 cases in the series. The median estimated blood loss was 307 mL and the median length of hospital stay was 10 days. The median number of lymph nodes resected was 20. Five patients (24%) were converted to open procedure. Five patients (24%) had major complications. One (5%) died of complications on postoperative day 70, and 3 (14%) had clinically significant anastomotic leaks. Three patients (14%) in this early experience developed airway fistulas. The authors concluded that four-arm robotic esophagectomy may offer advantages over standard minimally invasive esophagectomy approaches, its adoption in a structured program, with critical evaluation of adverse events and subsequent adjustment of technique, is paramount to maximize patient safety, minimize complications and improve the conduct of operation early in the learning curve.

The feasibility and safety of robot-assisted thoracoscopic esophagectomy for esophageal cancer in the prone position was assessed by Kim DJ et al.[8] Twenty-one patients underwent robot-assisted thoracoscopic esophagectomy in the prone position by a surgical oncologist who had no prior experience with thoracoscopic esophagectomy. The principal finding of this study was the potential role of a robotic system to achieve an adequate learning curve by a low-volume surgeon who had no prior experience with thoracoscopic esophagectomy.

Most of these studies have demonstrated the safety and feasibility of robotic assisted esophagectomy. However, further trials are required to establish its superiority as compared to open and thoracoscopic procedures.

At present, no prospective data comparing robotic esophagectomy with standard laparoscopic or open procedures exists. Most reports have described transthoracic esophagectomy and have demonstrated the feasibility and safety of esophagectomy using the surgical robot.

At the Memorial Sloan-Kettering Cancer Center, Sarkaria and Rizk[9] are actively accruing a prospective quality-of-life and outcomes trial comparing robotic assisted minimal invasive esophagectomy (RAMIE) with open esophagectomy (ClinicalTrials.gov: NCT01558648). In addition, a prospective, randomized controlled trial comparing complications and outcomes in robotic esophagectomy versus open transthoracic esophagectomy (also known as the ROBOT trial) is under way in the Netherlands, with an expected completion in 2015.

Robotic-assisted esophageal surgery is an evolving field. However, Level 1 evidence supporting a robotic approach when compared with other approaches is lacking. The benefits are not very clear when compared with a conventional laparoscopic or thoracoscopic approach. Prolonged operative times together with high costs are obstacles to wide acceptance of these techniques. Further research in the field of robotic surgery leading to better technology and reduced costs will likely generate more interest and acceptance increasing its role in esophageal surgery in the near future.

REFERENCES

1. Horgan S, Berger RA, Elli EF, Espat NJ. Robotic-assisted minimally invasive transhiatal esophagectomy. Am Surg. 2003;69(7):624-6.
2. Kernstine KH, DeArmond DT, Shamoun DM, Campos JH. The first series of completely robotic esophagectomies with three-field lymphadenectomy: initial experience. Surg Endosc. 2007; 21(12):2285-92.

3. Boone J, Schipper ME, Moojen WA, Borel Rinkes IH, Cromheecke GJ, van Hillegersberg R. Robot-assisted thoracoscopic oesophagectomy for cancer. Br J Surg. 2009;96(8):878-86.
4. Puntambekar SP, Rayate N, Joshi S, Agarwal G. Robotic transthoracic esophagectomy in the prone position: experience with 32 patients with esophageal cancer. J Thorac Cardiovasc Surg. 2011;142(5):1283-4.
5. Cerfolio RJ, Bryant AS, Hawn MT. Technical aspects and early results of robotic esophagectomy with chest anastomosis. J Thorac Cardiovasc Surg. 2012 Aug 18. [Epub ahead of print]
6. Dunn DH, Johnson EM, Morphew JA, Dilworth HP, Krueger JL, Banerji N. Robot-assisted transhiatal esophagectomy: a 3-year single-center experience. Dis Esophagus. 2012 Mar 6. doi: 10.1111/j.1442-2050.2012.01325.x. [Epub ahead of print]
7. Sarkaria IS, Rizk NP, Finley DJ, Bains MS, Adusumilli PS, Huang J, Rusch VW. Combined thoracoscopic and laparoscopic robotic-assisted minimally invasive esophagectomy using a four-arm platform: experience, technique and cautions during early procedure development. Eur J Cardiothorac Surg. 2013 May;43(5):e107-15. doi: 10.1093/ejcts/ezt013. Epub 2013 Jan 30.
8. Kim DJ, Hyung WJ, Lee CY, Lee JG, Haam SJ, Park IK, Chung KY. Thoracoscopic esophagectomy for esophageal cancer: feasibility and safety of robotic assistance in the prone position. J Thorac Cardiovasc Surg. 2010;139(1):53-59.e1.
9. Sarkaria IS, Rizk NP. Robotic-assisted minimally invasive esophagectomy: The Ivor Lewis approach. Thorac Surg Clin. 2014;24:211–22.

CHAPTER

13

Vascular Surgery

Arvind Kumar, Belal Bin Asaf

INTRODUCTION

Vascular surgery of the aorta has evolved progressively, and several report of minimally invasive aortic surgery for aneurysm and atherosclerotic occlusive disease have been reported from centers around the world.[1,2] One of the largest reported series comes from Czechoslovakia by Peter Stadler et al.[3] who have reported a series of 150 cases including aortofemoral reconstructions and surgery on aneurysms of the abdominal aorta, the pelvic arteries and the splenic artery. The technical difficulties faced in performing a vascular anastomosis using laparoscopic instruments are the major roadblock preventing widespread use of laparoscopic techniques for such surgeries. The daVinci surgical system may offer a solution to this problem by making the intra-corporeal suturing relatively easier.

We started our robotic vascular program with Dr Peter Stadler and are now routinely performing aortobifemoral bypass using the da Vinci surgical system. Till date we have done 18 cases of aortobifemoral bypass.

ANESTHESIA AND POSITIONING

The procedure is carried out in general anesthesia. The patient is placed in semi right lateral decubitus with a 45° angle. The left upper limb is placed along the patient's side and the right arm is kept outstretched. A Trendelenburg position is used.

From this point on the procedure can be divided into three distinct stages.

Stage 1: Exposure of femoral arteries in both groins

5–6 cm incisions are given in bilateral groin to expose the femoral artery which is dissected and looped in preparation of the graft-femoral artery anastomosis later in the operation.

Stage 2: Robotic assisted laparoscopic aortograft anastomosis.

Stage 3: Graft femoral artery anastomosis in both groins.

After the patient is positioned and secured with straps. The operating table is tilted towards left and to achieve a near supine position required for groin exploration. Once the femoral arteries on both sides have been explored both the groins are covered with sterile drapes and the patient is brought back to right semilateral decubitus by tilting the table to it neutral lie.

Pneumoperitoneum was created through the subcostal incision in the anterior axillary line. We use six ports for the procedure. Three ports of 12 mm in the anterior axillary line. The cranial port for robotic instrument arm 1, middle for the robotic camera arm and the caudal for robotic instrument arm 2. Three additional ports are placed to the left of the previously described ports for the proximal and distal aortic clamps with the middle port being the assistant port. The small bowel and omentum is moved to the right upper quadrant. The robot is now docked from the right side for robot assisted dissection of the aorta and iliacs. We use the 12 mm 30° down telescope. The exposure of aorta is begun by incising the retroperitoneum to the left of aorta and exposing the aorta from the left renal vein alongside the left gonadal vein. The posterior peritoneum along with pre-aortic fat is lifted off the aorta up to its right side and is sutured to the parietal peritoneum. The lumbar arteries in the region of proposed aortotomy are dissected and clipped. Tunneling is performed from both the groins under direct laparoscopic view using a long curved vascular clamp. A knitted Dacron vascular prostheses graft with attached shortened CV-3 Gore-Tex Suture is inserted into the abdomen through the assistant port. The right and left limbs of the y-graft are pulled out into the groin. The distal and proximal aortic clamps are applied. An aortotomy is made using the robotic scissors. Thromboendartrectomy is done where required followed by the aorto-graft anastomosis. The endowristed robotic instruments provide unparalleled freedom of movement which makes the creation of anastomosis; essentially the most difficult part of laparoscopic aortobifemoral surgery; relatively easier. After the completion of anastomosis, the clamps are released and any leak from the anastomotic site controlled. The posterior peritoneum is sutured back completely covering the anastomosis. The y-limbs of the prostheses are subsequently anastomosed to respective femoral arteries and the operation is completed.

STATUS OF ROBOTIC AORTIC SURGERY

Laparoscopy has substantially improved the postoperative course of patients suffering from a variety of gastrointestinal disorders like hepatobiliary, gastric, or colonic diseases. An important advantage of minimal invasive approach instead of a laparotomy is the decrease in postoperative pain, which diminishes cardiopulmonary complications. Patients with aortoiliac atherosclerotic disease are at high risk for postoperative complications, and a minimally invasive procedure may favorably affect their postoperative recovery.

In a comparison of laparoscopic and open aortobifemoral bypass in the treatment of aortoiliac disease, analysis of results revealed statistically significant advantages in the majority of patients in terms of decreased blood loss, faster post-operative recovery and shorter hospital stay.[4,5] Despite the presence of numerous series on laparoscopic aortic surgery demonstrating its advantages over open surgery, it is yet not widely accepted. Laparoscopic dissection and exposure of the aorto-iliac region was found to be extremely difficult an the aorto-graft anastomosis required advanced laparoscopic skills which inherently come with a prolonged learning curve.[6] The fact that laparoscopic surgery involves use of long instruments with the surgeons working off their central line in a counter-intuitive fashion, makes the surgery ergonomically difficult. At the same time majority of the vascular surgeons have either no or very limited laparoscopic skills. This leads to a much longer learning curve and more so for the vascular surgeons. The robotic system, with its state of the art high definition 3D vision combined with unparalleled freedom of movements provided by the endowrist technology, has removed the basic limitations of conventional laparoscopic surgery namely 2D vision with its attendant lack of depth perception, counterintuitive movements and surgeon ergonomics. With these improvements surgeons can perform complex surgeries in a manner very close to conventional open surgery, albeit without the large laparotomy incision and its attendant morbidities.

The first report of the use of robotic surgical system for the aortobifemoral bypass came from Wisselink W et al.[7] Robot-assisted vascular surgery can be of value in overcoming the long learning curve required for laparoscopic suturing of vascular anastomoses.[8] In their reported total laparoscopic procedures by Stadler et al. the mean operating time was 259 minutes (150–420 minutes), and the aortic cross-clamping time was 69 minutes (35–150 minutes).[9] When compared with Robot-assisted vascular surgery, the times taken for the procedures were much longer in case of laparoscopic cases.[10]

In the largest series of robotic aortoiliac surgery by Stadler P et al.[11] Ninety-seven of 100 procedures (97%) were successfully completed robotically, while conversions were necessary in three patients (3%). The median operating time was 235 minutes (150–360 minutes), with a median clamp-time of 42 minutes (25–120 minutes). The median anastomosis time was 29 minutes (12–60 minutes) and median blood loss was 430 mL (50–1500 mL). The median intensive care unit stay was 1.7 days and the median hospital stay was 5.1 days. A regular oral diet was resumed after a mean of 2.4 days. Thirty-day survival was 100% and non-lethal postoperative complications were observed in three patients (3%).

There have been no randomized controlled trials comparing the long-term outcomes of these procedures. But initial experience with robotic assisted aorto-bifemoral bypass has been encouraging in terms of better technical accuracy, improved surgeon ergonomics and lesser patient morbidity. It results in surgical outcomes equivalent to that of open surgery with less morbidity. The robotic surgical system will encourage more vascular surgeons to consider it in their armamentarium for patients not fit for endovascular approach. However, further studies are required to prove its long-term outcomes and benefits.

REFERENCES

1. Dion YM, Griselli F, Douville Y, Langis P. Early and mid-term results of totally laparoscopic surgery for aortoiliac disease: lessons learned. Surg Laparosc Endosc Percutan Tech. 2004;14:328-34.
2. Olinde AJ, McNeil JW, Sam A, Hebert SA, Frusha JD. Totally laparoscopic aortobifemoral bypass: a review of 22 cases. J Vasc Surg. 2005;42:27-34.
3. Stádler P, Dvoracek L, Vitasek P, Matous P. Robotic vascular surgery, 150 cases. Int J Med Robot. 2010;6(4):394-8.
4. Bruls S, Quaniers J, Tromme P, Lavigne JP, Van Damme H, Defraigne JO. Comparison of laparoscopic and open aortobifemoral bypass in the treatment of aortoiliac disease. Results of a contemporary series (2003-2009). Acta Chir Belg. 2012;112(1):51-8.
5. Tiek J, Remy P, Sabbe T, D'hont C, Houthoofd S, Daenens K, Fourneau I. Laparoscopic versus open approach for aortobifemoral bypass for severe aorto-iliac occlusive disease—a multicentre randomised controlled trial. Eur J Vasc Endovasc Surg. 2012;43(6):711-5.
6. Dion YM, Garcia CR. A new technique for laparoscopic aortobifemoral grafting in occlusive aortoiliac disease. J Vasc Surg. 1997;26:685-92.
7. Wisselink W1, Cuesta MA, Gracia C, Rauwerda JA. Robot-assisted laparoscopic aortobifemoral bypass for aortoiliac occlusive disease: a report of two cases. J Vasc Surg. 2002;36(5):1079-82.
8. Novotný T, Dvorák M, Staffa R. The learning curve of robot-assisted laparoscopic aortofemoral bypass grafting for aortoiliac occlusive disease. J Vasc Surg. 2011;53(2):414-20.
9. Stadler P, Sebesta P, Vitasek P, Matous P, El Samman K. A modified technique of transperitoneal direct approach for totally laparoscopic aortoiliac surgery. Eur J Vasc Endovasc Surg. 2006; 32:266-9.
10. Stadler P, Matous P, Vitasek P, Spacek M. Robot-assisted aortoiliac reconstruction: A review of 30 cases. J Vasc Surg. 2006; 44(5):915-9.
11. Stádler P, Dvorácek L, Vitásek P, Matous P. Is robotic surgery appropriate for vascular procedures? Report of 100 aortoiliac cases. Eur J Vasc Endovasc Surg. 2008;36(4):401-4. doi: 10.1016/j.ejvs.2008.06.028. Epub 2008 Aug 21.

SECTION 4

Gynecology

- **Myomectomy**
  Rooma Sinha, Madhumati S, B Rupa
- **Challenges in Robotic Myomectomy**
  Kiranabala Dash, SB Khanna
- **Robotics in Benign Gynecology**
  Mala Srivastava, Ankita Srivastava
- **Sentinel Node Mapping in Gynecological Cancers**
  Anupama Rajanbabu
- **Robotic Staging Surgery for Endometrial Cancer**
  Anupama Rajanbabu
- **Endometrial Cancer and Cervical Cancer**
  Sabhyata Gupta, Shradha Chaudhari
- **Ovarian Cystectomy**
  Neelam Suri

CHAPTER

14

Myomectomy

Rooma Sinha, Madhumati S, B Rupa

INTRODUCTION

Fibroid is a common problem in women of reproductive age group. Myomectomy is an important option for fertility and uterine preservation in young women. While uterine artery embolization and MRI-guided focused ultrasound are also methods that are becoming popular in managing fibroid uterus, myomectomy remains the gold standard method. Myomectomy was first described by Bonney, and has now become a part of management for decade. We also have long-term data of good reproductive outcome following it. With advent of minimally invasive techniques, laparoscopic myomectomy becomes the obvious method of choice for its minimal access and comfort. The data published by Cochrane Review in 2014 states that myomectomy by laparoscopy is a less painful procedure compared with open surgery. A significantly lower risk of postoperative fever was observed in the laparoscopic myomectomy group compared with groups treated with all types of open myomectomy (OR 0.44, 95% CI 0.26–0.77, $I^2 = 0\%$, six studies, 635 women). Women undergoing laparoscopic surgery have shorter hospital stay compared with all types of open myomectomy.[1] Despite these advantages, the question remains—why still so many open myomectomies are being performed all over the world? Laparoscopic myomectomy is a technically challenging surgery and good outcomes are possible only by high volume surgeons who have exceptional skills. The need for extensive suturing in myomectomy is the main limitation in its wide spread acceptance by surgeons. Most literature reports about 50% myomectomies being performed via open method. There is no doubt that a laparoscopic approach is more advantageous than laparotomy, however laparoscopic suturing is more demanding. This can be overcome by robotic-assisted laparoscopic myomectomy.[2] Robotic surgery is a natural progress in the field of minimally invasive surgery. As robotic surgery allows surgeon to perform detailed surgery due to magnified 3D vision and deep reach into the pelvis. Therefore a new technology of computer assistance in laparoscopic surgery is slowly gaining ground. The da Vici system has EndoWrist technology with increased instrument range of motion (7°) enabling the surgeon to mimic open surgical techniques. The fact that robotic arms helps the surgeon to follow open surgical steps, addresses the technical challenges of conventional laparoscopic suturing and knot-tying. But the robotic technology cannot simplify all the challenges that myoma's pose. Although robotic assistance has improved the adoption of endoscopic myomectomy, the da Vinci system requires an experienced gynecologic endoscopic surgeon with good knowledge of surgical anatomy. Compared with open abdominal myomectomy, the robot-assisted laparoscopic approach is associated with less blood loss, lower complication rates, and shorter hospitalization.[3] A retrospective case study from the Cleveland Clinic confirmed these findings when investigators compared surgical outcomes between the robot-assisted laparoscopic approach, standard laparoscopy, and open myomectomy. In an assessment of 575 cases (393 open, 93 laparoscopic, and 89 robot-assisted), they found the robot-assisted laparoscopic approach to be associated with the removal of significantly larger myomas (as compared to standard laparoscopy), as well as lower blood loss and shorter hospitalization when compared to open myomectomy.[4]

Today robotic assisted myomectomy is slowly becoming the gold standard approach and is one of our favorite surgeries. The reasons for this are that *myomectomy is a suture-intensive surgery and assistance with robotic arms makes suturing simple and easy. Robotic myomectomy guarantees a procedure that is as effective as a classic open myomectomy. Robotic assisted surgery is as safe and acceptable as a laparoscopic operation.* This article discusses the principles and techniques of doing robotic assisted laparoscopic myomectomy in a systematic, safe, and efficient manner.

The chapter is divided as follows:

- Preoperative assessment and the role MRI
- Role of intrauterine manipulation
- Port placement, positioning and docking
- Methods of blood loss control
- Hysterotomy
- Enucleation
- Suturing
- Adhesion prevention
- Hybrid procedure
- Fibroid retrieval.

PREOPERATIVE ASSESSMENT AND ROLE OF MAGNETIC RESONANCE IMAGING

Careful patient selection and a good preoperative assessment for size, location and number of fibroids are vital for the success of the minimally invasive myomectomy. It is difficult to assess this on a 2 D scan and even on 3 D scan if the fibroids are multiple and constitute large volume. Preoperative MRI of the pelvis is suggested before robotic myomectomy and this is a routine in our unit. In fact we also suggest reviewing the MRI scan at the console with an experienced radiology colleague and create a mental picture of the location and number of fibroids before starting the surgery. The da Vinci system provides an opportunity to review the MRI film along with the surgical picture at the console (Tile pro technology). MRI is an excellent tool to differentiate between fibroids and adenomyosis and this avoids surprised during operation. This information also helps in the counseling session before surgery, as women with solitary fibroid or a few large fibroids, or pedunculated fibroids are good candidates and full clearance is possible **(Fig. 14.1)**. Diffuse fibromas, adenomyoma, adenomyosis with very little normal myometrium, are poor surgical candidates and these should be identified preoperatively **(Fig. 14.2)**. Although there are no limits on the number of fibroids that can be removed (maximum of 9 fibroids in our series), multiple seedlings disseminated throughout the uterus are not the right candidates for myomectomy. Adenomyomectomy is also possible with symptomatic women with the help of robotic assistance. Preopertaive MRI gives an opportunity to take a decision for hybrid procedure.

ROLE OF INTRAUTERINE MANIPULATION

This is an important step in completing the procedure in minimally invasive way. The role of the person who manipulates this instrument is equally important as the surgeon in robotic surgery is far from the patient and it is not possible for him to manually manipulate (as it is possible in routine laparoscopic procedures). Various types of uterine manipulators available and the selection depends on the surgeon's choice and experience. The manipulator helps the assistant to present the fibroid to the surgeon especially when there are multiple fibroids, can hold the uterus within the pelvis, improving the field of vision. A downward pull on the uterus can prove as counter traction during enucleation.

PORT PLACEMENT, POSITIONING AND DOCKING

The primary port is placed in the midline. We place this port by open technique however it can be placed in classical method with veress insufflation. The initial port (12 mm XL trocar-Ethicon Endo-Surgery) can be at the umbilicus or above (2–5 cm), depending on the size of the fibroid. As shown in the figure the primary port is 5 cm above the umbilicus as the upper border of the fibroid is 5 cm above the pubic symphysis **(Fig. 14.3)**. The rest of the 8 mm telerobotic trocar ports are placed as shown in the figure, in an inverted "W" so that there is about 10 cm space (one hands breadth—**Fig. 14.4**) between the ports. Selection of port placement is important to prevent clashing of the robotic arms as this can hinder the movements of the instruments. The next step is the selection of instruments in each port. We recommend the hot shears in arm 1, bipolar forceps in arm 2 and tenaculum in arm 3 **(Fig. 14.5)**. Once the myoma enucleation is complete we change the hot shears in arm 1 and 2 to needle drivers. The tenaculum can be changed to a prograsp in arm 3 for the myoma bed suturing. The assistant port can be used for suction-irrigation, passage of needle and for morcellation in the end. The bedside assistant also does the instrument exchanges on the robotic arms. The recommendation was

Fig. 14.1: T2 sagittal image showing solitary myoma (8 × 7 cm) in anterior wall of the uterus. The uterus is retroverted, bladder is compressed and endometrial lining seen posterior to myoma

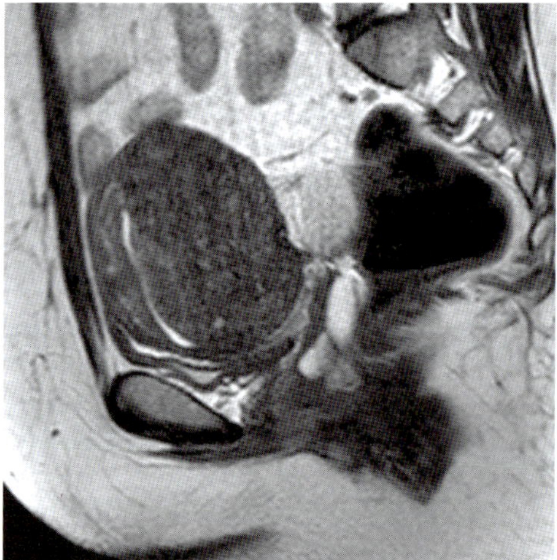

Fig. 14.2: T2 sagittal image showing diffuse posterior wall thickening with multiple cystic spaces suggestive of posterior wall adenomyosis. There is ill-defined posterior junctional zone

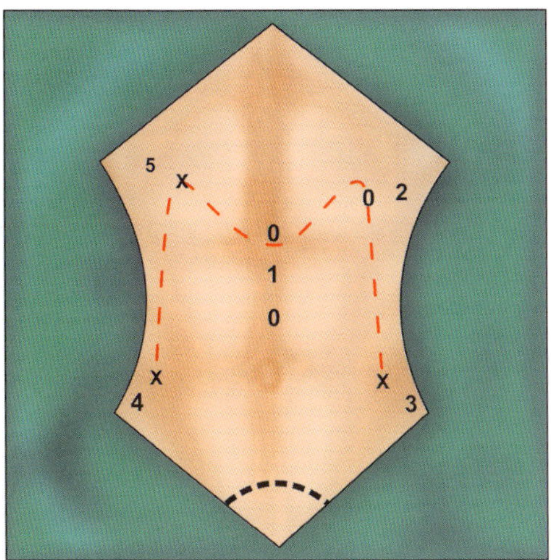

Fig. 14.3: Diagramatic representation of surface anatomy of port locations in robotic myomectomy. Port 1 is the 12 mm camera port. Port 2 is the 11 mm assistant port. Ports 3, 4 and 5 are the 8 mm telerobotic ports. The level of the fibrois is depicted in suprapubic region

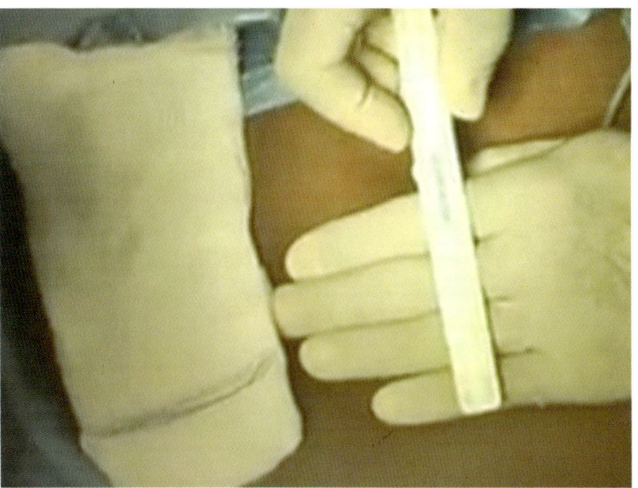

Fig. 14.4: Distance of one hand's breadth that measures 10 cm as distance between ports. This prevents collision between the arms

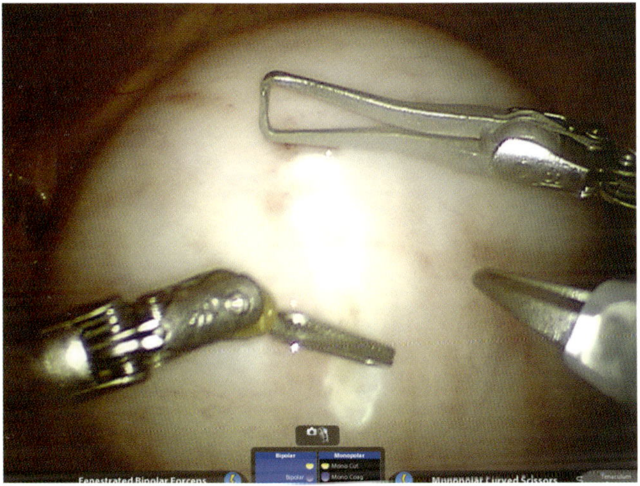

Fig. 14.5: Initial picture with the insertion of the three instruments—hot shears, tenaculum and bipolar forceps

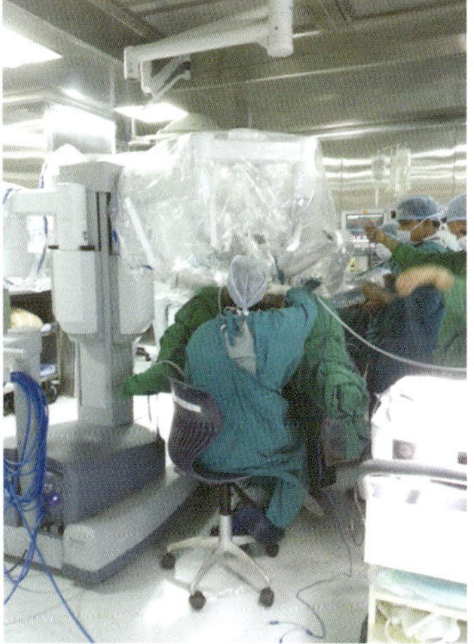

Fig. 14.6: Right side docking of the da Vinci robot enabling space for uterine manipulation by the assistant

to put the patients in deep trendelenburg position (30°), however with experience now we perform myomectomy with 15-20° tilt. Next step is to dock the patient-side cart with robotic arms. This cart is moved to the right side of the patient for side docking in our operating room, thus keeping the area between the patient's legs for uterine manipulation free **(Fig. 14.6)** Each robotic arm is connected to one trocar and the instruments are then inserted.

TECHNIQUES TO REDUCE BLOOD LOSS

Uterus with fibroids has increased number arterioles and venules and can cause significant blood loss during myomectomy. The average volume of blood loss during abdominal myomectomy performed is 200-800 mL and for laparoscopic myomectomy is 80-250 mL.[5] There are some reports for using GnRH agonists prior to myomectomy, however we do not suggest using GnRH agonist pretreatment for women undergoing myomectomy, as evidence does not support benefit in the procedure. One can use GnRH agents in large fibroids to reduce their bulk in order to allow a transverse rather than a vertical incision during myomectomy in order to prevent damage to cornual ends of the tube. Our recommendation is to use intramyometrial injection of vasopressin before each uterine incision. 20 units diluted in 100 mL saline are used to inject into the capsule. Repeated withdrawal should be done to check for any inadvertent direct vascular injection. Either an aspiration

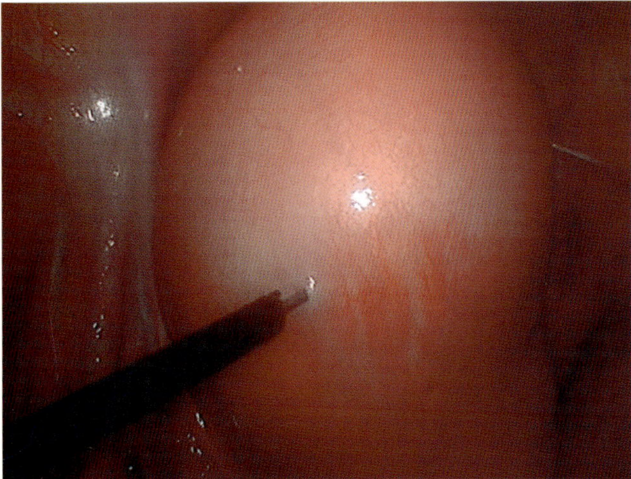

Fig. 14.7: Aspiration needle being used to inject dilute vasopressin into the myoma capsule

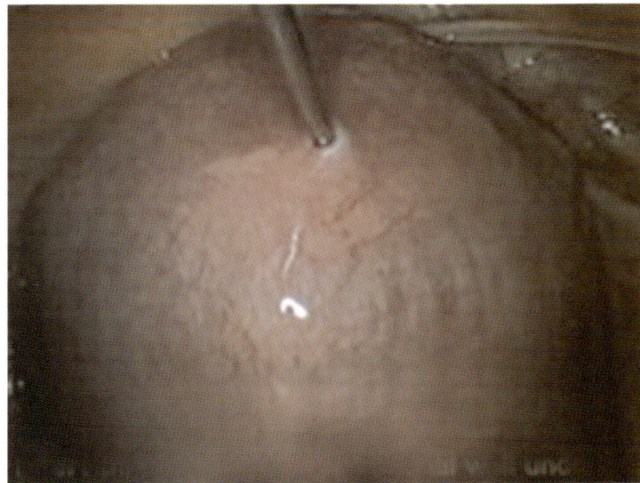

Fig. 14.8: Spinal needle or Veress needle through abdominal wall inserted under vision for injecting dilute vasopressin

needle **(Fig. 14.7)** through the assistant port or a direct insertion of spinal needle or veress needle **(Fig. 14.8)** under visual guidance can be used for this injection. Vasopressin acts by causing vasospasm of arterioles and contraction of uterine muscle. One must be careful as rare cases of life threating hypotension, pulmonary edema, bradycardia and cardiac arrest have been reported in the literature especially with intravascular injection of vasopressin. Some authors mention skillful use of misoprostol in reduction of blood loss. A randomized trial compared vaginal misoprostol (400 mcg, one hour before surgery) with placebo and found that the cases with misoprostol had significantly less blood loss.[6] It is neither our practice nor recommendation to use tourniquets or clamps to occlude the uterine blood supply.

HYSTEROTOMY

Hysterotomy is begun by first locating the fibroid with visual inspection of the uterus by hot shears **(Fig. 14.9)**. The initial incision on the uterus can be either vertical or transverse. This is usually made on the most prominent part of the fibroid. Uterus has ascending blood supply from the uterine arteries and descending blood supply from the ovarian arteries, which pass through the infundibulopelvic ligaments. The uterine and ovarian vessels anastomose to perfuse the uterus. Arcuate arteries run transversely within the uterine wall and radial arteries penetrate into the myometrium. Fibroids when present can distort the normal vascular architecture and the arcuate arteries can run in any axis and not in the predicted transverse fashion.[7] Therefore, it does not matter whether the incision is vertical or transverse, as it may still transect the arcuate arteries. The presence of vascular pedicle at the base of the fibroid is a concept no longer accepted. A study using vascular corrosion casting and electron microscopy revealed that fibroids are surrounded completely by a dense vascular layer supplying the fibroids, which is separated from the

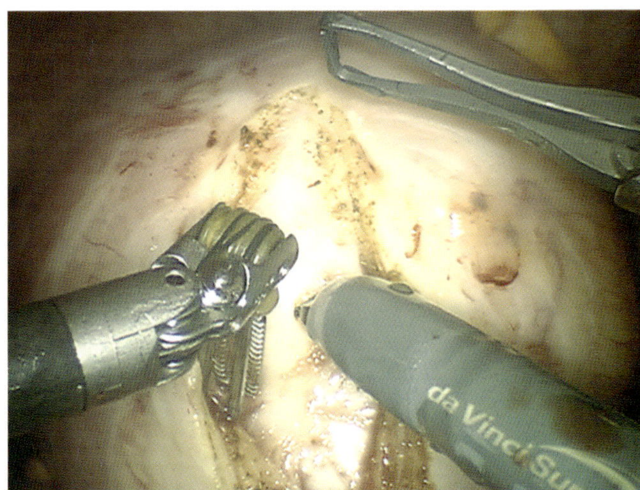

Fig. 14.9: Initial incision over the myoma made with hot shears

myometrium by a narrow avascular cleft.[8] Two points need to be kept in mind during hysterotomy. Firstly, adequate length of the incision and secondly, precise depth to be able to reach the pseudo capsule. The length is important for easy enucleation as with a small incision one can struggle to get the myoma out. Correct depth allows intracapsular myomectomy preserving the capsule enabling good healing.

ENUCLEATION

Once the incision is made, robotic tenaculum is used to grasp the fibroid **(Fig. 14.10)** and traction is given. This step helps to expose the capsule and presents the leading edge of the fibroid. We recommend a Pull-Spread-Toggle (PST) technique to enucleate the fibroid. The tenaculum in arm 3 pulls the fibroid away from the uterus, the bipolar in arm 2 spreads the space between normal myometrium and the

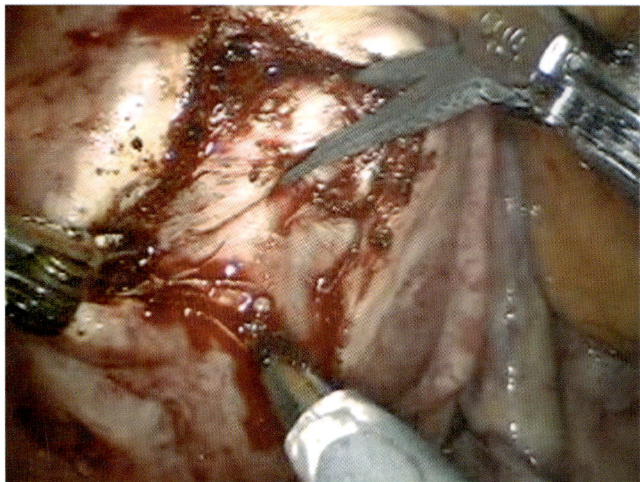

Fig. 14.10: Pull on the myoma using the robotic tenaculum

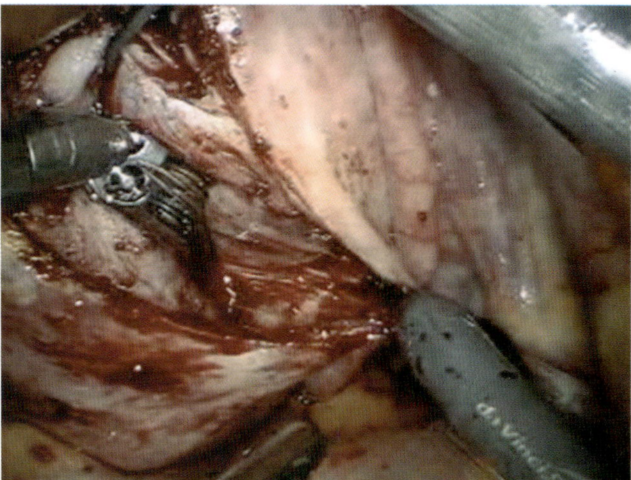

Fig. 14.11: The bipolar forceps being used for spreading the layer between myoma and the normal myometrium

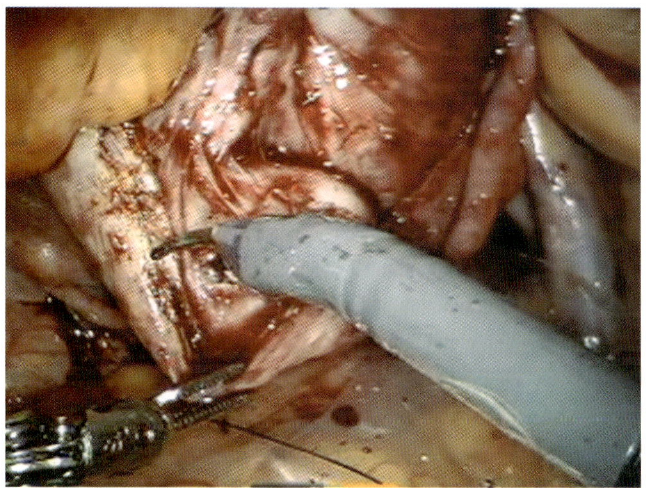

Fig. 14.12: Hot shears used to toggle and release the myoma from the bed, thus rolling out the myoma

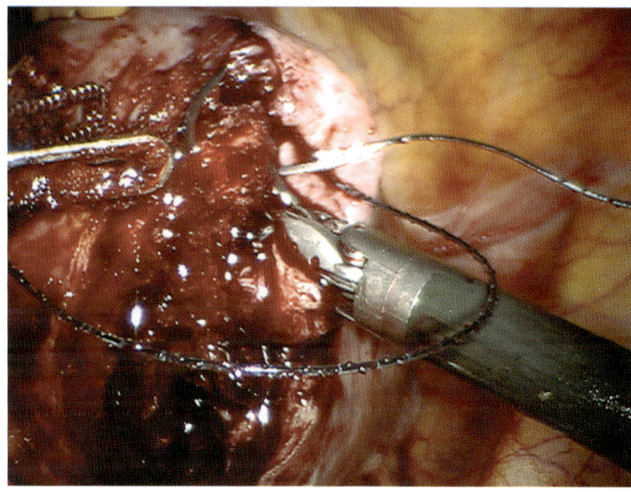

Fig. 14.13: Suturing in progress of the myoma bed

capsule **(Fig. 14.11)** and the hot shears in arm 1 toggle with monopolar energy to enucleate fibroid from within the capsule **(Fig. 14.12)**. However one must minimize the use of monopolar current as use of excessive electrical energy is linked with poor wound healing. The bedside assistant can provide additional pull on the fibroid with the help of myoma screw or laparoscopic tenaculum. As we progress in enucleation, the fibroid is regrapsed closer to the leading edge; this maneuver helps in rolling out the myoma. Fibroids that are close to cavity deserve more precise dissection, as they need to be lifted up from the endometrial layer preventing the damage to the endometrium.

SUTURING TECHNIQUES

By the time we start suturing, the effect of vasopressin usually wanes off, with slight oozing from the myometrial edges. We use V Loc 0 30 cm, (Covidien) for this procedure. This length although long at the beginning, we find that one suture is often sufficient for multilayer closure of small defects. There are fewer needle passes and cost is also less. Curve of the needle helps to take good deep bites for proper approximation **(Fig. 14.13)**. The use of unidirectional knotless barbed suture facilitates closure of uterine defects during robotic myomectomy enabling multiple layers in shorter time as they hold the edges of myoma bed together with adequate tension for suturing.[9] Barbed suture are used safely for gynecology, surgery including myomectomy.[10] With arm 1 and 2 actively *used* for suturing, arm three with prograsp forceps can be used to keep adequate tension on the suture. Hence, robotic platform enables skillful use of all the 3 arms for quick and effective suturing and is identical to that of an open myomectomy. The last layer is inverted (baseball) suture to invert the raw edges **(Fig. 14.14)**.

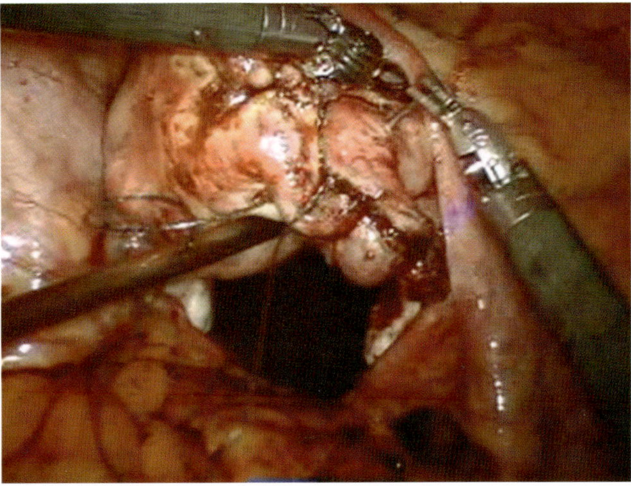

Fig. 14.14: Baseball suturing at the end to invert the raw edges

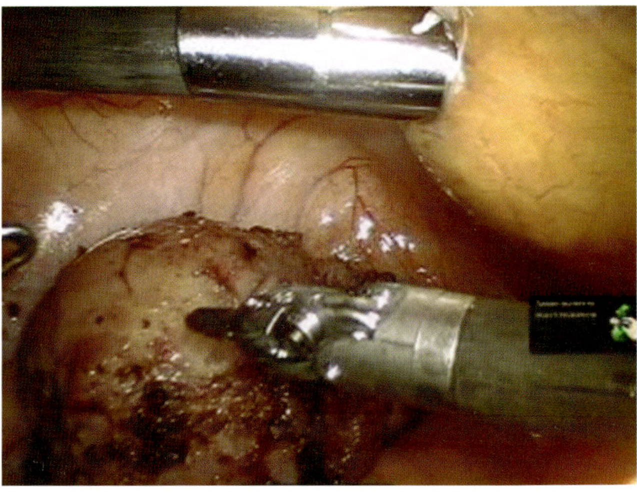

Fig. 14.15: Myoma parked in the right para-colic gutter while suturing is being performed

ADHESION PREVENTION

Myomectomy is known to have adhesions in the postoperative period. Good microsurgical techniques like gentle tissue handling and effective hemostasis including minimally invasive approach can be the first step in good outcome, however this approach alone cannot guarantee absence of adhesions as high insufflation pressures can itself increase risk of adhesions. While enucleation, keeping the tissues hydrated with saline prevents tissue desiccation and postoperative adhesion.[11] Oxidized regenerated cellulose (ORC-interceed) is absorbed over 5–7 days enabling fibrin clot dissolution and regeneration of the peritoneum. A systematic review and meta analysis identified 11 trials using ORC in gynecologic surgery and found that ORC significantly reduced risk of adhesions.[12] Based on these evidence we suggest use of these barriers for adhesion prevention but the peritoneal cavity should not be having free fluid at the end of the surgery.

FIBROID RETREIVAL

Anesthesia team in our operating room maintains the precise count of removed myomas. Collecting and keeping the fibroids can be a challenge, as the fibroids tend to run into upper abdomen due to deep Trendelenburg position. If large in size we keep them either in pouch of Douglas or in right paracolic gutter **(Fig. 14.15)**. If there are multiple small fibroids, we insert a bag at the beginning of the surgery and keep collecting them in the bag for retrieval later. Some surgeons thread all the small myomas like a necklace through a suture. In the end morcellation can be done using power morcellator (be aware of FDA warning). Alternatively we use scalpel for cold morcellation of these fibroids via the umbilical port or through posterior fornix.

HYBRID TECHNIQUE

A technique in which conventional laparoscopic enucleation of the myoma is followed by reconstruction with the da Vinci robot. Can be used when myomas are 10 cm or more as these are often beyond pelvis. Deep intramural myomas or highly vascular myomas can also be tackled by this technique. Hybrid technique preserves tactile sensation (Lacking in da Vinci surgical system) helping in enucleation at times. Rigid (not articulated) myoma screw and suction cannula can help mechanically to remove myomas. It is also effective in manipulation outside the pelvis and into the upper abdominal quadrants.[13] We use arm 2 and assistant port on the left side for hybrid procedure as using ipsilateral ports is easier to handle and operate. Once myomectomy is done, the robot is swiftly docked and suturing of the uterus done. This technique has a time lag between the myoma enucleation and the time when the surgeon starts suturing. This 'docking time' should be as minimal as possible and this depends on the team's coordination and efficiency. Hybrid robotic myomectomy is regarded as an advanced robotic technique.

CONCLUSION

In the years to come there will be various techniques to perform myomectomy, however one fact is clear that most surgeons will prefer minimally invasive technique for obvious advantages. Robotic platform will be of great help in replacing open myomectomy with minimally invasive. The use of robotic technology is a means to facilitate the laparoscopic completion of a myomectomy.[14] Robotic approach will help surgeons to extend their boundaries in terms of the size and number of myomas that can be removed. This also helps to remove myomas in odd locations. Reduced cost and miniaturization of the equipment along with addition of haptic feedback will improve acceptance. Single incision applications will further add to the benefits of robotic technology in gynecological surgeries.

REFERENCES

1. Chittawar PB. Minimally invasive surgical techniques versus open myomectomy for uterine fibroids (Review). The Cochrane Collaboration, 2014.
2. Agdi M, Tulandi T. Minimally invasive approach for myomectomy. Semin Reprod Med. 2010;28(3):228-34.
3. Quaas AM, Einarsson JI, Srouji S, Gargiulo AR. Robotic Myomectomy: A Review of Indication and Techniques. Reviews in Obstetrics and Gynecology. 2010;3(4).
4. Barakat EE, Bedaiwy MA, Zimberg S, Nutter B, Nosseir M, Falcone T. Robotic-assisted, laparoscopic, and abdominal myomectomy: a comparison of surgical outcomes. Obstet Gynecol. 2011;117(2 Pt 1):256-65.
5. Sawin SW, Pilevsky ND, Berlin JA, et al. Comparability of perioperative morbidity between abdominal myomectomy and hysterectomy for women with uterine leiomyomas. Am J Obstet Gynecol. 2000;183:1448.
6. Celik H, Sapmaz E. Use of a single preoperative dose of misoprostol is efficacious for patients who undergo abdominal myomectomy. Fertil Steril. 2003;79:1207.
7. Discepola F, Valenti DA, Reinhold C, et al. Analysis of arterial blood vessels surrounding the myoma: relevance to myomectomy. Obstet Gynecol. 2007;110:1301.
8. Walocha JA, Litwin JA, Miodoński AJ. Vascular system of intramural leiomyomata revealed by corrosion casting and scanning electron microscopy. Hum Reprod. 2003;18:1088.
9. Soto E1, Flyckt R2, Falcone T2. Minimally invasive myomectomy using unidirectional knotless barbed suture. J Minim Invasive Gynecol. 2014;21(1):27.
10. Angioli R, Plotti F, Montera R, et al. A new type of absorbable barbed suture for use in laparoscopic myomectomy. Int J Gynaecol Obstet. 2012;117(3):220-3.
11. Practice Committee of the American Society for Reproductive Medicine, Society of Reproductive Surgeons. Pathogenesis, consequences, and control of peritoneal adhesions in gynecologic surgery. Fertil Steril. 2007;88:21.
12. ten Broek RP, Stommel MW, Strik C, et al. Benefits and harms of adhesion barriers for abdominal surgery: a systematic review and meta-analysis. Lancet. 2014;383:48.
13. Quaas AM, Einarsson JI, Serene S, Gargiulo AR. Robotic myomectomy: a review of indication and techniques. Rev Obstet Gynecol. 2010;3(4).
14. Advincula AP, Xu X, Goudeau S 4th, Ransom SB. Robot-assisted laparoscopic myomectomy versus abdominal myomectomy: a comparison of short-term surgical outcomes and immediate costs. J Minim Invasive Gynecol. 2007;14(6):698-705.

CHAPTER

15

Challenges in Robotic Myomectomy

Kiranabala Dash, SB Khanna

INTRODUCTION

Uterine fibroids are the most common benign tumors in women, and are the most common indications for hysterectomy. The incidence varies from 5 to 21% between the ages of 35 and 49 years.[1] Incidence of fibroids in Caucasian women is 40% by the age of 35, which increases to 70% by the age of 50 where as in African-American women the incidence is 60% by the age 35 and >80% by the age 50.[2]

Majority of women with uterine fibroids are asymptomatic. Symptoms associated with fibroids are menorrhagia, dysmenorrhea, pelvic pain, pressure symptoms, infertility, pelvic mass and in some recurrent miscarriages. The treatment done traditionally was removal of fibroids by laparotomy or vaginally in women desiring uterine conservation particularly to retain future fertility. Since last few decades, laparoscopy has been evolved as a minimal access surgery, which has the advantages like short hospital stay, less postoperative pain, cosmetic benefits and faster recovery.

In 2005, the da Vinci surgical system was the first robort approved by the US Food and Drug Administration (FDA) for gynecological surgeries. The advantages with this newer technique have shown numerous benefits over the conventional laparoscopic surgery in the form of a three-dimensional image, superior instrument articulation and comfort for the surgeon. In addition to these benefits, in myomectomy, the multilayered suturing becomes easier by Robotic than by laparoscopic approach.

PREOPERATIVE PREPARATION AND PRECAUTIONS

Preoperative assessment of the number, size and location of the fibroids is very important. Although a good ultrasound can determine, an magnetic resonance imaging (MRI) pelvis should be done which confirms the information and also rules out adenomyosis. Also should be done are the tests like serum lactate dehydrogenase (LDH), cancer antigen 125 (CA 125), positron emission tomography-magnetic resonance imaging (PET-MRI) with 17-β estradiol in selected cases where one is suspicious of leiomyosarcoma (LMS) due to abnormal configuration of myoma on ultrasonography (USG). Other blood investigations are done as required before any other procedure requiring general anesthesia. Certain drugs like aspirin and antiplatelet drugs should be stopped at least 3 days prior to surgery. A physician and preanesthetic checkup are done. One day prior to surgery bowel preparation is done with peglec.

Patient and relatives should be counseled regarding blood loss, infection, injury to uterus, bladder and bowel, conversion to laparotomy and may be a need for hysterectomy.

ANESTHESIA AND PORT PLACEMENT

After general anesthesia, the patient is put in a low dorsal lithotomy position and the arms being padded, tucked by the side of the patient. Sequential compression device (SCD) pumps are applied as the prophylactic thromboprophylaxis measure. Shoulder guards are applied in order to avoid patient slippage during positioning. Orogastric tube is put to decompress the stomach. A Foley's catheter is inserted into the bladder and uterine manipulator is introduced into the uterine cavity. A 12-mm camera port is created at 10 cm above the upper border of uterus, in the midline above the umbilicus. Two 8 mm telerobotic ports are inserted 8 cm lateral and 2 cm below the camera port. In some patients, a third telerobotic side port is used on left side at least one hand's breadth below and lateral to left upper port. A 12-mm assistant port is placed on right side a hand's breadth below the right side port and above and lateral to anterior superior iliac spine. This port is used by the assistant for use for suction and irrigation, introducing needle holders and sutures and later for morcellation. Then steep Trendelenburg position is given and Robot docking is done from the left side of the patient. Some surgeons use docking in the middle and some use right side docking also. A 30° scope is used for the procedure.

After positioning and docking of the Robot the surgeon sits near the console unit and surgery is started.

STEPS OF SURGERY

Steps of myomectomy is very much like open myomectomy. Dilute Vasopressin (20 units in 100–200 mL of saline) is injected into the subcapsular area of fibroids. The instruments used for the procedure include monopolor scissors, bipolar forceps and a grasper or tenaculum and sometimes a hook. With the monopolor scissors/hook an incision is made over the myoma. Mostly a transverse incision is given, but sometimes longitudinal incision can be given. The myoma is enucleated in similar fashion as in open myomectomy. Even the assistant can provide traction using a laparoscopic myoma screw or a tenaculum.

The enucleated fibroid is then placed in the pouch of Douglas (POD). If multiple, all the myomas are first enucleated. A multilayer closure is performed using No 1 V-LOC barbed suture though 1-0 vicryl can be used.

Some surgeons use a running baseball stich that utilizes 3-0 vicryl to close the uterine serosa, once the deeper layers are approximated.

The myoma is then morcellated through the assistant port by power morcellator. Complete hemostasis is ensured. Anti-adhesive barrier is put on this suture area to prevent future scar tissue formation and adhesions.

In hybrid robotic technique, the enucleation of myoma(s) is done by conventional laparoscopy and suturing is done by docking the robot quickly. We have not used the hybrid technique for any patients. The robot is then de-docked and all the port areas are sutured.

Postoperative Care

Like laparoscopic procedures, the postoperative care in robotic myomectomy includes early ambulation, catheter removal and early oral feeds and discharge within or after 24 hours.

Complications and Their Management

Although the surgeon, anesthesist and the team are very careful and work hard to make the surgery safe, some complications may happen. If detected timely, these are dealt with accordingly.

Possible Complications

- *Bleeding:* If there is excessive bleeding the patient will require blood transfusion.
- Injury to bladder, uterus and bowel may occur in less than 1% of surgeries. If detected intraoperatively are repaired during the procedure only.
- *Conversion to laparaotomy:* Sometimes because of bleeding or technical difficulties, one may need to convert the procedure to laparotomy.
- *Hysterectomy:* As in open myomectomy there is always a minimal risk of converting to hysterectomy.

Postoperative Complications

As in other surgeries, the following complications may happen:

- Thromboembolism
- Intestinal obstructions
- Urinary infection
- Port site infection.

Late Complications

- Hernia
- Decrease fertility
- Pregnancy complications
- Morcellenomas.

Personal Experience Tips and the Challenges

At Indraprastha Apollo Hospital in last 2 years and 8 months total number of 98 gyne procedures were done by robotic surgery, which includes 26 robotic myomectomies.

The clinical profile of patients who underwent robotic myomectomy is:

- Grossly obese-picture No. 1
- Nullipara
- Unmarried
- Women working in corporate institutes
- Height of funds uteri up to or just above umbilicus
- Mostly a big posterior wall fibroid.

In our experience, average time taken for surgery was 3–4 hours with an average blood loss of 150–200 mL. Average blood transfusion of one unit each was given in ten patients. Conversion to laparotomy to take out the fibroid was done in 5 cases.

There are many challenges involved in this surgery.

First of all the challenge includes higher costs incurred on robotic myomectomy in comparison to laparoscopic procedure. Studies have shown that the outcome for routine myomectomy does not improve with higher cost equipment.[3]
The challenges during surgery are:
When there are multiple myomas:

- Dissection of myomas properly from its bed to reduce blood loss
- Multilayer suturing of the myoma bed, and eventually no uterine rupture during the pregnancy. Since the reported uterine scar rupture postmyomectomy is reported to be about 1%,[4] the appropriate multilayer suturing is important, which is often performed by expert laparoscopic surgeons only, during laparoscopic myomectomy but done better by Robotic assistance.

An important challenge during the robotic myomectomy is to find all the myomas during surgery which were not obvious preoperatively. The absence of haptic feedback is the limiting factor for it, as well to, determine the appropriate strength during suturing to avoid the breaking of the suture.

Another important challenge for the procedure has lately been erupted is the power morcellation for hysterectomy and myomectomy. This has become a matter of concern after an unsuspected leiomyosarcoma (LMS) morcellation during routine hysterectomy progressed to Stage IV uterine cancer. The FDA response to this issue in 2014 was that "If laparoscopic power morcellation is performed in women with unsuspected uterine sarcoma there is risk that the procedure will spread the cancerous tissue within the abdomen and pelvis, significantly worsening the patients likelihood of long-term survival. For this reason, and because there is no reliable method of predicting whether a woman with fibroids may have a uterine sarcoma the FDA discourages the use of laparoscopic power morcellation during hysterectomy or myomectomy for uterine fibroids". After this advisory power morcellators were withdrawn from the market by Johnson & Johnson.[5] This big challenge still continues as there is no definitive diagnostic modality to diagnose preoperative malignancy in a leiomyoma (LM). This also questions[3] (i) whether only open myomectomy is the treatment of choice for fibroids and (ii) should other treatment modalities such as uterine artery embolization, infection of gonadotropin-releasing hormone (GnRH) analogs, USG-guided ablation by high-intensity focus ultrasound (HIFU) on endometrial ablation be banned?

The various institutions in the west have evolved their own protocols for this morcellation. At Temple University Hospital, USA, the Department of OBGYN, no morcellation is done outside of an isolation bag to prevent spillage of tumor/tissue. Fibroid uteri smaller than 10–12 weeks size are delivered vaginally without morcellation, fibroid uteri of larger than 16–18 weeks are operated only by laparotomy and between 12–16 week size delivered by morcellation in a bag or through minilaparotomy incision. For other hysterectomies for any benign condition there has to be normal cervical cytology and endometrial biopsy done before morcellation can be done during robotic hysterectomy.

The American College of Obstetricians and Gynecologists (ACOG) statement of May 2014[6] addresses both the risks and benefits of morcellation. Some of the excerpts from this statement are:

"Minimal invasive surgery, including the use of power morcellation, should still be an option for some women undergoing hysterectomy or myomectomy. Women with known uterine cancer or for whom there is high suspicion of it, should not receive power morcellation. Women for power morcellation should have careful preoperative evaluation for occult malignancy and patients require counseling about the risks, benefits and alternatives to treatment with morcellation. Informed consent should be taken."

The American Association of Gynecologic Laparoscopists (AAGL) statement of July 2014[7] regarding the FDA safety communication includes the following:

"It is the AAGL's position that we should improve but not abandon power morcellation and that power morcellation with appropriate informed consent should remain available to appropriately screened, low risk women."

Finally, it means that one has to thoroughly do preoperative evaluation for LMS. The incidence of leiomyosarcoms in uterine leiomyomas is estimated to be between 0.13 and 0.29%. However, the exact incidence of leiomyosarcoma in uteri removed for benign uterine myoma has not been reported. According to FDA the incidence is 1:352 for sarcoma and 1:458 for leiomyosarcoma whereas Leibsohn et al.[8] found the incidence of 1% (8 of 817) of leiomyosarcoma, between the ages of 40–60 years, in preoperatively presumed benign leiomyomas. Our own incidence in Apollo Hospital has been about 1 in 130 for last 10 years.

Recently a 35 years old lady presented with a 26 weeks size uterine fibroids, and underwent open myomectomy. The histopathology report was suggestive of smooth muscle tumor of undetermined malignant potential. Her pre-operative serum LDH was normal and MRI pelvis was suggestive of leiomyoma only. This again warrants that proper case selection is the most important challenge before planning for Robotic myomectomy.

The risk factors for uterine sarcoma are as follows:

- Postmenopausal age
- Tamoxifen use for 5 years or more
- History of pelvic irradiation
- Hereditary leiomyomatosis and renal cell carcinoma syndrome
- Survival of childhood retinoblastoma
- History of prolonged unopposed estrogen in post-menopausal women
- Failure of myoma to respond to GnRH analogs, and uterine artery embolization and magnetic resonance-guided focused ultrasound (UAE and MRgFUS).
- Quickly growing myomas
- On USG-absence of calcification and ill-defined margins, mixed or poor echogenicity and central necrosis
- On Doppler velocimetry-irregular vessel distribution, low impedance flow and high peak systolic velocity.

The most important modality for preoperative diagnosis of uterine malignancy is MRI. The findings suggestive of LMS include large heterogeneous masses and hemorrhage or cystic necrosis.[9] The contrast MRI with gadolinium and serum LDH and CA-125 levels are supposed to differentiate between leiomyoma and LMS. The PET-MRI with 16 × 18F (Fluro-17β ostradiol shows high uptake in LMS than LM.[10]

For all cases, we are doing MRI pelvis, serum LDH, serum CA-125 levels. But we could not do PET-MRI with since the availability of the agent was not there. Now we are in the process of making it available and in future hope to take the PET-MRI which will gives us a more definitive diagnosis.

REFERENCES

1. Marino JL, Eskenazi B, Warner M, Samuels S, Vercellini P, Gavoni N, and Olive D. Uterine leiomyoma and menstrual cycle characteristics in a population-based cohort study. Human Reprod. 2004;19(10):2350-5.

2. Day Baird D, Dunson DB, Hill MC, Cousins D, Schectman JM. High cumulative incidence of uterine leiomyoma in black and white women: ultrasound evidence. Am J Obstet Gynecol. 2003;188(1):100-107.
3. Nezhat C, Lavie O, Hsus, et al. Robotic assisted laparoscopic myomectomy compared with standard laparoscopic myomectomy: a retrospective matched control study. Fertil Steril. 2009;91:556-9(Pub Med).
4. Dubuisson J, Fauconnier A, Deffarges J, Norgaard C, Kreiker G, Chapron C. Pregnancy outcome and deliveries following laparoscopic myomectomy. Hum Reprod. 2000;15:869-73.
5. *www.fda.gov/medicaldevcies/safety/alertsandnotice/4cm 393576. htm.*
6. ACOG-*www.medscape.com/viewarticle/825043#vp-4.*
7. AAGL-*www.aagl.org/aaglnews/aagl-statements to-the fda-on-power-morcellation/*
8. Leibsohn, S, d'Ablaing, G, Mishell, Dr Jr and Schlaerth, JB leiomyosarcoma in a series of hysterectomies performed for presumed uterine leiomyomas. Am J Obstet Gynecol. 1990; 162(4):968-74.
9. Tanaka YO, Nishida M, Tsunoda H, Okamoto Y and Yoshikawa H. Smooth muscle tumors of uncertain malignant potential and leiomyosarcomas of the uterus: MR findings. Journal of Magnetic Resonance Imaging. 2004;20(6):998-1007.
10. Goto S, Takeuchi K, Sugimura and Maruo T. Usefulness of Gd-DTPA contrast enhanced dynamic MRI and serum determination of LDH and its isozymes in the differential diagnosis of leiomyosarcoma from degenerated leiomyoma of the uterus. International Journal of Gynecological Cancer. 2002; 12(4):354-61.

CHAPTER

16

Robotics in Benign Gynecology

Mala Srivastava, Ankita Srivastava

SURGICAL EVOLUTION IS NOTHING NEW

"There are numerous technologies outside the immediate interest or view of surgeons, which will either require surgeons to implement or which will impact upon the way surgery is performed or possibly even replaced."

—Dr Freidrich Trendelenburg, 1885

Minimally invasive surgery (MIS) has revolutionized the management of gynecologic disorders over the last 30 years. However, the most substantial improvements have come with the advent of robotic surgery.[1]

Laparoscopy was introduced in gynecology in the 1940s for diagnostic purpose and later on for tubal ligations. It was not until 1988 that the first laparoscopic-assisted vaginal hysterectomy was performed by Harry Reich in Pennsylvania.[2]

However, not all surgeons are comfortable with the laparoscopic approach due to its steep learning curve, nor are all patients and procedures amenable to traditional laparoscopy. The first application of robotics in laparoscopic procedures was as a surgical assistant and functioned as a laparoscope holder. The device was known as Automated Endoscopic System for Optimal Positioning or AESOP (Computer Motion Inc., Coleta, CA). The world's first robot assisted gynecological procedure reported was a case of tubal reanastomosis with the ZEUS Robotic System (Computer Motioni, Goleta, CA, USA) in 1993. The first robotic system that integrated the control of both the laparoscope and surgical instruments into a single unit is the da Vinci Robotic Surgical System (Intuitive Surgical, Inc., Mountain View, CA, USA).

There are many advantages of robotic laparoscopic surgery versus conventional laparoscopy[3]

In robotic surgery:

- The surgeon sees a three-dimensional view of the operating field, which gives a feeling of immersion without peripheral distraction.
- The surgeon is able to control the stereo endoscope using the operating arms and foot pedal and is not reliant on an assistant.
- The stereo endoscope remains motionless unless purposely moved by the surgeon.
- The motionless field of view enables increased magnification (× 10) of the surgical field. The fulcrum effect of straight-stick surgery (the hand moves the instrument to the left and the tip moves to the right) is lost in robotic surgery, with the instruments mimicking exactly the movement of the surgeon's hands.
- Different sensitivity settings on the console enable the surgeon to choose the degree of movement of the instrument tips relative to hand movements depending on the type of surgery being undertaken. The movements of the surgeon are digitalized, scaled at 1/1, 1/3, or 1/5, and transmitted by computer to the intra-abdominal instruments without noticeable delay.
- The surgeon is seated with arms rested, decreasing surgeon fatigue.
- The da Vinci Si system has three operating arms, all of which are controlled by the surgeon, who is able to switch between each instrument using the control pedal. On disengaging one arm to use another, the nonoperating arm remains stationary but will still maintain tension on grasped tissue.
- The EndoWrist laparoscopic instruments used in the da Vinci system allows seven degrees of movement, thereby mimicking the full range of the surgeon's hand, compared with four degrees of movement with straight-stick surgery.
- The robot cart holds the surgical trocars so that the fulcrum point is directly on the abdominal wall, decreasing the movement on the abdominal wall and reducing local trauma.
- The EndoWrist instrument tips and stereo endoscope are disengaged from control if the surgeon's head is removed from the console and they remain stationary. This is advantageous in teaching scenarios where a trainer may wish to demonstrate or assist a trainee during the procedure. The newest version of the da Vinci system, the SiHD, has the potential for using dual consoles where the trainer can operate with the trainee simultaneously.

- Changing operating instruments can be done at speed, as the newly replaced instrument returns to exactly the same place as the removed instrument and does not need to be tracked into the pelvis with the endoscope.
- The console concept offers the potential for telesurgery, where the surgeon is at an unlimited distance from the patient.

Disadvantages of the da Vinci System

- Cost is the biggest disadvantage. There can be an initial outlay costs, as well as the yearly service charge and instrument costs. The EndoWrist instruments are proprietary and each can only be used 10 or 20 times before being replaced.
- The robot takes time to set up but if it is done while the woman is being anesthetized, it does not add significantly to the overall operating theater time. Docking of the robot does add to overall surgical time; however, docking time can be reduced to less than 5 minutes with experience.
- Although the system can be folded away when not in use, it still occupies floor space and it does decrease the room available in the operating room.

INDICATIONS

Robotic gynecologic surgery has indications similar to conventional laparoscopy. Because of the increased setup time, indications for robotic gynecologic surgery are primarily operative, as opposed to a diagnostic laparoscopy.[4]

- Hysterectomy
- Myomectomy
- Tubal reanastomosis
- Sacrocolpopexy
- Endometriosis
- VVF repair
- Cervical cercalage.

Patients scheduled for gynecologic procedures of short duration and low complexity are unlikely to benefit from robotic-assisted surgery.[5]

- Tubal ligation
- Simple ovarian cystectomy
- Surgical management of ectopic pregnancy
- Prophylactic bilateral salpingo-oophorectomy.

HYSTERECTOMY

The hysterectomy is the most commonly performed gynecologic surgery, with approximately 600,000 performed annually.[6] Ninety percent of these are performed for benign indications, including fibroids, abnormal uterine bleeding, endometriosis, and chronic pelvic pain. Several approaches are available, including abdominal, vaginal, laparoscopic (total laparoscopic hysterectomy [TLH], laparoscopic-assisted vaginal hysterectomy [LAVH], laparoscopic supracervical hysterectomy [LSH]), and robotic-assisted laparoscopic hysterectomy (RALH).

In 2002, only 10% of hysterectomies were performed in a minimally invasive fashion. Wu et al. evaluated 538,722 hysterectomies performed during this year for benign indications. Of these, 66.1% were performed abdominally, 21.8% were performed vaginally, and only 11.8% were performed laparoscopically.[7] The American Association of Gynecologic Laparoscopists (AAGL) released a statement in November 2010 stating that hysterectomies should be performed in as minimally invasive manner as far as possible.[8]

Robot-assisted gynecologic surgery can be performed safely in centers with experienced surgeons. This minimally invasive approach could be considered for procedures that might otherwise require laparotomy.

In 2010, 30.5% of benign hysterectomies were performed laparoscopically. 0.5% of all hysterectomies performed robotically in 2007 compared with 9.5% in 2010. No differences in blood loss, length of stay, type or number of complications, postoperative pain levels, analgesic use, or recovery time were found.[5]

Analysis of US surgical data in 2003 showed that abdominal hysterectomy is performed in 66% of cases, vaginal hysterectomy in 22% of cases, and laparoscopic hysterectomy in 12% of cases. The feasibility and safety of the robotic-assisted laparoscopic hysterectomy has been demonstrated in multiple retrospective case series. Robotic-assisted laparoscopy was found to be safe and effective for hysterectomy in the initial experiences.

Blood loss, length of stay, and postoperative complications were comparable. Surgeons reported that they enjoyed the better ergonomics of robotic instruments, and did not find lack of haptic feedback to be a disadvantage.

In summary, the number of abdominal hysterectomies has decreased, and this is due to an increase in the adoption of minimally invasive approaches, both conventional laparoscopic and robotic-assisted laparoscopic hysterectomies.[9]

A large cohort study analyzed 264,758 women who underwent hysterectomy for benign gynecologic disorders in United States from 2007 to 2010. Robot-assisted hysterectomy was associated with significantly lower risk of hospitalization longer than 2 days. But at a significantly higher total cost.[5]

In a large retrospective review of robotic versus laparoscopic hysterectomies published in 2010, few clinical differences in perioperative or postoperative events were observed. This study reviewed data from 358 hospitals for a total of 36,188 hysterectomies, 95% (34,527) of which were performed with conventional laparoscopy. Although there were few clinical differences, the cost of the robotic approach was significantly increased.[10] Paraiso et al. performed a randomized controlled trial comparing laparoscopic versus robotic hysterectomies for benign indications. They compared 27 women undergoing a laparoscopic hysterectomy and 26 women undergoing a robotic hysterectomy. They concluded that conventional laparoscopy has a significantly shorter operating room time versus robotic (171.6 +/- 75.8 minutes vs 245.8 +/- 117.1 minutes, respectively). In addition, they concluded there was no difference in perioperative complications or postoperative pain and return to work.[11]

MYOMECTOMY

Women with symptomatic fibroids may undergo a myomectomy to preserve fertility. The robotic approach can be used to treat myoma in a minimally invasive manner in young women. It is associated with a shorter recovery time. Obstacles with robotic myomectomy include difficulty enucleating leiomyomas, performing adequate multilayer closure, and the concern for uterine rupture with subsequent pregnancies. Nonetheless, a review of articles regarding robotic-assisted laparoscopic myomectomy reports favorable outcomes. Laparoscopic myomectomy decrease postoperative morbidity and allows faster recovery. The robotic system may help overcome limitations, such as unfavorable myoma location, patient obesity and aid in meticulous suturing of the myoma bed. Blood loss, change in hematocrit, length of stay, and febrile morbidity were decreased in the robotic-assisted laparoscopic group, while operative time was increased compared with laparotomy and laparoscopic myomectomy.[12]

In 2004, Advincula et al. reported a series of 35 patients with an average of 1.6 myomas who underwent robotic myomectomy. The mean operating time was 230.8 minutes, the estimated blood loss (EBL) was 169 mL, and the conversion rate was 8.6%. Two conversions were due to difficult enucleations caused by absent haptic feedback.[13] In 2007, a retrospective case analysis by Advincula et al. compared myomectomies performed robotically or via a laparotomy. They had 29 patients in both the robotic and open arms. Robotic myomectomy resulted in decreased EBL, length of stay, and complications. However, a longer operative time was reported.[14] No major advantage of robotic over laparoscopic myomectomy was identified in a retrospective case study by Nezhat et al. in 2009, but the operative time was 234 minutes for robotic cases versus 203 minutes for standard laparoscopic myomectomies. This study compared 15 robotic versus 35 laparoscopic myomectomies.[15] Another large retrospective data review that compared 575 myomectomies performed abdominally (68.3%), laparoscopically (16.2%), and robotically (15.5%) showed decreased length of stay and decreased EBL in the robotic-assisted group. In this review, heavier myomas were removed more often via abdominal (average, 263 g) than robotic-assisted (average, 223 g) and laparoscopic approaches (average, 96.65 g). EBL was highest in abdominal myomectomy (200 mL vs 150 mL robotic vs 100 mL laparoscopic). Operative time was the longest in the robotic group (181 minutes vs 155 minutes laparoscopic vs 125 minutes abdominal).[16] A retrospective data review in a community-based hospital compared surgical outcomes in 77 patients who underwent robotic-assisted laparoscopic myomectomy to those in 30 patients who underwent open myomectomy. The body mass index (BMI) and specimen weight were comparable, but the robotic modality resulted in significantly less EBL (125 ± 106 mL vs 353 ± 373 mL), a shorter hospital stay (1.4 vs 2.69 days), and a longer operative time for robotic myomectomy than open myomectomy (212 ± 88 minutes vs 136 ± 53 minutes).[17]

Although additional data are needed, the first case report of an uncomplicated full-term pregnancy after laparoscopic myomectomy with the assistance of the da Vinci robotic system was published in 2007 and supports the suturing capabilities of the robot.[18]

TUBAL REANASTOMOSIS

Tubal sterilization is a common and accepted method for permanent contraception. However, there are request for reversal of tubal ligation for various reasons like remarriage, loss of children or simply a change of heart. Tubal reanastomosis has a success rate about 67.6% in open surgery with 5.6% incidence of ectopic pregnancy in subsequent conception after reversal.[19] In 1998, a study was first conducted in animal models to demonstrate that the robotic technology could safely be used in microsurgical anastomosis using the Zeus® Surgical System.[20] A pilot study was then done in 1999 to perform laparoscopic tubal anastomosis.[21] The procedure was successfully completed in all patients without complications. The pregnancy was reported in 2 out of 8 patients at 4 months following the surgery. A feasibility study done in University of Alabama in 2004, Dharia[22] compared open microsurgical technique with the da Vinci surgical system for tubal anastomosis in 18 patients. Robotic-assisted procedures greatly increased operative time, however the length of hospital stay, recovery time, and time to return to normal activities were significantly shorter in robotic group.[23] Robotic assisted reanastomosis has the advantage of delicate manipulation of tubes and good visualization of anatomical layers for excellent suturing. However, long-term comparative studies are needed to determine if robotic surgery will be beneficial for sterilization reversal in terms of patient satisfaction and pregnancy outcome.

A tubal recanalization is a procedure to restore fertility after a woman has had a tubal ligation. During the tubal recanalization, four robotic ports are made, the blocked segments of the fallopian tubes are cut and edges are freshened. The cut ends are re-anastomosed using 6'O vicryl to the remainder of the fallopian tubes. The procedure is repeated on the other side. This may allow ovum to again move through the tubes and sperm to travel up the fallopian tubes.

Sterilization procedures that cause the minimal damage to the fallopian tubes are the most likely candidates for successful tubal recanalization for examples sterilization with tubal clips or rings. Procedures that cause scarring of the fallopian tubes, such as the Essure or Adiana systems, cannot be reversed.

A tubal recanalization is not appropriate for everyone. There are several factors to determine if tubal ligation reversal is likely to be successful, such as:

- Age and body mass index
- The type of tubal ligation
- The extent of the damage to the fallopian tubes
- Remaining healthy tubal length
- Other fertility factors, such as sperm and egg quality.

SACROCOLPOPEXY

Pelvic organ prolapse is increasing as the female life expectancy increases. Sacrocolpopexy for prolapse is an advanced surgery that requires suturing with dissection of the presacral space and suturing of mesh from the vagina to the sacral promontory, which has prohibited its popularity in conventional laparoscopy. Traditionally, this procedure is performed abdominally owing to the technical difficulty associated with dissection of these spaces.

Robotic-assisted sacrocolpopexy is an alternative to the abdominal approach and conventional laparoscopy. It helps in effectively and efficiently dissect these spaces and suture while providing a minimally invasive modality with faster recovery time.

Sacrocolpopexy is a technique for repairing pelvic organ prolapse. The treatment approach is chosen in accordance with the type and degree of pelvic organ prolapse, as well as the severity of symptoms.

A graft is used to support the vaginal wall and suspend the apical vault to the sacral promontory.

Sacrocolpopexy is intended to repair apical or vaginal vault prolapse in women. Reconstruction is achieved either by an open abdominal technique or with the use of minimally invasive surgery, such as laparoscopy or robotic-assisted surgery. The salient component of reconstruction is suspension of the apical portion of vagina in a manner that recreates the natural anatomic support that the uterosacral and cardinal ligaments provide, by tacking it to the sacral promontory. In postmenopausal women with uterine prolapse, hysterectomy can be performed at the time of surgical repair. Uterine sparing techniques have also been described.

Pelvic organ prolapse is the symptomatic descent of one or more of components of the vaginal wall, including the anterior wall, posterior wall, and the vaginal apex, which could lead to descent of the cervix and uterus or the vaginal cuff following hysterectomy.[24,25]

The degree of prolapse is assessed using a quantification system, such as the Pelvic Organ Prolapse Quantification (POPQ) or the Baden-Walker system.

Epidemiology

The prevalence of pelvic organ prolapse varies between studies, but has been reported in larger observational studies of menopausal women in the range of 31–41.1%.[26,27]

In a multicenter observational study of women presenting to an outpatient gynecology clinic, the distribution of prolapse according to a POPQ assessment was 24% with stage 0 prolapse, 38% with stage I, 35% with stage II, 2% with stage III, and 0% with stage IV.[28]

Nygaard et al. studied a smaller population that was a subset of those enrolled in the Women's Health Initiative Hormone Replacement Therapy trial. They found 2.3% with stage 0 prolapse, 33% with stage I, 62.9% with stage II, 1.9% with stage III, and 0% with stage IV.[29] The lifetime risk of undergoing an operation for pelvic organ prolapse is reported to be 11–19%.[30,31]

Etiology

Pelvic organ prolapse can be considered as herniation of pelvic or abdominal contents into the structural weaknesses in the support of the pelvic floor. The etiology of the fascial defects that leads to prolapse is multifactorial and involves genetics, environmental factors, comorbidities, and lifetime events such as the number of vaginal births.

Risk factors for pelvic organ prolapse include the following:
- Increasing age
- Increasing body mass index (obesity)
- Increasing gravidity
- Increasing parity
- Number of vaginal deliveries
- Macrosomic delivery
- Chronic obstructive pulmonary disease
- Constipation
- Strenuous activity, weight bearing, or strenuous labor.

Nygaard and colleagues studied patients enrolled in the WHI Hormone Replacement Therapy trial and found varying risk factors for prolapse depending on the definition of prolapse itself. Education level, the number of vaginal deliveries, and the weight of the infant were significant factors in distinguishing patients with Stage II prolapse or greater.[29]

Consideration for surgical repair of apical (vaginal vault) or uterine prolapse is based on adequate assessment of the patient's symptoms and degree of bother, as well as a standard method to quantify prolapse.

Symptoms may include the following:
- Vaginal bulge
- Pelvic pressure
- Bleeding
- Infection
- Splinting or digitation (the need to manually assist in reducing prolapse, often to void or defecate)
- Back pain.

Concomitant symptoms may include the following:[32,33]
- Urinary incontinence symptoms, such as stress, urgency, or postural incontinence
- Bladder storage symptoms, such as frequency, urgency, or overactive bladder syndrome
- Voiding symptoms, such as hesitancy, slow stream, straining, incomplete emptying, or position-dependent voiding
- Sexual dysfunction symptoms, such as dyspareunia or obstructed intercourse
- Anorectal dysfunction, such as fecal incontinence, flatal incontinence, fecal urgency, straining to defecate, constipation, and incomplete evacuation.

Many of the general contraindications to sacral colpopexy are the same for any surgical procedure. These may include the following:

- Anemia
- Bleeding diathesis or the need for anticoagulation
- Significant cardiac or pulmonary comorbidities
- Active infection such as cystitis, bacterial or fungal vaginal infection, pelvic inflammatory disease, or active sexually transmitted disease
- Active venous thromboembolism
- Uncontrolled hyperglycemia.

Other contraindications specific to sacral colpopexy include the following:

- Vaginal cancer, cervical cancer, or uterine cancer that is untreated or cannot be adequately treated due to advanced stage
- Fistulas such as vesicovaginal, rectovaginal, vesico-utero, or urethral fistulas
- Previous pelvic prolapse repairs with infected or exposed foreign material and erosions.

Relative contraindications include the following:

- Pelvic irradiation
- Previous pelvic surgery or prolapse repair, depending on the nature of the operation and their pathology, side effects, or complications
- Concomitant cystocele, rectocele, or urinary incontinence which may require additional surgery, a vaginal approach, or a combined approach.

Prevention of Complications

Immediate perioperative complications include bowel obstruction, peritonitis, urine leak from missed intraoperative recognition of a cystotomy, dehiscence, and infection. Most of these complications occur rarely but they must be included in the differential diagnosis when symptoms occur. Delayed bleeding is also a rare complication.

In the modified lithotomy position for sacral colpopexy, femoral nerve injury can occur by hyperextension at the hip. Perineal nerve injury may result from compression against the stirrup if not properly positioned.

Prophylactic measures including placement of sequential compression devices or antiembolic compression stockings prior to anesthesia induction, early postoperative ambulation, and prophylactic doses of heparin or low-molecular weight heparin in those with increased risks of thromboembolic events.

Mesh erosion is a late complication of abdominal sacral colpopexy with a reported rate of 3–7.6%.[34-37]

Lower rates of erosion have been identified with monofilament polypropylene mesh.[35] Concurrent hysterectomy was associated with increased erosion rates in one study.[35] Another study did not find associated risk factors or demonstrate increased erosions with concurrent hysterectomy.[38] Symptoms include persistent dyspareunia, vaginal discharge, or bleeding.[35,38] The time from surgery to erosion varies but has been reported on an average to be between 5 and 14 months.[35,38]

Postoperative Care

Any strenuous activity or heavy lifting should be avoided in the immediate postoperative period, i.e. 6–8 weeks, to allow adequate time for scar tissue formation. Activities that cause perineal strain or trauma, such as bicycle riding, squatting should be avoided.

Imaging

The role of medical imaging in evaluating women with pelvic organ prolapse is not standardized. An overall 7.7% prevalence of hydronephrosis has been identified in women undergoing prolapse surgery.[39] The prevalence was higher in those with worsening prolapse.[39] A preoperative renal ultrasound may identify patients who may require additional assessment of urinary system or changes in management.

Gellar et al. compared 73 robotic sacrocolpopexies versus 108 open sacrocolpopexies and demonstrated increased operative times, decreased EBL, decreased length of hospital stays, and similar vaginal vault support in the robotic arm after a 6-week postoperative follow-up.[40] Elliott et al. reported high patient satisfaction with the robotic approach and one recurrent vaginal vault prolapse in 12 months of follow-up of patients with posthysterectomy vaginal vault prolapse who underwent robotic sacrocolpopexy.[41]

Paraiso et al. performed a randomized controlled trial comparing conventional versus robotic sacrocolpopexies. They included 38 in the laparoscopic group and 40 in the robotic group. The robotic group had a longer operating time, procedure time, and suturing time. They also suggested that robotic procedures had more postoperative pain, requiring more NSAID. In addition, the robotic group had a greater cost, with a mean difference of $1,936. Both groups had improvement in their vaginal support, and there were no differences in functional outcomes after 1 year.[42]

An observational study from Mayo clinic describes and demonstrates the use and benefit of robot-assisted laparoscopic sacrocolpopexy in the treatment of post-hysterectomy vaginal vault prolapse in obese patients along with mid-urethral sling application.[43] Cost and operating time are double with robotic procedures, but sexual function and improvement of pelvic support tend to be better under robotic manipulation.[44]

ENDOMETRIOSIS

Endometriosis affects approximately 10% of reproductive-aged women. The disease significantly impairs a women's quality of life, owing to chronic pelvic pain, dysmenorrhea, dyspareunia, and bowel disturbances. Superficial, ovarian, and deep infiltrating endometriosis can be treated with surgical resection. Laparoscopy is the standard for diagnosis of this condition. Robotic surgery provides a means to perform difficult procedures in deep infiltrating endometriosis and a frozen pelvis.

Laparoscopy, considered the gold standard for diagnosis of endometriosis, is also recognized as subsequent management when conservative therapy fails. Recently, the robot has been used to aid in the management of endometriosis by allowing the surgeons to see more endometriosis, though this has not been shown in any published reports. One retrospective cohort study by Nezhat et al.[45] compared robotic-assisted laparoscopy with conventional laparoscopic surgery for the treatment of endometriosis in 78 patients. Operative time was longer for the robotic-assisted laparoscopy compared with conventional laparoscopy (191 vs 159 minutes). There were no significant differences in blood loss, hospitalization, or intraoperative and postoperative complications. There were no conversions to laparotomy. To date, there are no studies showing the differences in outcomes for endometriosis and course of the disease between robotic-assisted and conventional laparoscopic surgery. There are limited studies evaluating the role of robotic-assisted surgery for endometriosis.

Siesta et al. performed a 5-year retrospective cohort study to assess the feasibility of using robotic surgery to resect deep infiltrating endometriosis. They evaluated 19 bowel resections, 23 removals of rectovaginal septum nodules, and 5 bladder resections. They did not have any intraoperative complications and reported one anastomotic leak.[46]

In addition, Nezhat et al. compared robotic versus conventional laparoscopy for the treatment of endometriosis. Forty patients were in the robotic group and 38 were in the conventional group. Both groups had similar age, BMI, and stage of endometriosis. There were no significant differences in the 2 groups in terms of blood loss, days in the hospital, and perioperative complications. The mean operating time of the robotic group was slightly higher than the conventional laparoscopy group (191 minutes vs 159 minutes).[47]

VESICOVAGINAL FISTULA

Vesicovaginal fistula (VVF) is a type of female urogenital fistula (UGF). VVF is an abnormal fistulous tract extending between the bladder and the vagina that allows the continuous involuntary discharge of urine into the vaginal vault.

James Marion Sims published his famous discourse on the treatment of VVF in 1852.[48] Sims achieved success on his 30th surgical attempt on a slave named Anarcha.

During the early 20th century, several techniques were used to improve outcome for the repair of VVF. An accurate diagnosis is essential before consideration of repair.

Frequency

In developing countries, the predominant cause of VVF is prolonged obstructed labor (97%). VVFs are associated with marked pressure necrosis, edema, tissue sloughing, and cicatrization. In 1991, the World Health Organization identified the following geographic areas where obstetric fistula prevalence is high: virtually all of Africa and south Asia, the less-developed parts of Oceana, Latin America, the Middle East, remote regions of Central Asia, and isolated areas of the former Soviet Union and Soviet-dominated eastern Europe.[49,50]

The majority of UGFs in developed countries are a consequence of gynecological surgery. Consequently, the incidence may change as surgical management changes. Most authors quote an incidence rate of VVF after total abdominal hysterectomy (TAH) of 0.5–2%, others suggest only a 0.05% incidence rate of injury to either the bladder or ureter. So if injuries to the bladder and ureters occur in roughly 1% of major gynecologic procedures, and approximately 75% are associated with hysterectomy, and if there are about 500,000 hysterectomies performed each year then about 5,000 women will experience an injury.

Lee, in a series of 35,000 hysterectomies, found more than 80% of genitourinary fistulas arose from gynecological surgery for benign disease. Uncomplicated TAH accounted for more than 70% of these surgeries.

Numerous factors contribute to the development of VVF in developing countries, marriage and conception at a young age. In addition, few women are attended by qualified health care professionals or have access to medical facilities during childbirth; their obstructed labor may be protracted for days or weeks.[49,50]

The effect of prolonged impaction of the fetal presenting part in the pelvis is one of the causes of widespread tissue edema, hypoxia, necrosis, and sloughing resulting from prolonged pressure on the soft tissues of the vagina, bladder base, and urethra. Typically in these countries, the UGF is large and involves the bladder, urethra, bladder trigone, and the anterior cervix.

VVFs in developing countries are attributed predominantly to inadvertent bladder injury during pelvic surgery (90%). They involve a relatively small bladder injury leading to smaller VVFs than are observed in developing countries. Such injuries include unrecognized intraoperative injury of the bladder, bladder wall injury from electrocautery or mechanical crushing, and the dissection of the bladder into an incorrect plane, causing avascular necrosis.

The risk of formation of a hematoma or avascular necrosis after a suture is placed through the bladder wall can lead to infection, abscess, and subsequent suture erosion through the bladder wall. This wall defect permits the escape of urine into the vagina. Gynecologic procedures are the most common iatrogenic factor. Symmonds evaluated 800 genitourinary fistulas over a 30-year period at the Mayo Clinic. Of these, 85% of the VVFs were related to pelvic operations and 75% were related to hysterectomy, with more than 50% being secondary to simple uncomplicated total abdominal or vaginal hysterectomy. Symmonds also found that 5% of these VVFs were obstetric and 10% occurred after radiotherapy. Obstetric UGFs in modern centers include vaginal lacerations from forceps rotations, cesarean delivery, hysterectomy, and ruptured uterus.

The other types of pelvic surgery also contribute to the incidence of VVFs; such surgeries include suburethral sling procedures, surgical repair of urethral diverticulum, electrocautery of bladder papilloma, and surgery for pelvic carcinomas. Other less common causes of VVFs include pelvic infections (e.g. tuberculosis, syphilis, lymphogranuloma venereum), vaginal trauma, and vaginal erosion with foreign objects (e.g. neglected pessary). Lastly, a congenital urogenital abnormality may exist that includes a VVF.

Tancer found prior cesarean delivery to be the most common factor predisposing to vault fistula after abdominal surgery in his series of 110 cases; here, 29% were associated with prior cesarean delivery.[51]

Procedure

Robotic assisted VVF repair is done by making four robotic ports. The edges of VVF are freshened; bladder mobilized and separated from vagina. The vagina repaired and bladder repaired separately and in between the omentum is interposed, to prevent residual VVF and recurrence. Post-operative care includes continuous catheterization for 14 days and avoidance of infection. In next pregnancy patient should have elective cesarean section to avoid recurrence of fistula.

CERVICAL CERCLAGE

Cervical insufficiency is a condition which is characterized with painless cervical dilatation and is an important factor causing second trimester pregnancy loss. Cervical insufficiency occurs in 0.5–1% of all pregnancies.[52] Extensive cervical conization, routine dilation and curettage for diagnostic and therapeutic purposes, traumatic cervical lacerations during deliveries, and congenital or DES exposure-related abnormalities may lead to cervical insufficiency.[53]

The vaginal route is the most used surgical method for cervical cerclage. The abdominal approach is usually done if the cervix is too short to attempt a standard cerclage, or if a vaginal cerclage has failed or is not possible. The minimal invasive techniques, such as laparoscopy, have been considered for the abdominal cerclage in the last few years.[54-56] Due to technical difficulties and limitations of the laparoscopic surgery, laparoscopic abdominal cerclage has not gained widespread popularity. Robotic surgery gives the opportunity to surgeons to perform operations requiring advanced suturing techniques and helps to eliminate the technical limitations of the laparoscopic surgery.[57] In robotic assisted abdominal cerclage. da Vinci Si surgical system—four-trocar transperitoneal approach is used for the procedure. The surgical technique is as follows. The vesicouterine peritoneal flap is created and taken down, and then visualization of the uterine vessels bilaterally is done. An avascular area between the uterus and the bifurcation of the uterine artery is prepared. A 5 mm mersilene tape with a flattened needle is sent to the abdominal cavity and is passed medially to the uterine artery from the anterior to the posterior direction. The same procedure is performed at the other side. The passed tape is tied firmly posteriorly. The operation time and console time is approximately 67 and 41 minutes, respectively.

The placement of a transabdominal cervical cerclage has been regarded as considerably more morbid than a transvaginal cerclage. Minimal invasive techniques such as laparoscopy and robotic assisted surgery in the treatment of an incompetent cervix are promising options.[54,58] Barmat et al. reported a case which included the first robotic assisted abdominal cerclage in a nonpregnant woman.[58] In this report, there was no information about the follow-up of the patient to know either of further pregnancy status or successful live birth to assess the success of the robotic abdominal cerclage.

The first robotic-assisted laparoscopic cerclage in a pregnant patient was performed by Fechner et al. in 2009.[59]

The most comprehensive study including robotic assisted abdominal cerclage was reported by Moore et al. in which a total of 24 nonpregnant patients underwent robotic procedure.[60] Only in one case conversion to laparotomy due to dense adhesions was done. The mean operation and console times were reported to be 118 and 58 minutes, respectively. The mean length of hospital stay was less than one day. The robotic surgical outcomes with laparoscopy were compared and found that although the robotic procedure takes additional time to complete and requires longer exposure to anesthesia (155 minutes in robotic group vs 103 minutes in laparoscopy), recovery time (21 hours in robotic group vs 50 hours in laparoscopy group) and blood loss (50 mL in robot vs 150 mL in laparoscopy) reveal a less invasive operation.

There are two reports of robotic-assisted laparoscopic cervical cercalage in the literature. Barmat et al.[58] first reported robotic-assisted laparoscopic placement of an abdominal cercalage. Subsequently robotically placed merselene tape was reported by Fechner in a series of seven patients.[61] Gocmen[62] reported two successful live births after robotic-assisted abdominal cercalage performed in two non-pregnant women.

CONCLUSION

The goal of robotic gynecologic surgery is to use a minimally invasive approach to perform procedures which are generally performed by laparotomy or are too complex for conventional laparoscopy or surgeons who are novices in laparoscopic surgery.

Advantages of robotic over conventional laparoscopy include three-dimensional (3D) imaging, mechanical improvement (e.g. instruments with seven degrees of freedom), stabilization of instruments within the surgical field, and improved ergonomics. The major advantage to the patient is a potentially shorter hospital stay, and more rapid postoperative recovery and return to full function.

The limitations of robotic technology include high costs and increased operating room time, lack of tactile feedback, large size of the devices, and risk of mechanical failure.

Surgical simulation, telementoring (guidance given to the surgeon by another surgeon who is not in the operating room), and telepresence surgery (surgery performed via a robot by a surgeon who is not in the operating room) are potential novel benefits of robotic technology. So, besides using robotic assistance in gynecological malignancies there are many indications to use it for benign gynecological conditions.

REFERENCES

1. Lori Weinberg, Rao S, Escobar PF. Robotic Surgery in Gynecology: An updated systematic Review. Obstetrics and Gynecology International vol. 2011, 29 pages.
2. Sutton C. Past, present, and future of hysterectomy. J Minim Invasive Gynecol. 2010;17(4):421-35.
3. Hewitt M, O'Carroll M, O'Reilly B. Robot-assisted surgery in gynaecology. The Obstetrician & Gynaecologist. 2011;13: 183-8.
4. Gecsi KS, Rivlin ME. Robotic Surgery in Benign Gynecologic Indications, 2015.
5. ACOG Committee Opinion No.628.
6. Hysterectomy Surveillance—United States, 1994-1999. Available at *http://www.cdc.gov/mmwr/preview/mmwrhtml/ss5105a1.htm.*
7. Wu JM, Wechter ME, Geller EJ, Nguyen TV, Visco AG. Hysterectomy rates in the United States, 2003. Obstet Gynecol. 2007;110(5):1091-5. [Medline].
8. AAGL position statement: route of hysterectomy to treat benign uterine disease. J Minim Invasive Gynecol. 2011;18(1):1-3. [Medline].
9. Matthews CA, Reid N, Ramakrishnan V, Hull K, Cohen S. Evaluation of the introduction of robotic technology on route of hysterectomy and complications in the first year of use. Am J Obstet Gynecol. 2010;203: 499.e1-499.e5 (Class II-3).
10. Pasic RP, Rizzo JA, Fang H, Ross S, Moore M, Gunnarsson C. Comparing robot-assisted with conventional laparoscopic hysterectomy: impact on cost and clinical outcomes. J Minim Invasive Gynecol. 2010;17(6):730-8. [Medline].
11. Paraiso MF, Ridgeway B, Park AJ, et al. A randomized trial comparing conventional and robotically assisted total laparoscopic hysterectomy. Am J Obstet Gynecol. 2013;208(5):368.e1-7. [Medline].
12. Journal of Minimally Invasive Gynecology, Vol 20, No 1, January/February 2013.
13. Advincula AP, Song A, Burke W, Reynolds RK. Preliminary experience with robot-assisted laparoscopic myomectomy. J Am Assoc Gynecol Laparosc. 2004;11(4):511-8. [Medline].
14. Advincula AP, Xu X, Goudeau S 4th, Ransom SB. Robot-assisted laparoscopic myomectomy versus abdominal myomectomy: a comparison of short-term surgical outcomes and immediate costs. J Minim Invasive Gynecol. 2007;14(6):698-705. [Medline].
15. Nezhat C, Lavie O, Hsu S, Watson J, Barnett O, Lemyre M. Robotic-assisted laparoscopic myomectomy compared with standard laparoscopic myomectomy—a retrospective matched control study. Fertil Steril. 2009;91(2):556-9. [Medline].
16. Barakat EE, Bedaiwy MA, Zimberg S, Nutter B, Nosseir M, Falcone T. Robotic-assisted, laparoscopic, and abdominal myomectomy: a comparison of surgical outcomes. Obstet Gynecol. 2011;117(2 Pt 1):256-65. [Medline].
17. George A, Eisenstein D, Wegienka G. Analysis of the impact of body mass index on the surgical outcomes after robot-assisted laparoscopic myomectomy. J Minim Invasive Gynecol. 2009;16(6):730-3. [Medline].
18. Bocca S, Stadtmauer L, Oehninger S. Uncomplicated full term pregnancy after da Vinci-assisted laparoscopic myomectomy. Reprod Biomed Online. 2007;14(2):246-9. [Medline].
19. Abelha Mde C, Costa RR, Lopes VM, Reis RC, Silva CM. Tubal reanastomosis: Analysis of the results of 30 years of treatment. Rev Bras Ginecol Obstet. 2008;30:294-9.
20. Margossian H, Garcia-Ruiz A, Falcone T, Goldberg JM, Attaran M, Gagner M. Robotically assisted laparoscopic microsurgical uterine horn anastomosis. Fertil Steril. 1998;70:530-4.
21. Degueldre M, Vandromme J, Huong PT, Cadière GB. Robotically assisted laparoscopic microsurgical tubal reanastomosis: A feasibility study. Fertil Steril. 2000;74:1020-3.
22. Dharia SP, Steinkampf M, Whitten SJ. ESHRE Annual Meeting. Berlin, Germany: 2004. Robotically assisted tubal reanastomosis in a Fellowship Training program (Abstract)
23. Rodgers AK, Goldberg JM, Hammel JP, Falcone T. Tubal anastomosis by robotic compared with outpatient minilaparotomy. Obstet Gynecol. 2007;109:1375-80.
24. Haylen BT, de Ridder D, Freeman RM, Swift SE, Berghmans B, Lee J, et al. An International Urogynecological Association (IUGA)/International Continence Society (ICS) joint report on the terminology for female pelvic floor dysfunction. Neurourol Urodyn. 2010;29(1):4-20.
25. Abrams P, Andersson KE, Birder L, Brubaker L, Cardozo L, Chapple C, et al. Fourth International Consultation on Incontinence Recommendations of the International Scientific Committee: Evaluation and treatment of urinary incontinence, pelvic organ prolapse, and fecal incontinence. Neurourol Urodyn. 2010;29(1):213-40.
26. Handa VL, Garrett E, Hendrix S, Gold E, Robbins J. Progression and remission of pelvic organ prolapse: a longitudinal study of menopausal women. Am J Obstet Gynecol. 2004;190(1):27-32.
27. Hendrix SL, Clark A, Nygaard I, Aragaki A, Barnabei V, McTiernan A. Pelvic organ prolapse in the Women's Health Initiative: gravity and gravidity. Am J Obstet Gynecol. 2002;186(6):1160-6.
28. Swift S, Woodman P, O'Boyle A, Kahn M, Valley M, Bland D, et al. Pelvic Organ Support Study (POSST): the distribution, clinical definition, and epidemiologic condition of pelvic organ support defects. Am J Obstet Gynecol. 2005;192(3):795-806.
29. Nygaard I, Bradley C, Brandt D. Pelvic organ prolapse in older women: prevalence and risk factors. Obstet Gynecol. 2004;104(3):489-97.
30. Olsen AL, Smith VJ, Bergstrom JO, Colling JC, Clark AL. Epidemiology of surgically managed pelvic organ prolapse and urinary incontinence. Obstet Gynecol. 1997;89(4):501-6.
31. Smith FJ, Holman CD, Moorin RE, Tsokos N. Lifetime risk of undergoing surgery for pelvic organ prolapse. Obstet Gynecol. 2010;116(5):1096-100.
32. Haylen BT, de Ridder D, Freeman RM, Swift SE, Berghmans B, Lee J, et al. An International Urogynecological Association (IUGA)/International Continence Society (ICS) joint report on the terminology for female pelvic floor dysfunction. Neurourol Urodyn. 2010;29(1):4-20.
33. Weber AM, Richter HE. Pelvic organ prolapse. Obstet Gynecol. 2005;106(3):615-34.
34. Brubaker L, Nygaard I, Richter HE, Visco A, Weber AM, Cundiff GW, et al. Two-year outcomes after sacrocolpopexy with and without burch to prevent stress urinary incontinence. Obstet Gynecol. 2008;112(1):49-55.
35. Begley JS, Kupferman SP, Kuznetsov DD, Kobashi KC, Govier FE, McGonigle KF, et al. Incidence and management of abdominal sacrocolpopexy mesh erosions. Am J Obstet Gynecol. 2005;192(6):1956-62.

36. Nygaard IE, McCreery R, Brubaker L, Connolly A, Cundiff G, Weber AM, et al. Abdominal sacrocolpopexy: a comprehensive review. Obstet Gynecol. 2004;104(4):805-23.
37. Ferry P, Sedille L, Roncheau V. Rectal Mesh Exposure Following Laparoscopic Sacrocolpopexy. J Minim Invasive Gynecol. 2013.
38. Kohli N, Walsh PM, Roat TW, Karram MM. Mesh erosion after abdominal sacrocolpopexy. Obstet Gynecol. 1998;92(6): 999-1004.
39. Beverly CM, Walters MD, Weber AM, Piedmonte MR, Ballard LA. Prevalence of hydronephrosis in patients undergoing surgery for pelvic organ prolapse. Obstet Gynecol. 1997;90(1):37-41.
40. Geller EJ, Siddiqui NY, Wu JM, Visco AG. Short-term outcomes of robotic sacrocolpopexy compared with abdominal sacrocolpopexy. Obstet Gynecol. 2008;112(6):1201-6. [Medline].
41. Elliott DS, Frank I, Dimarco DS, Chow GK. Gynecologic use of robotically assisted laparoscopy: Sacrocolpopexy for the treatment of high-grade vaginal vault prolapse. Am J Surg. 2004; 188(4A Suppl):52S-56S. [Medline].
42. Paraiso MF, Jelovsek JE, Frick A, Chen CC, Barber MD. Laparoscopic compared with robotic sacrocolpopexy for vaginal prolapse: a randomized controlled trial. Obstet Gynecol. 2011;118(5):1005-13. [Medline].
43. Ramavath KK, Murthy PS. Robotic sacrocolpopexy: An observational experience at mayoclinic, USA. J Gynecol Endosc Surg. 2011;2:53-7.
44. Akl MN, Long JB, Giles DL, Cornella JL, Pettit PD, Chen AH, et al. Robotic-assisted sacrocolpopexy: Technique and learing curve. Surg Endosc. 2009;23:2390-4.
45. Nezhat C, Lewis M, Kotikela S, Veeraswamy A, Saadat L, Hajhosseini B. Robotic versus standard laparoscopy for the treatment of endometriosis. Fertil Steril. 2010;94:2758-60 (Class II-2).
46. Siesto G, Ieda N, Rosati R, Vitobello D. Robotic surgery for deep endometriosis: a paradigm shift. Int J Med Robot. 2013;[Medline].
47. Nezhat C, Lewis M, Kotikela S, et al. Robotic versus standard laparoscopy for the treatment of endometriosis. Fertil Steril. 2010;94(7):2758-60. [Medline].
48. Sims JM. On the treatment of vesico-vaginal fistula. 1852. Int Urogynecol J Pelvic Floor Dysfunct. 1998;9(4):236-48. [Medline].
49. Capes T, Ascher-Walsh C, Abdoulaye I, Brodman M. Obstetric fistula in low and middle income countries. Mt Sinai J Med. 2011; 78(3):352-61. [Medline].
50. Tebeu PM, Fomulu JN, Khaddaj S, de Bernis L, Delvaux T, Rochat CH. Risk factors for obstetric fistula: a clinical review. Int Urogynecol J. 2011 [Medline].
51. Tancer ML. Observations on prevention and management of vesicovaginal fistula after total hysterectomy. Surg Gynecol Obstet. 1992;175(6):501-6. [Medline].
52. DaCosta V, Wynter S, Harriott J, Christie L, Frederick J, Frederick-Johnston S. Laparoscopic cervicoisthmic cerclage for the treatment of cervical incompetence: case reports. West Indian Medical Journal. 2011;60(5):590-3.
53. Anum EA, Brown HL, Strauss III JF. Health disparities in risk for cervical insufficiency. Human Reproduction. 2010;25(11): 2894-2900.
54. Al-Fadhli R, Tulandi T. Laparoscopic abdominal cerclage," Obstetrics and Gynecology Clinics of North America. 2004;31(3): 497-504.
55. Ghomi A, Rodgers B. Laparoscopic abdominal cerclage during pregnancy: a case report and a review of the described operative techniques," J Mini Inv Gynec. 2006;13(4):337-41.
56. Carter JF, Soper DE. Laparoscopic abdominal cerclage. Journal of the Society of Laparoendoscopic Surgeons. 2005;9(4):491-3.
57. Schreuder HWR, Verheijen RHM. Robotic surgery. An Int J Obs Gyn. 2009;116(2):198-213.
58. Barmat L, Glaser G, Davis G, Craparo F. Da Vinci-assisted abdominal cerclage. Fertil Steril. 2007;88:1437.
59. Fechner AJ, Alvarez M, Smith DH, Al-Khan A. Robotic-assisted laparoscopic cerclage in a pregnant patient. Am J Obs Gyn. 2008; 200(2):e10-e11.
60. Moore ES, Foster TL, McHugh K, Addleman RN, Sumners JE. Robotic-assisted transabdominal cerclage (RoboTAC) in the non-pregnant patient. J Obs Gyn. 2012;32(7):643-7.
61. Fechner AJ, Alvarez M, Smith DH, Al-Khan A. Robotic-assisted laparoscopic cerclage in a pregnant patient. Am J Obstet Gynecol. 2009;200:e10-1.
62. Göçmen A, Sanlýkan F. Two Live Births following Robotic-Assisted Abdominal Cerclage in Nonpregnant Women. Case Rep Obstet Gynecol. 2013;2013:256972.

CHAPTER

17

Sentinel Node Mapping in Gynecological Cancers

Anupama Rajanbabu

INTRODUCTION

Lymph node status is one of the most important prognostic factors in early cervical and endometrial cancers. But lymphadenectomy is associated with increased operating time, intraoperative complications such as vessel and nerve injury as well as long-term complications like lymphedema and lymph cyst formation. Sentinel lymph node (SLN) is the first node to which an organ drains and it will be the first node to which metastatic disease will spread from the primary tumor. SLN mapping and biopsy will enable the clinician to get the necessary prognostic information about lymph nodal involvement while reducing the surgical and long-term morbidity associated with a complete lymphadenectomy. SLN mapping is an accepted technique in the management of breast cancer and melanoma. In Gynecologic cancers, SLN mapping is accepted for vulvar cancers and is now being increasingly utilized in the management of cervical and uterine cancer. This chapter will be dealing with the technique and evidence for robotic sentinel node mapping in cervical and endometrial cancers.

BACKGROUND

Complete pelvic lymphadenectomy is the current standard of care in surgery for cervical cancer. In inoperable cervical cancers the rate of lymph node involvement is 0–4.8% in Stage I A, and 17% in Stage I B.[1] So, over 80% of women who undergo lymphadenectomy do not benefit from the procedure and may suffer the adverse affects related to it.

Lymphadenectomy in endometrial cancer is a topic of ongoing debate. In endometrial cancer, practice of lymphadenectomy is variable worldwide ranging from no lymphadenectomy or selective nodal sampling to pelvic lymphadenectomy alone, or complete pelvic and para-aortic lymphadenectomy up to the level of renal vessels. Though retrospective series have shown survival advantage for lymphadenectomy,[2] the two randomized clinical trials that looked into systematic lymphadenectomy failed to show any survival advantage.[3-5]

Use of sentinel node mapping was first described by Cabanas in the management of penile cancer.[1] It was widely used after the study on melanoma by Morton et al.[6] and is currently approved and accepted in the management of breast cancer, vulvar cancer and melanomas. In early cervical and endometrial cancers sentinel node mapping has been tried with blue dye (methylene blue or isosulphan blue) and radioactive technetium alone or in combination with detection rates of about 80%.[7-9] Recently, immunofluorescent imaging using indocyanine green (ICG) injection and near infrared (NIR) fluorescent imaging using endoscopic/robotic fluorescent imaging system has been used which gave detection rates above 95%.[10,11] In addition to the high detection rates it has excellent sensitivity and high negative predictive value.[12] Since 2014 the NCCN guidelines have incorporated sentinel node mapping in the surgical management of endometrial cancer provided the algorithm by Barlin et al. is adhered to.[13] This algorithm developed at Memorial Sloan Kettering Cancer Centre, New York, states that any enlarged or suspicious looking nodes should be removed irrespective to whether they are mapped or not, and if sentinel node is not mapped on one side, complete lymphadenectomy should be done on that side.

Another advantage of identifying and removing the sentinel nodes is that, during histopathology examination, these nodes can be ultra staged. Ultra staging is a technique where multiple serial sections are taken perpendicular to the long axis of the node and stained with cytokeratin for immunohistochemistry in addition to the hematoxylin and eosin (H & E) stain. This helps in the identification of micrometastasis which otherwise would not have been detected in the routine H & E stain.

TECHNIQUE OF SENTINEL LYMPH NODE MAPPING USING INDOCYANINE GREEN

Preparing ICG Dye for Injection

Indocyanine green (ICG) dye is available as a sterile powder vial with each vial containing 25 mg of ICG. It is diluted

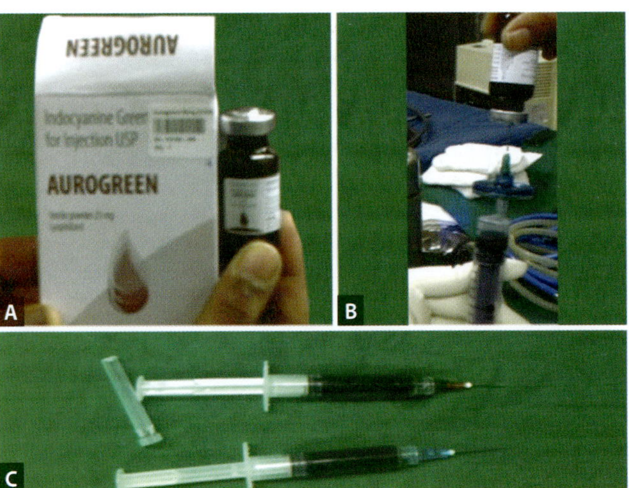

Figs 17.1A to C: (A) Indocyanine green dye; (B) Dilution to 0.5% solution; (C) Loaded for injection

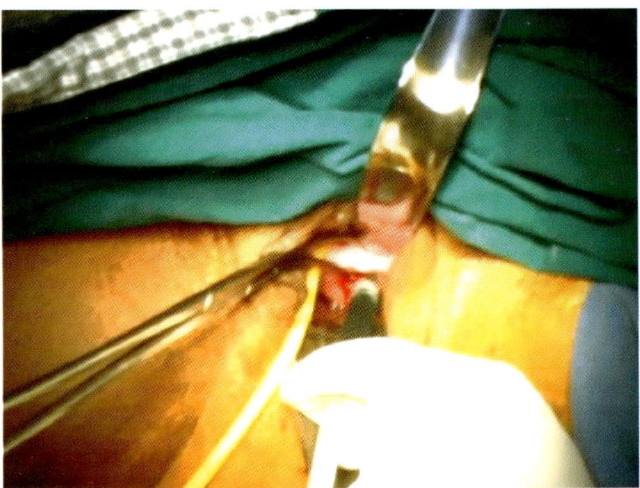

Fig. 17.2: Indocyanine green dye being injected into the cervix at 3 o'clock position

with aqueous sterile water to get the desired concentration **(Figs 17.1A to C)**. Researchers have used different concentrations ranging from 0.5 to 1.25 mg/mL. In our experience a concentration of 0.5 mg/mL gives adequate immunofluorescence for detecting the sentinel nodes. No studies have reported any adverse reactions from using ICG dye for SLN mapping. ICG contains sodium iodide and use is not recommended in patients allergic to iodides.

Site of Injection

Traditionally, the dye for SLN mapping is injected around the tumor. In case of endometrial cancers, the tumor is not visible from outside and in the initial phases, hysteroscopic injections and injection to the uterine fundus was tried in addition to cervical injection in order to improve detection rates. Studies have now shown that injection into the deep cervical stroma results in diffusion of dye throughout the uterus and can give an accurate assessment of the uterine sentinel nodes.[12] With a 22 Gauge spinal needle, 1 mL each of dye is injected at 3o'clock and 9o'clock position in the cervix superficially and also deep into the cervical stroma **(Fig. 17.2)**. We do the injection after induction of anesthesia and placement of all robotic ports. If a uterine manipulator is used, it can be placed after the injection. We apply an anchoring stich on the cervix with a No.1 prolene and apply a vaginal tube.

SLN Mapping

After docking and placing the robotic instruments, the peritoneal cavity is inspected. The NIR imaging is activated to see any fluorescent lymphatic or nodes. It will be possible to see the fluorescent lymphatics and nodes through undissected tissue in thin patients. Then the retroperitoneal spaces are opened up. These steps usually take about 15–30 minutes. Any enlarged suspicious lymph nodes are noted. The NIR imaging system (Firefly system) is activated. The lymphatics will be seen traversing the parametrium from the site of injection to the regional nodes **(Figs 17.3A and B)**. Careful inspection must be made at this point to identify the first draining node, which will be the sentinel node **(Figs 17.4A and B)**. If a pelvic sentinel is not seen, thorough inspection of the para-aortic area and also unusual areas of sentinel node like pre sacral area are done under fluorescence imaging. If sentinel node cannot be identified bilaterally or unilaterally, complete node dissection of the side where it was not seen must be done. In addition any enlarged or suspicious looking nodes are removed.

Sentinel Node Mapping Using Blue and/or Technetium-99

Methylene blue or Isosulphan blue alone or in combination with radioactive technetium is also being used. The injection is done on the cervix in the same way as described above for ICG. The blue color can be identified after dissection of the retroperitoneal spaces. Laparoscopic gamma probe inserted through the assistant trocar site can be helpful in identifying the radioactivity. Study comparing all three modalities has shown that ICG has a better detection rate when compared to blue dye and similar detection rates as compared to Technetium-99.[13]

Advantages of ICG

Blue dye can cause allergic reactions and even anaphylaxis and Tc-99 is a radioactive product, ICG is safer and so far no allergic reactions have been reported with its use for sentinel node mapping. ICG stays in the lymph node better than blue dye and does not leak out while dissecting. In obese patients ICG with its bright green color offers better visualization that blue dye.

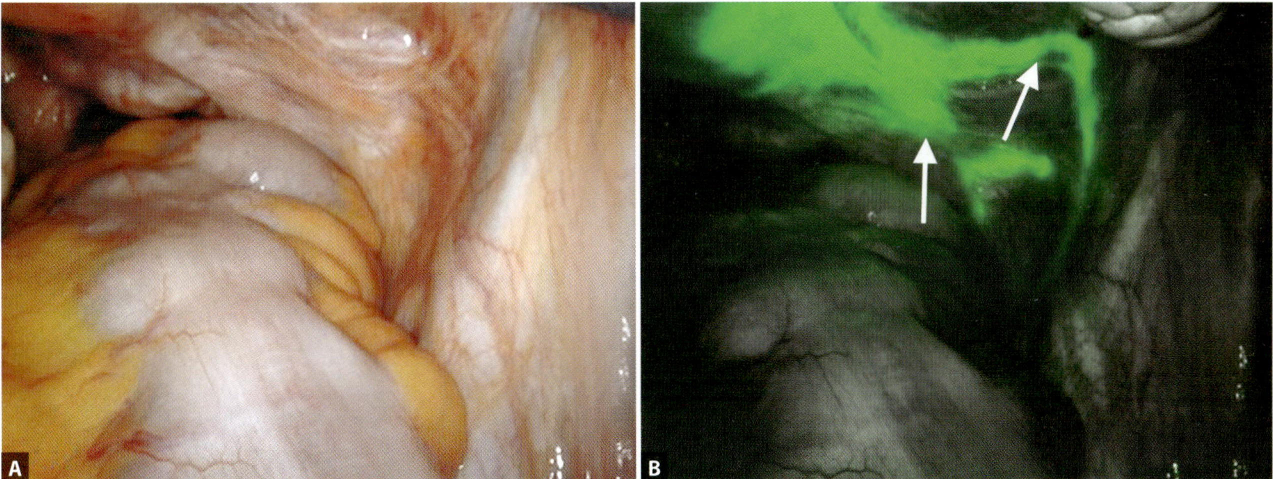

Figs 17.3A to B: Right parametrium under normal light (A) and with NIR imaging; (B) showing fluorescent lymphatics

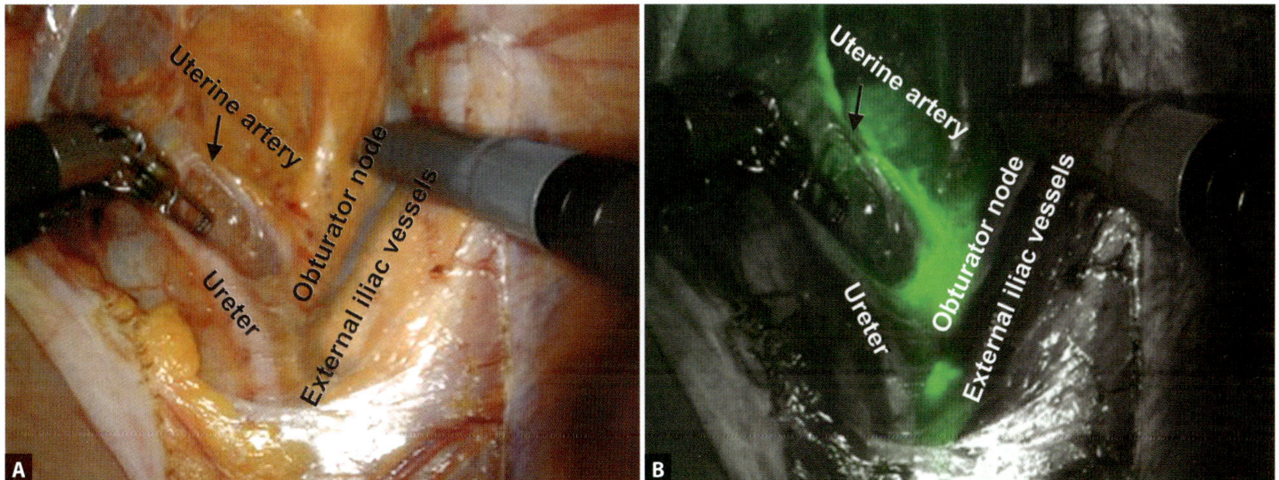

Figs 17.4A and B: Right obturator sentinel node and lymphatics traveling along uterine artery seen

LEARNING CURVE

As for any procedure, there is a learning curve associated with SLN mapping also. Khoury-Collado F et al.[14] has shown that SLN mapping has got a learning curve of at least 30 cases. Although the learning may vary from surgeon to surgeon, in the initial learning curve it is advisable not to deviate from the standard surgical protocols for lymph node mapping. When we started SLN mapping, we completed the lymphadenectomy even if the nodes did not light up. After 20 cases, our analysis showed a detection rate of 90% with 100% sensitivity to detect affected nodes.

SUMMARY

Sentinel node mapping is emerging as a technique that can replace complete lymphadenectomy in early cervical or endometrial cancer patients undergoing surgical staging. It can help decrease the complications due to lymphadenectomies and also help the pathologist to focus on a smaller number of nodes and detect micro metastasis with the help of ultra staging. ICG dye has got good safety profile and the technique of intracervical ICG injection followed by fluorescent imaging is simple and easy to reproduce and has high detection rates with excellent sensitivity and negative predictive value.

REFERENCES

1. Wu Y, Li Z, Wu H, Yu J. Sentinel lymph node biopsy in cervical cancer: A meta-analysis. Molecular and Clinical Oncology. 2013;1(6):1025-30.
2. Chino JP, Jones E, Berchuck A, et al. The influence of radiation modality and lymph node dissection on survival in early – stage endometrial cancer. Int J Radiation Oncology Biol. 2012; 82(5):1872-9.

3. Kitchener H, Swart AM, Qian Q, Amos C, Parmar MK. Efficacy of systematic pelvic lymphadenectomy in endometrial cancer (MRC ASTEC trial): a randomised study. Lancet. 2009;373:125-36.
4. Benedetti Panici P, Basile S, Maneschi F, et al. Systematic pelvic lymphadenectomy vs no lymphadenectomy in early-stage endometrial carcinoma: randomized clinical trial. J Natl Cancer Inst. 2008;100:1707-16.
5. Cabanas RM. An approach for the treatment of penile carcinoma. Cancer. 1977;39:456-66.
6. Morton DL, Wen DR, Wong JH, Economou JS, Cagle LA, Storm FK, et al. Technical details of intraoperative lymphatic mapping for early stage melanoma. Arch Surg. 1992;127:392-9.
7. Pieterse QD, Kenter GG, Gaarenstroom KN, Peters AA, Willems SM, Fleuren GJ, et al. The number of pelvic lymph nodes in the quality control and prognosis of radical hysterectomy for the treatment of cervical cancer. Eur J Surg Oncol. 2007;33:216-21.
8. Ballester M, Dubernard G, Rouzier R, Barranger E, Darai E. Use of the sentinel node procedure to stage endometrial cancer. Ann Surg Oncol. 2008;15:1523-9.
9. Schneider A. The sentinel concept in patients with cervical cancer. J Surg Oncol. 2007;96:337-41.
10. Jewell EL, Huang JJ, Abu-Rustum NR, Gardner GJ, Brown CL, Sonoda Y, Leitao MM. Detection of sentinel lymph nodes in minimally invasive surgery using indocyanine green and near-infrared fluorescence imaging for uterine and cervical malignancies. Gynecologic Oncology. 2014;133(2):274-7.
11. Plante M, Touhami O, Trinh XB, Renaud MC, Sebastianelli A, Grondin K, Gregoire J. Sentinel node mapping with indocyanine green and endoscopic near-infrared fluorescence imaging in endometrial cancer: A pilot study and review of the literature. Gynecologic Oncology. 2015;137(3):443-7.
12. How J, Gotlieb WH, Press JZ, et al. Comparing indocyanine green, technetium, and blue dye for sentinel lymph node mapping in endometrial cancer. Gynecologic Oncology. 2015;137(3):436-42.
13. The National Comprehensive Cancer Network guidelines. Uterine Neoplasms. Available at: http://www.nccn.org. Retrieved September 16, 2015.
14. Khoury-Collado F, Glaser GE, Zivanovic O, Sonoda Y, Levine DA, Chi DS, et al. Improving sentinel lymph node detection rates in endometrial cancer: how many cases are needed? Gynecol Oncol. 2009;115(3):453-5.

CHAPTER

18

Robotic Staging Surgery for Endometrial Cancer

Anupama Rajanbabu

INTRODUCTION

Endometrial cancer is the seventh most common cancer in women worldwide.[1] The incidence of endometrial cancer though low in India as compared to the western population, is steadily rising due to urbanization and changes in lifestyle.[2] Approximately 34,000 women will be affected with endometrial cancer in India by 2020.[2] Presently endometrial cancers are surgically staged according to the joint 2010 International Federation of Gynecology and Obstetrics (FIGO)/Tumor Node Metastases (TNM) classification system.[3,4] The surgical staging includes total hysterectomy (radical hysterectomy in case of cervical involvement), bilateral salpingo-oophorectomy, pelvic and para-aortic lymphadenectomy and omentectomy with peritoneal biopsies for serous and clear cell histologic types.[5]

Minimally invasive surgery for endometrial cancer began in 1993, with Childers, et al. describing laparoscopic hysterectomy with pelvic and para-aortic lymphadenectomy for endometrial cancer.[6] The landmark Gynecologic Oncology Group (GOG) LAP2 randomized trial showed that laparoscopy can give the same surgical clearance as laparotomy in endometrial cancers with similar survival rates and a superior quality of life.[7-9] However, there is a steep learning curve associated with advanced laparoscopic surgery. Laparoscopy has therefore, been used in a lesser proportion of patients with endometrial cancers.[10]

In USA, the Food and Drug Administration (FDA) approved the use of robots for gynecological surgeries in 2005. In contrast to laparoscopy, the robot became more universally accepted and by 2010 about 50% of the endometrial cancer staging procedures in USA were being done with robotic assistance.[11] Another significant advantage that robotic-assisted surgery had over laparoscopy was a reduced conversion rate to laparotomy.[12]

PREOPERATIVE EVALUATION AND PREPARATION

Most of the patients who are candidates for open staging surgery will be eligible to undergo robotic staging surgery. Imaging of the pelvis and abdomen (Ultrasonography/computed tomography/magnetic resonance imaging [USG/CT/MRI]) is helpful to rule out extra uterine disease and cervical involvement.

The patient is allowed to have a normal diet until the midnight prior to the day of surgery. Bowel preparation is limited to a proctoclysis enema on the morning of surgery. Thromboprophylaxis is started on the night prior to surgery with low molecular weight heparin in a weight-adjusted dose. Prophylactic antibiotic is given at the time of induction of anesthesia.

PATIENT POSITIONING

After induction of anesthesia, patient is placed in dorsal lithotomy position with buttocks just beyond the edge of the table and legs placed in Allen stirrups. Thromboembolic deterrent (TED) stockings and pneumatic compression devices on legs can help prevent venous stasis and thrombosis in legs.

Both arms of the patient are tucked by her sides. This allows maximum space for the robotic arms and the patient side surgeon. After tucking of the arms, care must be taken to ensure that intravenous catheters placed on the arms are functioning well, as it may be difficult to gain access to them once the robotic arms are docked.

For pelvic surgeries, the patient is kept in a steep Trendelenburg position with a 20–30° tilt of the table. It is important to take precautions, so that patient does not slide of the operating table.

The following precautions can be used:

- Reusable gel mattress on the operating table which reduces patient sliding
- Shoulder braces with gel pads
- 'Memory' foam, 'Eggcrate' foam or vaccuum 'bean bag' mattresses
- Strapping the patient to the operating table over cotton pads kept over the chest and upper arms. The strapping can be done with cloth straps or leucoplast **(Figs 18.1A to C)**.

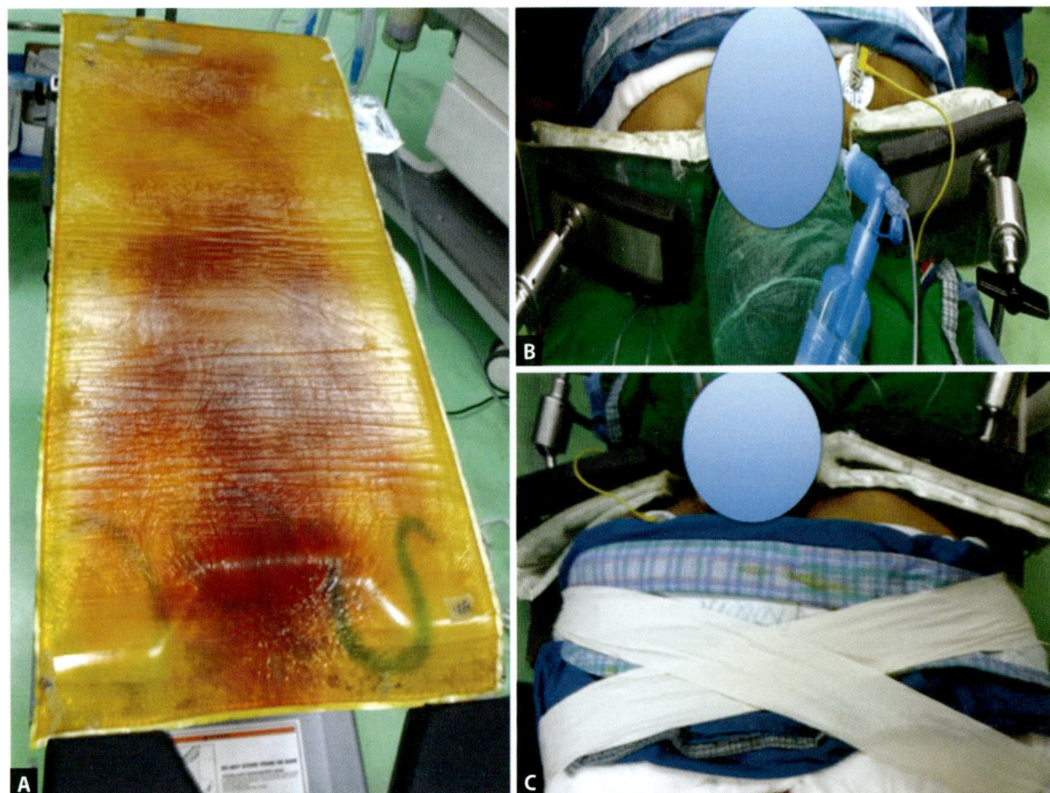

Figs 18.1A to C: (A) Gel mattress on operating table; (B) Shoulder braces; (C) Patient strapping technique

Before the start of surgery, it might be prudent to ensure that a vascular set is kept ready in the operating room, so that in case of any inadvertent vascular injury, speedy action can be taken.

UTERINE MANIPULATOR

A good uterine manipulator is a great help in uterine surgery. It can give good retraction for parametrial dissection and also, the vaginal cup when pushed in, will help the surgeon in colpotomy. The use of uterine manipulator in endometrial cancer patients was thought to disseminate cancer cells from the endometrial cavity through fallopian tubes into the peritoneum. Many surgeons practice sealing of the fallopian tubes at the beginning of surgery although there is no definite evidence to support the incidence of peritoneal seeding through manipulation.[13] Different manipulators are available. Among them, the most popular are: V Care (Vaginal-Cervical Ahluwalia Retractor Elevator), Clermont-Ferrant manipulator and ZUMI with KOH rings. Surgery can be done without an intrauterine manipulator in which case the prograsp forceps is used to retract the uterus during surgery. We do not use an intrauterine manipulator during endometrial cancer surgery. Instead, No.1 prolene stitch placed on the cervix anchors the specimen and a vaginal tube aids colpotomy.

PORT PLACEMENT

We start by placing the assistant trocar at Palmer's point using an Optiview trocar. Before port placement, the port site is anesthetized with 0.5% bupivacaine solution (pre-emptive analgesia). After making a skin incision, the trocar is inserted under direct camera vision into the peritoneal cavity. Once placed intraperitoneally, CO_2 insufflation is done to a pressure of 15 mm Hg. Alternatively, pneumoperitoneum can be created using a Verres needle before trocar placement.

The da Vinci Xi surgical system has four 8 mm trocars. The camera trocar is the first robotic trocar to be inserted and should be ideally placed 10–15 cm from target anatomy. This will approximately be just above the level of the umbilicus in a normal sized uterus. The camera port can be placed higher up if para-aortic lymphadenectomy is planned. All the ports are placed in a straight-line lateral to the camera ports to create the maximum working space in the Xi system. Two ports are placed to the right of the camera port keeping a distance of 6–8 cm between them. The markings for the placement of ports are done after CO_2 insufflation. On the left side, one 8 mm port is placed at a distance of 6–8 cm from the camera port and at least 8 cm away from the assistant port. All the ports should be 2 cm or more away from bony prominences and they should not be placed between the target anatomy and other ports **(Figs 18.2 and 18.3)**.

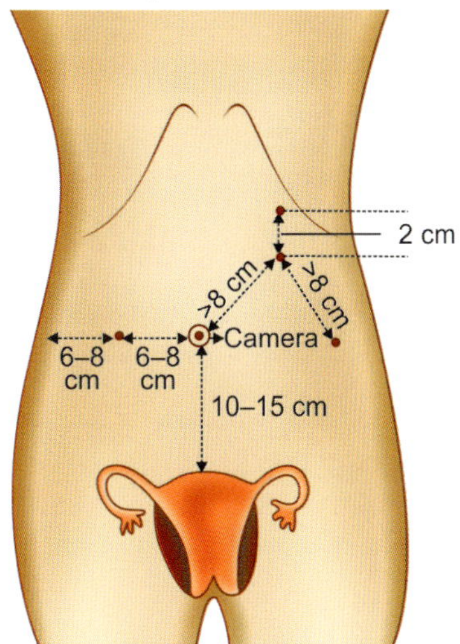

Fig. 18.2: Port placement for gynec surgery in da Vinci Xi

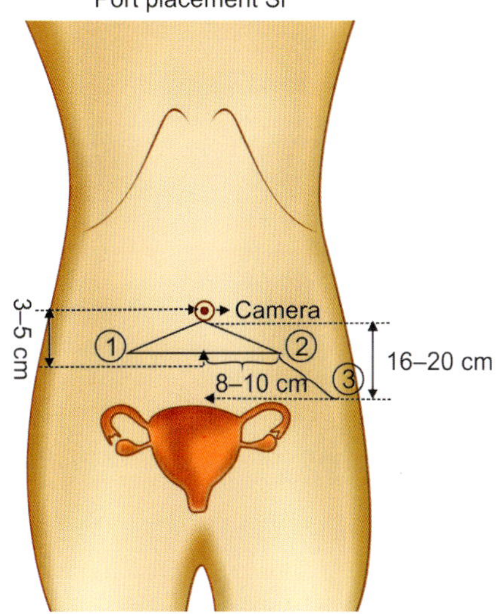

Fig. 18.3: Port placement for gynec surgery in da Vinci Si

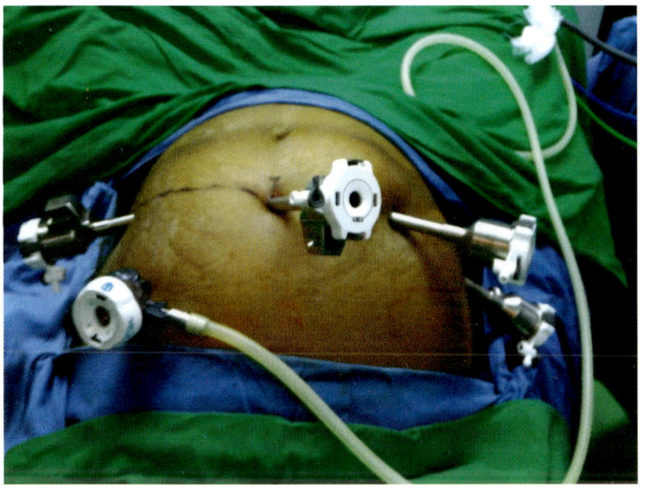

Fig. 18.4: Port placement in the patient in da Vinci Xi

If a da Vinci Si or S system is used, the 12 mm camera port is placed at a distance of 16–20 cm from target anatomy. Arm 1, is placed on the patient's right side 8–10 cm lateral and 3–5 cm inferior to the camera port. The second instrument arm is placed on the patients' left side 8–10 cm lateral and 3–5 cm inferior to the camera port. The third instrument port is placed 8–10 cm from the left instrument port in a diagonal line, 1–2 cm superior to the anterior superior iliac spine **(Fig. 18.4)**.

The remote center on the robotic cannula must be placed at the level of peritoneum. Once all the ports are inserted, complete visual inspection of the abdominal cavity is done and the patient is placed in a steep Trendelenburg position with adequate tilt as to keep the bowel loops away from pelvis. Small bowel loops are flipped over to the upper abdomen, fully exposing the line of mesenteric attachment and aortic bifurcation. The flipping and eversion of bowel on its mesenteric attachment prevents the bowel from falling down into the pelvis. A 5″ × 5″ surgical gauze can be kept as a sling around the root of mesentery if the bowel tends to fall back. However, this is tricky as, if displaced, may be difficult to find in the brand life. If you do keep it, ensure that the circulating reverse has made a note of it and informs you at this end of the procedure the intra-abdominal pressure is reduced to 12 mm Hg after this step. Pelvic washings are given and fluid taken for cytology.

DOCKING

The da Vinci Xi patient cart can be docked from the right or the left side of the patient depending upon the space available in the operating room (OR). Ideally the docking side must be opposite to where the assistant trocar is placed, but same side docking as the assistant trocar is also feasible. Central docking is not usually done, as we need space for uterine manipulation and removal of the specimen. The table height is adjusted to as low as possible and the Trendelenburg position with optimum tilt for bowel retraction maintained. The patient cart is then 'deployed' for docking, its arms raised to clear the patient legs and driven to position the green laser crosshairs on the camera port. Before connecting the Arm 2 to the camera port ensure that the arm is between the letters L and E of the overhead beam with FLEX written on it **(Fig. 18.5)**. This allows for optimal movement of the robotic arms during surgery. 'Targeting' is performed after docking and inserting the robotic camera. The remaining arms are then docked and patient clearance and instrument clearance are adjusted as optimally as possible to allow maximum range of motion to the robotic arms without a clash. Adjustment of the robotic arms is done in such a way that the arms are close together but not touching each other during

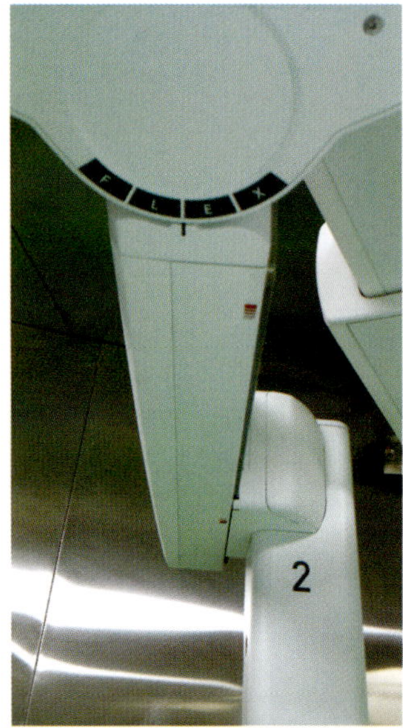

Fig. 18.5: Camera arm positioned between L and E

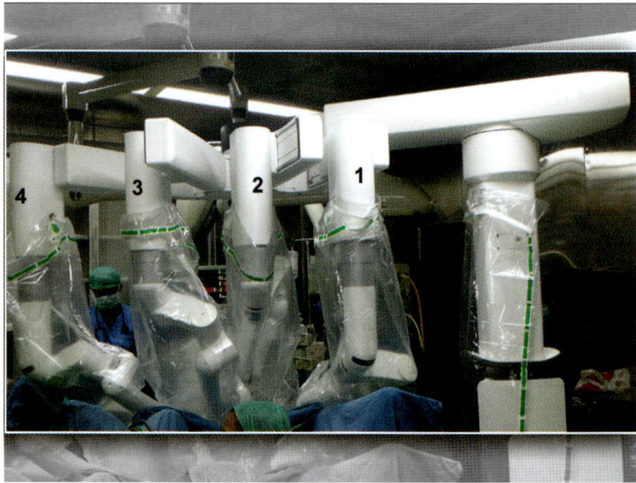

Fig. 18.6: Robotic arms after docking in da Vinci Xi

movement **(Fig. 18.6)**. This is in contrast to that of Si system where after docking, maximum space is ensured between the patient arms. For doing a high para-aortic lymphadenectomy, the arms are undocked; the boom is rotated towards the new target organ, following which the new anatomic area is targeted and the machine docked again.

INSTRUMENT PLACEMENT

The instruments used for robotic staging surgery are: monopolar curved scissors (hot shears), fenestrated bipolar forceps or Maryland bipolar forceps, prograsp forceps and a large or Megacut needle driver. For hysterectomy, a 0 or 30° scope can be used but for pelvic and para-aortic lymphadenectomy, the 30° scope is better. In the Xi system for pelvic surgery, the bipolar forceps is placed on Arm 1 to the left of camera; monopolar scissors comes in Arm 3 and prograsp forceps on Arm 4 **(Fig. 18.7)**. During high para-aortic node dissection, after docking for upper abdomen, the camera is placed in Arm 2, prograsp in Arm 1, Maryland bipolar in Arm 3 and monopolar scissors in Arm 4 for optimum use. In the Si system, for pelvic surgery, hot shears are used in Arm 1, bipolar forceps in Arm 2 and prograsp forceps in Arm 3.

CAUTERY SETTINGS

The da Vinci Xi system uses the ERBE VIO dV electrosurgery system. The following settings were found to give optimal results during surgery:

- Bipolar kept at 'Soft Coag' with a strength of 3
- Monopolar cutting kept on 'Dry Cut' with a strength of 4 and
- Monopolar coagulation kept on 'Swift Coag' with a strength of 4.

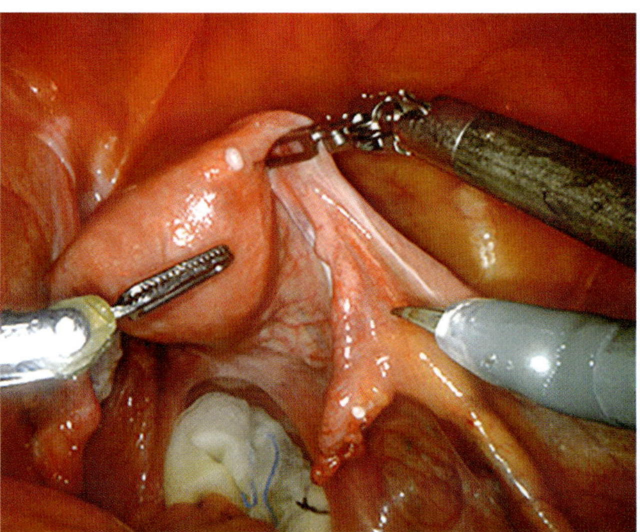

Fig. 18.7: Placement of arms for hysterectomy

SURGICAL TECHNIQUE

Uterus is retracted to one side with the help of uterine retractor and prograsp forceps holding the round ligament close to the uterine cornua. This stretches out the peritoneum nicely which forms a triangle with round ligament anteriorly, infundibulopelvic and ovarian ligament medially and the external iliac vessels laterally. The stretched peritoneum is incised and the incision is carried parallel to the infundibulopelvic ligament opening up the retroperitoneal space.

The next step is developing the paravesical and pararectal spaces. Pararectal space is bounded by the ureter medially, internal iliac vessels laterally, uterine artery anteriorly and the sacrum posteriorly. The opened up retroperitoneal space is developed further with gentle traction and counter traction similar to that of open surgery. The amount of traction exerted should be guided by the visual feedback due to the lack of haptics in the robotic system. A steady traction on the broad ligament medially close to the ureter by the assistant will help in the development of pararectal space. The dissection is carried on to develop the paravesical space which is bounded by the obliterated umbilical artery medially, external iliac vessels and obturator area laterally, pubis anteriorly and uterine artery posteriorly. The obliterated umbilical artery can be held with prograsp forceps and moved medially to expose the area and as for pararectal space. After the development of both the spaces, uterine artery will be nicely seen originating from the internal iliac artery and it can be coagulated/clipped and divided if radical hysterectomy is planned.

HYSTERECTOMY

A window is made on the medial leaf of the broad ligament below the ovarian vessels and above the ureters, and the ovarian vessels are coagulated with bipolar forceps and divided with monopolar scissors. The peritoneum on the medial half of the broad ligament is incised with monopolar scissors and the cut is extended downwards, medial to the ureters and taken to the posterior surface of the uterus over the uterosacrals.

The round ligament is cauterized and divided near the lateral pelvic wall and the anterior leaf of the broad ligament is divided medially up to the lateral uterovesical junction. Same steps are repeated on the opposite side.

The uterus is kept in the midline and in a slightly retroverted position with the help of either a uterine manipulator or a prograsp forceps. The vesicouterine peritoneum is stretched with the bipolar grasper and opened with monopolar scissors. With traction on the bladder peritoneum, the plane between the bladder and uterus will be well exposed and the bladder can be dissected away from the uterus.

With the prograsp forceps, the uterine cornua is firmly grabbed and stretched to left side exposing the uterine arteries close to uterus on the right side. The vaginal tube or colpotomy ring if pushed in by the assistant at this point will help expose the uterine arteries better. Uterine arteries are coagulated with bipolar cautery below the level of internal os and divided with hot shears. The same steps are repeated on the other side.

The colpotomy ring is pushed in, colpotomy completed and the uterus is delivered through the vagina. A 8″ × 8″ gauze pack mop placed within a surgical glove can maintain the pneumoperitoneum. After removal of all specimens vaginal cuff closure is done with a 2-0 Barbed wire or 2-0 Vicryl on CT-1 needle cut to 15″ length. During suturing full thickness vaginal bites should be taken to avoid vault dehiscence.

PELVIC LYMPHADENECTOMY

The role of lymphadenectomy in endometrial cancer is a matter of much debate with randomized studies showing no added benefit for lymphadenectomy.[14,15] But lymph nodal involvement is one of the most important prognostic factors in endometrial cancer and adjuvant treatment based only on uterine factors may lead to over or under treatment with radiation and/or chemotherapy. Sentinel node mapping is an alternative, which is described in detail in Chapter 17.

The pelvic nodal dissection is carried out from the distal half of common iliac artery down to where the deep circumflex iliac vein crosses external iliac artery. Lateral and medial boundaries are the genitofemoral nerve and the obliterated umbilical artery respectively. The dissection is carried out to the level of obturator nerve inferiorly. The zero degree scope used for port insertion is changed to a 30° scope at the start of lymphadenectomy.

The obliterated umbilical artery is grasped distally with the prograsp forceps and retracted medially. The nodal tissue is separated from it using monopolar scissors. The nodal tissue around the external iliac vein is dissected from the lateral side starting at the proximal limit. The bipolar forceps can hold the dissected nodal tissue to give traction making it easier for the hot shears to dissect it from the vessels. Once the distal limit is reached, the nodal tissue is retracted medially and obturator nodes are dissected off exposing the pubic ramus, part of the obturator internus muscle and the obturator nerve. The dissected nodes are then retracted downwards and medially, and the dissection is carried back proximally to dissect the nodal tissue over the iliac bifurcation and the internal iliac vessels. Removed nodal tissue is kept in a small endobag on which the side is marked and removed through the vagina.

Para-aortic Node Dissection

Para-aortic lymphadenectomy is carried out for high-risk patients (deep myometrial invasion, Grade 3 tumor, high risk pathologies like papillary serous or clear cell types). Before para aortic dissection, the robot is undocked and the boom is rotated to target the upper abdomen. The prograsp is changed to Arm 1, bipolar forceps to Arm 3 and hot shears to Arm 4. Renal vessels form the upper boundary and common iliac vessels, the lower boundary of the para-aortic nodal basin. Both the ureters are considered as the lateral margins. Incising the peritoneum over the right common iliac artery starts the para-aortic node dissection. The peritoneal edge is held with prograsp forceps and the incision is extended along the common iliac artery and parallel to the aorta to the level of duodenum. The peritoneum is mobilized laterally to expose the inferior vena cava, psoas muscle and the ovarian vessels. It is stretched with the help of prograsp forceps and assistant's grasper and the duodenum is gently mobilized upwards. This will give access to the right para-aortic nodal basin. This dissection is extended to the left side and the descending colon and rectosigmoid mesocolon are mobilized to expose the left psoas muscle and ureter. The inferior mesenteric artery on this side and needs to be retracted to complete the dissection up to the level of renal veins.

Skin Closure

All the trocar sites are closed with subcuticular stitches and after closure local anesthetic infiltration is done in the wound for postoperative pain relief.

Postoperative Care

Patient is shifted to the room after 4 hours, oral feeds started, Foley's catheter is removed and she can be discharged home on the same day as the surgery.

SUMMARY

Minimally invasive surgery has almost become the standard of care in the management of uterine cancers. The use of laparoscopy was low among gynecologic oncologists, but the advent of robotic surgery has increased the use of minimally invasive surgery in gynecologic oncology. The aim of any treatment is to offer maximum benefit with minimum morbidity and robotic surgery seems to be doing that by enabling more number of surgeons to do minimally invasive surgery.

REFERENCES

1. Peter Boyle and Bernard Levin, World Cancer Report 2008. WHO LEON; 2008. p.428.
2. Time trends in Cancer Incidence Rates 1982-2010. Indian Council of Medical Research. 2013;93.
3. Creasman W. Revised FIGO staging carcinoma of the endometrium. Int J Gynaecol Obstet. 2009;105:109.
4. American Joint Committee on Cancer. Corpus Uteri, AJCC Staging Manual. 7th edition. New York: Springer; 2010. p. 403.
5. The National Comprehensive Cancer Network Guidelines. Uterine Neoplasms. Available at: *http://www.nccn.org*. Retrieved July 16, 2015.
6. Childers JM, Surwit EA. Combined laparoscopic and vaginal surgery for the management of two cases of stage I endometrial cancer. Gynecol Oncol. 1992;45(1):46-51.
7. Walker JL, Piedmonte MR, Spirtos NM, Eisenkop SM, Schlaerth JB, Mannel RS, et al. Laparoscopy compared with laparotomy for comprehensive surgical staging of uterine cancer: Gynecologic Oncology Group Study LAP2. J Clin Oncol. 2009;27(32):5331-6.
8. Walker JL, Piedmonte MR, Spirtos NM, Eisenkop SM, Schlaerth JB, Mannel RS, et al. Recurrence and survival after random assignment to laparoscopy versus laparotomy for comprehensive surgical staging of uterine cancer: Gynecologic Oncology Group LAP2 Study. J Clin Oncol. 2012;30(7):695-700.
9. Kornblith AB, Huang HQ, Walker JL, Spirtos NM, Rotmensch J, Cella D. Quality of life of patients with endometrial cancer undergoing laparoscopic International Federation of Gynecology and Obstetrics staging compared with laparotomy: a Gynecologic Oncology Group study. J Clin Oncol. 2009;27(32):5337-42 .
10. Leitao Jr MM, Bartashnik A, Wagner I, Lee SJ, Caroline A, Hoskins WJ, et al. Cost-effectiveness analysis of robotically assisted laparoscopy for newly diagnosed uterine cancers. Obstet Gynecol. 2014;123(5):1031-7.
11. Holloway RW, Ahmad S. Robotic-assisted surgery in the management of endometrial cancer. J Obstet Gynaecol Res. 2012;38(1):1-8.
12. Turunen H, Pakarinen P, Sjoberg J, Loukovaara M. Laparoscopic vs robotic-assisted surgery for endometrial carcinoma in a centre with long laparoscopic experience. J Obstet Gynaecol. 2013;33(7):720-4.
13. Lim S, Kim HS, Lee KB, Yoo CW, Park SY, Seo SS. Does the use of a uterine manipulator with an intrauterine balloon in total laparoscopic hysterectomy facilitate tumor cell spillage into the peritoneal cavity in patients with endometrial cancer? Int J Gynecol Cancer. 2008;18(5):1145-9.
14. Kitchener H, Swart AM, Qian Q, Amos C, Parmar MK. Efficacy of systematic pelvic lymphadenectomy in endometrial cancer (MRC ASTEC trial): a randomised study. Lancet. 2009;373:125-36.
15. Benedetti Panici P, Basile S,Maneschi F, et al. Systematic pelvic lymphadenectomy vs no lymphadenectomy in early-stage endometrial carcinoma: randomized clinical trial. J Natl Cancer Inst. 2008;100:1707-16.

CHAPTER

19

Endometrial Cancer and Cervical Cancer

Sabhyata Gupta, Shradha Chaudhari

INTRODUCTION

Carcinoma endometrium is the most common gynecological cancer in females in western countries. The lifetime risk of developing this cancer is 2.5%. It accounts for 6% of all cancers in females in the west. Its rising incidence and prevalence amongst both pre- and post-menopausal women today has brought this disease to the limelight. Unlike ovarian cancer, which often reveals itself in late stages, endometrial carcinoma usually presents in early stages and treated patients show promising results. The five year survival rate for early stage disease is 96%. In case of regional spread, it drops to 67% and further to 17% in metastatic disease.

PRETREATMENT EVALUATION

A complete history and physical evaluation should be done to assess size and mobility of uterus, abdominal size and shape and presence of any enlarged lymph nodes. Histological diagnosis for type, grade and differentiation is made on an endometrial biopsy. To assess depth of myometrial invasion, parametrial/cervical involvement and lymphadenopathy, contrast enhanced MRI has been proved to be superior to PET scan, CT scan and transvaginal ultrasound.

Familial Lynch syndrome and another synchronous primary like ovarian malignancy must be ruled out. Measurement of CA 125 levels can be useful to look for extra uterine spread. Values greater than 40 units/mL have 78% sensitivity and 81% specificity for nodal disease.[1]

SURGICAL STAGING OVERVIEW

Mainstay of treatment is surgical and comprises of total extrafascial hysterectomy, bilateral salpingo-oopherectomy, peritoneal cytology with or without pelvic and para-aortic lymphadenectomy. Surgery alone is curative for low grade endometroid carcinoma with no myometrial invasion.

In cases with cervical involvement, radical hysterectomy is required. In the less common clear cell and serous histological variants, omentectomy is performed in addition to the rest of the surgery.

Once surgically staged, the patient may be given radiation and/or chemotherapy.

ROUTES OF SURGERY

Traditionally, open technique has been used since many years and proven as the standard of care for the staging endometrial carcinoma.

Laparoscopic route was adopted in benign gynecology very early on in its development. However, keyhole surgery was not popularised by gynecologists, unlike their contemporary surgeon colleagues, for surgery in malignant indications. The first laparoscopic surgery for endometrial carcinoma was reported by Childers in 1993.[2] Since then, this approach has been increasingly utilized by gynecologic oncologists. The Lap 2 protocol study confirmed that laparoscopic staging was feasible with acceptable complications and a superior quality of life as compared with the open approach.[3] Routine laparoscopic surgical staging, however, remains underutilized, because of the difficult learning curve, longer operative time, need for a well-trained surgical assistant, and technical issues. Urological surgeons have overcome many of the challenges posed by laparoscopic radical prostatectomy by incorporating robotic technology into surgical practice.[4]

A report with sample size of 235 cases operated by a single surgeon, mentioned 3% rate of conversion of laparoscopic endometrial carcinoma staging procedures to open technique. In patients with a body mass index of 40 or higher, conversion rates increased to 7%.[5]

Using laparoscopic route, it is difficult to dissect the para-aortic nodes above the inferior mesenteric artery (IMA). In a prospective series of cases with para-aortic metastatic disease, 77% of patients has presence of disease above the IMA.[6] Hence, para-aortic lymph node dissection is now performed superiorly to the level of the renal veins. To reach this level laparoscopically requires advanced skills, and possibly, special techniques.

Keeping in mind all factors, laparoscopic surgery for endometrial cancer may be routinely performed by a small subset of expert surgeons.

Robot-assisted Laparoscopy

Robot-assisted surgery has now emerged as the internationally accepted and preferred route of surgery for endometrial carcinoma staging for a large platform of surgeons.

Technique

Patient positioning: Steep Trendelenburg position with adequate cushioning of all pressure points and secure strapping of patient with legs in semi lithotomy position is mandatory for prolonged robotic surgery in endometrial cancers. Special attention must be paid while protecting the face which otherwise may receive trauma with the robotic camera. Preoperative thromboprophylaxis is a must for all such surgeries. Prior to strapping and positioning, the anesthetist secures good IV accesses for continuous access and monitoring throughout the procedure.

Different surgeons use different techniques for uterine manipulation. The Rumi's manipulator with a soft inflatable bulb is commonly used for cancer surgery. Some centers avoid instrumentation of the uterine cavity and adopt different techniques like cervical stitch prior to placing the cervical cup for uterine manipulation.

Docking: For gynecological surgery, uterine manipulation from the foot end plays an important role. Hence some centers routinely side dock the robot during the procedure which may or may not be continued during para-aortic lymphadenectomy. Other centers use central docking for the surgical staging. This limits vaginal access during hysterectomy which may be overcome with active use of the third arm.

Port placement: A 12 mm camera port is placed supraumbilically 5–10 cm above umbilicus and sometimes 3–5 cm right of the midline as per surgeon preference. Three robotic arm ports, 8 mm wide, are placed to make a W shaped port position to prevent arms clashing into each other during surgery. A 5 mm or 12 mm assistant port is placed either in the iliac fossa or higher up on right/left side based on surgical team's comfort. Once all ports are placed, the robot is docked **(Fig. 19.1)**.

Hysterectomy: Extrafascial hysterectomy is performed keeping in mind all oncological principles. Some surgeons cauterize Fallopian tubes prior to hysterectomy to prevent spill of cancer cells. Round ligaments and infundibulopelvic ligaments are cauterized with a fenestrated bipolar grasper and cut with monopolar hot shears. The UV fold is opened and bladder pushed caudally. Bilateral uterines are coagulated and cut. The uterosacrals are transected and vault is opened using monopolar hot shears. Overzealous use or cautery must be avoided at this step to prevent vault dehiscence in recovery phase **(Fig. 19.2)**.

Vault is closed using V loc/barbed/polyglactin suture. Prior to closure, some centers report removal of lymph nodes and uterus with adenexa in an endobag. This step may help decrease recurrence of the cancer at the vault or port site metastasis.

Pelvic and para-aortic lymphadenectomy: Lymphadenectomy may be started at caudal end and proceeded cranially along the external iliac, obturator and common iliac vessels **(Figs 19.3 and 19.4)**. En bloc specimens are preferred and retrieved in endobag through the assistant port or the vagina. Para-aortic lymph node dissection is performed after carefully displacing the colon out of the surgical field. Dissection must be performed till the renal vein so as to the stage the patient correctly **(Fig. 19.5)**.[7]

Important Considerations

Frozen section: As a matter of practice, all specimens must be examined for gross evaluation to assess the depth of myometrial invasion and tumor size. Intraoperative frozen section maybe performed to look for depth of myometrial

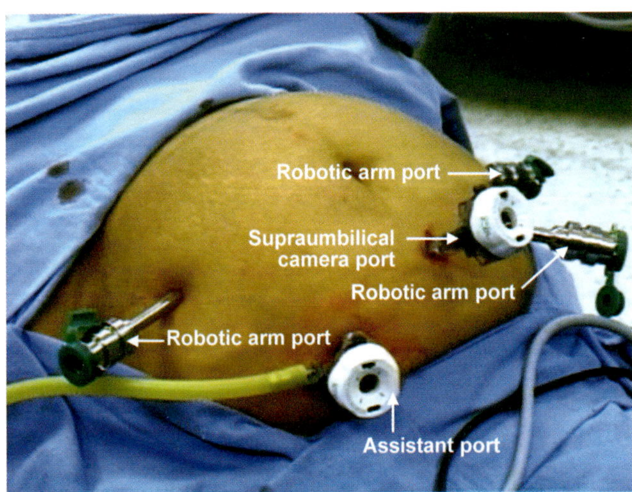

Fig. 19.1: Port placement

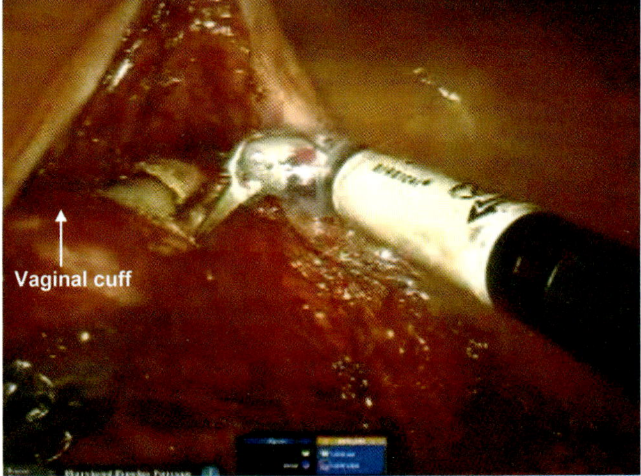

Fig. 19.2: Vaginal vault opening (*Courtesy:* Dr Sabhyata Gupta)

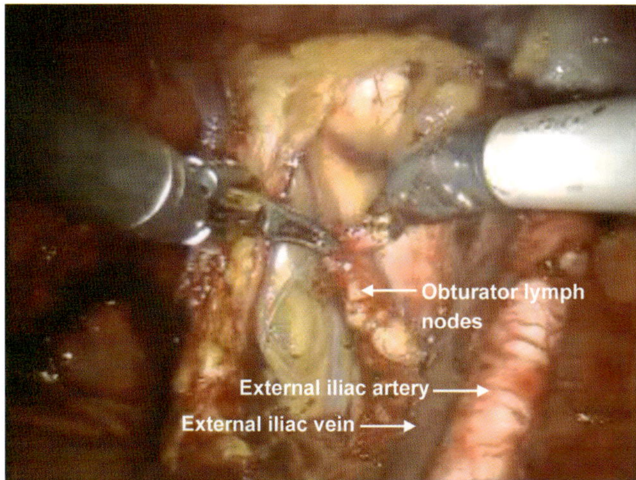

Fig. 19.3: Right pelvic lymphadenectomy
(*Courtesy:* Dr Sabhyata Gupta)

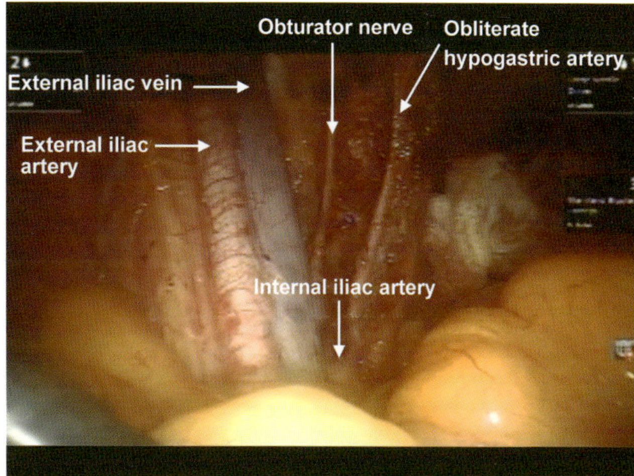

Fig. 19.4: Left pelvic retroperitoneal structures
(*Courtesy:* Dr Sabhyata Gupta)

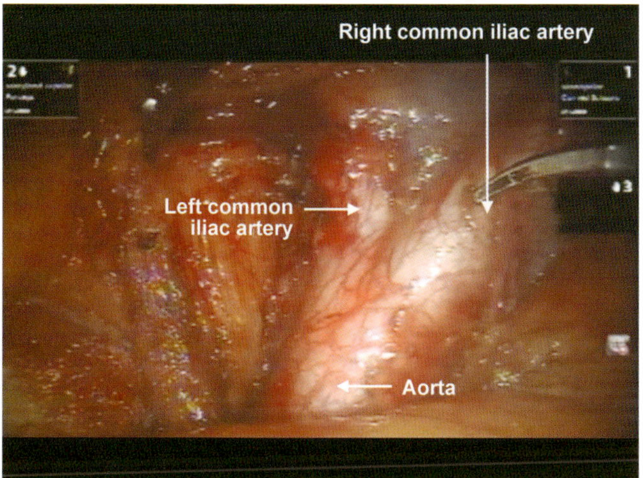

Fig. 19.5: Para-aortic and common iliac lymphadenectomy
(*Courtesy:* Dr Sabhyata Gupta)

invasion. In low grade endometroid tumors, staged as IA on frozen, lymphadenectomy maybe avoided.

Lymph node evaluation: There is controversy about requirement of lymphadenectomy or lymph node sampling for all endometrial cancer patients. Risk of nodal disease is 3–5% in well differentiated stage 1A endometroid variety and as high at 20% in poorly differentiated cancers or non-endometroid histologies.[8-10]

Sentinel node biopsy: Sentinel node biopsy is still investigational. Studies report 93% sensitivity in detection of nodal metastasis. Various dyes or tracers have been used like methylene blue dye, Indocyanine green (ICG) and technetium. Site of injection is also controversial. Sites used are peri-cervical, sub serosal and hysteroscopic guided in the endometrium.

In a recent publication by How J and Gotlieb et al, the authors concluded that intraoperative SLN mapping using cervical injection is feasible in patients with endometrial cancer and yields adequate detection rates. It allows mapping of SLNs in areas (pre-sacral, hypogastric vein, parametrial) not routinely sampled. Given the poorer performance of blue dye, surgeons may omit its use if a combination of ICG and technetium (A) is used.[11]

COMPARISON OF ROBOTIC ROUTE WITH OTHER ROUTES

Robot-assisted laparoscopic endometrial carcinoma staging was compared with conventional laparoscopy and laparotomy in a systematic review that included eight studies with a total of 589 patients.[12] The advantages of robotic procedures were mainly in comparison with laparotomy. Blood loss was significantly lower with robotic surgery than laparotomy (an average of 186 mL less) and conventional laparoscopy (an average of 86 mL less, a difference that is unlikely be clinically significant). The rate of transfusion was not significantly reduced compared with either laparotomy (OR 0.3, 95% CI 0.1–1.2) or conventional laparoscopy (OR 0.5, 95% CI 0.1–2.2), but the study was underpowered to detect significant improvements of this magnitude. The rate of wound and other complications (stroke, ileus, lymphedema, nerve palsy, acute renal failure, lymphocyst, urinary retention) were significantly reduced for robotic surgery compared with laparotomy (wound: OR 0.1, 95%CI 0.04–0.4 and other complications: OR 0.3, 95% CI 0.1–0.6), but not conventional laparoscopy. The primary disadvantage of robotic procedures was longer operative duration (an average of 89 minutes longer than laparotomy). Potential benefits of robotic technology include 3-dimensional, high-definition optics; instrumentation that allows greater range of motion, precision, and scaling; and surgeon autonomy.

CONCLUSION

Robotic surgery in endometrial cancers has gained worldwide acceptance and is a standard of care for endometrial cancers. Its shorter learning curve and machine benefits transmit to the surgeon and hence the patient. Blood loss and hospitalization rates are lesser than and oncological outcome comparable to open technique. Minimally invasive surgery renders the patient fit for future cancer therapy faster than with open route. Cost and hence availability are the only true limiting factors for this technique to take over open surgery for staging carcinoma endometrium as of today. In the future, with new robots expected to slash costs, robotic surgery may lead to minimal use of open surgery in endometrial cancers.

ROBOTIC SURGERY IN CERVICAL CANCERS

Introduction

Cervical cancer, a disease highly prevalent in the past, has shown decreasing trends and early stage diagnosis in today's times. In the future, with cervical cancer vaccination and better screening we hope to look forward to wiping out late stage presentation of this disease completely. A lot of scientific development relevant to this cancer has resulted in drop in incidence and early stage diagnosis. Similarly, treatments for early stage invasive disease are being redefined with new surgical armamentarium. Robotic surgery is applied to early stage, conventional and fertility sparing surgery and removal of metastatic disease in cervical cancers.

Pretreatment Evaluation

Prior to planning treatment for each individual, diagnostic workup needs to be performed. This includes tissue biopsy and clinical staging of the disease based on FIGO classification. Once histologically confirmed and clinically staged, treatment is tailored according to each individual case keeping in mind patients age, need for future childbearing, size and type of the tumor and presence of parametrial and nodal disease.

Surgical Treatment Overview

Standard Surgery

Standard treatment for operable (up to FIGO stage II A) cancer cervix is either extra fascial hysterectomy (Stage IA1 no LVSI) or radical hysterectomy with pelvic lymphadenectomy (Stages IA2, IB1, IIA1). Route of surgery traditionally was abdominal, vaginal or abdomino-vaginal route. Literature reports show increasing trend towards use of laparoscopic and now the robotic route for the radical hysterectomy and lymphadenectomy.

Fertility sparing surgical options include:
Conization with or without pelvic lymphadenectomy (FIGO Stage IA1 with or without LVSI).

Important considerations while performing conization are 3 mm negative margins of cone and absence of lymph vascular space invasion (LVSI). If margins of cone are positive, trachelectomy must be done. If H&E stain reveals lymph vascular space invasion, robotic or laparoscopic pelvic lymphadenectomy should be considered.

Simple/radical trachelectomy (robotic/laparoscopic/abdominal/vaginal routes) with pelvic lymphadenectomy (FIGO stage IA1 with LVSI, IA2, and IB1, less than 2 cm and squamous histology)

Simple trachelectomy is performed in stage IA1 cases and includes vaginal removal of the cervical stump. Vagina, parametria and the uterus are spared. In radical trachelectomy, surgeons adopt various routes like abdominal, robotic, laparoscopic and vaginal. To ensure good parametrial dissection, the first 3 approaches are more suitable. Surgery includes excision of the cervix, 1–2 cm vagina, and ureteric tunnel dissection, dividing the cardinal ligaments and the uterosacrals so as to obtain adequate parametrium and also perform nerve sparing surgery. Pelvic lymphadenectomy with or without para-aortic node sampling is performed to obtain nodal status. Sentinel node mapping and frozen section is performed in many centers.

Robotic Radical Trachelectomy

Robotic radical trachelectomy has been successfully performed since 2008, thus bridging the gap between traditional vaginal/abdominal route and recent laparoscopy.[13-19] The surgical principles of all the different routes must stay constant. Laparoscopic radical trachelectomy is difficult to replicate. Robotic route allows more number of practitioners to offer minimally invasive radical trachelectomy. Uterine artery preservation and nerve-sparing surgery have been performed. Feasibility for the same is increased due to benefits of better vision and dexterity, this allowing better understanding of anatomy and access to difficult pelvic structures.[14] Early literature suggests encouraging results. There is decreased morbidity, reduced intraoperative blood loss, and hospital stay is very short. However, one study reported conversion to radical hysterectomy for positive endocervical margin. This could be due to lack of haptic feedback and inability to palpate the lower uterine segment and the upper margin of the tumor. Thus, it is important to correctly identify exact level of amputation of the cervix in relation to the level of the tumor.[19] Robotic radical trachelectomy is a promising option for the selected patients and future trends will show increasing use of the technology in fertility sparing cervical cancer surgery.

ROBOT-ASSISTED RADICAL HYSTERECTOMY

Technique

As the term suggests, radical hysterectomy refers to en bloc resection of the uterus and cervix along with the parametrium and a portion of upper vagina depending upon the type of radical hysterectomy. A bilateral pelvic lymph node dissection is also required. The Querleu & Morrow and Piver-Rutledge-Smith classifications are most commonly used for classification of hysterectomy in cervical cancer.[20]

Anesthesia and Positioning

In pelvic cancer surgery (both gynecological and urological), principles of anesthesia and patient positioning remain the same. Preoperative thromboprophylaxis is recommended. The anesthetist secures good IV access and may secure arterial and central lines so as to monitor clinical parameters and requirement of intravenous fluids throughout the procedure. Once strapping and docking is done, peripheral extremities are covered and padded and IV access cannot be secured at a midpoint of surgery. For robotic procedure, special care is taken to pad all pressure points. Patient requires head low and semi lithotomy position for vaginal access. Yellow fin leg stirrups are used for simultaneous leg and foot padding and adjustment of leg position if need be in between the procedure. Some surgeons prefer uterine manipulation vaginally and may adopt different techniques for the same.

Docking

As in endometrial cancers, if the surgeon prefers vaginal access during surgery, side docking maybe preferred. Other surgeons prefer central docking for the ease during pelvic lymphadenectomy.

Port Placement

Robotic camera port may be placed about 5 cm above the umbilicus so as to allow a good lymphadenectomy procedure. The 3 robotic arms are placed either as an arc or as a 'W' or 'M' or 'C' to avoid clashing of arms during surgery. About 8 cm distance between ports allows easy maneuverability of the instruments. Assistant port can be 5 mm or 12 mm and placed in iliac fossa or higher and in line with the camera port on right of left side (depending where bedside assistant stands).

Procedure

The surgeon has a choice of robotic instruments including monopolar scissors, fenestrated bipolar forceps, prograsp forceps, harmonic and PK gyrus. Pelvic lymphadenectomy usually precedes the hysterectomy. It maybe started cranially or caudally. Caudal limit is the deep circumflex vein. The chain of nodes is lifted off the psoas muscle sparing the genitofemoral nerve. Lymph nodes in the pelvis are easily identified and classically run beside the vessels. They are dissected from lateral to medial aspect of the vessels allowing them to drop in the pelvis. The dissection is then carried further to dissecting nodes over the external iliac vein and thus entering the obturator fossa. The obturator nerve is identified and all the lymph tissue dissected from the area. Care must be taken to avoid injury to the obturator artery, vein and nerve. The accessory obturator vein present

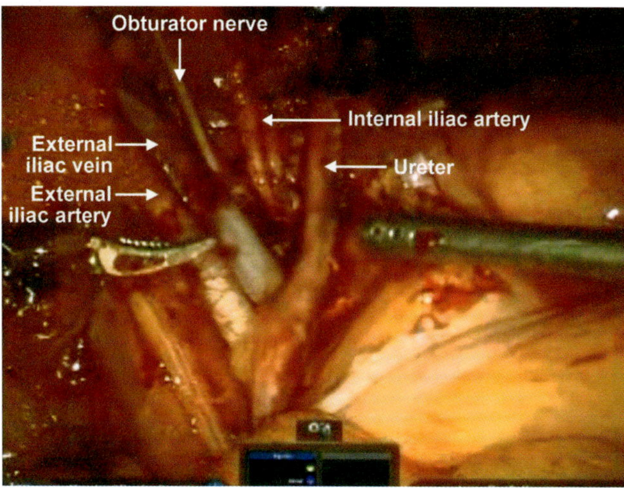

Fig. 19.6: Left pelvic retroperitoneal structures after lymphadenectomy (*Courtesy:* Dr Sabhyata Gupta)

in 30% of cases is commonly injured if not anticipated. The area or bifurcation of the common iliacs also must be cleanly dissected because metastatic disease if often here **(Fig. 19.6)**.

Radical hysterectomy is performed next. The round ligaments are separated at the present where point they enter the pelvis from the inguinal canal. The paravesical spaces and the pararectal spaces are developed. The ovaries are either preserved or retained and such pedicles thus taken. The UV fold is opened completely taking care to prevent vascular injuries. The superior vesical artery is identified and mobilised medially at this point. The ureteric dissection is next performed from the pelvic brim taking care to preserve its vascular supply. The uterine artery and veins are individually identified and cut at the origin. The ureter is then freed beyond the uterine pedicle and dissected from the ureteric tunnel. The rectum is mobilized and the posterior cul de sac opened. The uterosacral pedicles are taken as close to the rectum as possible. This is followed by dividing the cardinal ligaments and opening the vagina. Hysterectomy and lymphadenectomy specimens are removed vaginally in an endobag. The vault is closed. If patient requires pelvic radiation and also the preservation of ovarian function, then the ovaries must be transposed beyond the highest point of radiation.

COMPARISON OF ROBOTIC ROUTE TO LAPAROSCOPY AND OPEN ROUTE

Various studies show that robotic approach requires the same or less operative time than open surgery and conventional laparoscopy. The lymph node retrieval is comparable in all the routes. A meta-analysis of 26 studies concluded that the rate of blood transfusion and amount of blood loss and hospitalisation period is reduced in cases undergoing robotic surgery as compared to laparoscopy. Also, return to normal activity is the shortest with robotic route. Incidence of port site metastasis is higher in endoscopic route. Overall cancer survival and recurrence rates are comparable in all routes.[21-28]

CONCLUSION

Robotic technology for surgery in cervical cancers has paved its way to the forefront. Robotic technology incorporates benefits of both traditional laparotomy and conventional laparoscopy. A larger platform of surgeons may choose minimally invasive route for such skilled procedures. Currently, cost and availability are the main hindrances in increasing its popularity for its use in surgery for cervical cancer.

REFERENCES

1. Hsieh CH, ChangChien CC, Lin H, et al. Can a preoperative CA 125 level be a criterion for full pelvic lymphadenectomy in surgical staging of endometrial cancer? Gynecol Oncol. 2002;86:28.
2. Childers JM, Brzechffa PR, Hatch KD, Surwit EA. Laparoscopically assisted surgical staging (LASS) of endometrial cancer. Gynecol Oncol. 1993;51:33-8.
3. Walker J, Piedmonte M, Spirtos N, et al. Phase III trial of laparoscopy (scope) vs. laparotomy (open) for surgical resection and comprehensive surgical staging of uterine cancer: A Gynecologic Oncology Group (GOG) study funded by NCI. Paper presented at: 37th Annual Meeting of the Society of Gynecologic Oncologists; March 22-26, 2006; Palm Springs, CA.
4. Abbou CC, Hoznek A, Salomon L. Laparoscopic radical prostatectomy with a remote controlled robot. J Urol. 2001;165: 1964-6.
5. Fanning J, Hossler C. Laparoscopic conversion rate for uterine cancer surgical staging. Obstet Gynecol. 2010;116:1354.
6. Mariani A, Dowdy SC, Cliby WA, et al. Prospective assessment of lymphatic dissemination in endometrial cancer: a paradigm shift in surgical staging. Gynecol Oncol. 2008;109:11.
7. Dowdy SC, Aletti G, Cliby WA, et al. Extra-peritoneal laparoscopic para-aortic lymphadenectomy—a prospective cohort study of 293 patients with endometrial cancer. Gynecol Oncol. 2008; 111:418.
8. Creasman WT, Morrow CP, Bundy BN, et al. Surgical pathologic spread patterns of endometrial cancer: A Gynecologic Oncology Group Study. Cancer. 1987;60:2035.
9. Boronow RC, Morrow CP, Creasman WT, et al. Surgical staging in endometrial cancer: clinical-pathologic findings of a prospective study. Obstet Gynecol. 1984;63:825.
10. ASTEC study group, Kitchener H, Swart AM, et al. Efficacy of systematic pelvic lymphadenectomy in endometrial cancer (MRC ASTEC trial): a randomised study. Lancet. 2009;373:125.
11. How J, Gotlieb WH, Press JZ, Abitbol J, Pelmus M, Ferenczy A, Probst S, Gotlieb R, Brin S, Lau S. Comparing indocyanine green, technetium, and blue dye for sentinel lymph node mapping in endometrial cancer. Gynaecol oncol. 2015;137(3):436-42. doi: 10.1016/j.ygyno. 2015.04.004. Epub 2015 Apr 12.
12. Gaia G, Holloway RW, Santoro L, et al. Robotic-assisted hysterectomy for endometrial cancer compared with traditional laparoscopic and laparotomy approaches: a systematic review. Obstet Gynecol. 2010;116:1422.
13. Burnett AF, Stone PJ, Duckworth LA, Roman JJ. Robotic radical trachelectomy for preservation of fertility in early cervical cancer: case series and description of technique. J Minim Invasive Gynecol. 2009;16:569.
14. Hong DG, Lee YS, Park NY, et al. Robotic uterine artery preservation and nerve-sparing radical trachelectomy with bilateral pelvic lymphadenectomy in early-stage cervical cancer. Int J Gynecol Cancer. 2011;21:391.
15. Persson J, Imboden S, Reynisson P, et al. Reproducibility and accuracy of robot-assisted laparoscopic fertility sparing radical trachelectomy. Gynecol Oncol. 2012;127:484.
16. Persson J, Kannisto P, Bossmar T. Robot-assisted abdominal laparoscopic radical trachelectomy. Gynecol Oncol. 2008; 111:564.
17. Geisler JP, Orr CJ, Manahan KJ. Robotically assisted total laparoscopic radical trachelectomy for fertility sparing in stage IB1 adenosarcoma of the cervix. J Laparoendosc Adv Surg Tech A. 2008;18:727.
18. Chuang LT, Lerner DL, Liu CS, Nezhat FR. Fertility-sparing robotic-assisted radical trachelectomy and bilateral pelvic lymphadenectomy in early-stage cervical cancer. J Minim Invasive Gynecol. 2008;15:767.
19. Nick AM, Frumovitz MM, Soliman PT, et al. Fertility sparing surgery for treatment of early-stage cervical cancer: open vs. robotic radical trachelectomy. Gynecol Oncol. 2012;124:276.
20. Piver MS, Rutledge F, Smith JP. Five classes of extended hysterectomy for women with cervical cancer. Obstet Gynecol. 1974; 44:265.
21. Ramirez PT, Schmeler KM, Wolf JK, et al. Robotic radical parametrectomy and pelvic lymphadenectomy in patients with invasive cervical cancer. Gynecol Oncol. 2008; 111:18.
22. Sert B, Abeler V. Robotic radical hysterectomy in early-stage cervical carcinoma patients, comparing results with total laparoscopic radical hysterectomy cases. The future is now? Int J Med Robot. 2007;3:224.
23. Fanning J, Fenton B, Purohit M. Robotic radical hysterectomy. Am J Obstet Gynecol. 2008;198:649.e1.
24. Magrina JF, Kho RM, Weaver AL, et al. Robotic radical hysterectomy: comparison with laparoscopy and laparotomy. Gynecol Oncol. 2008;109:86.
25. Boggess JF, Gehrig PA, Cantrell L, et al. A case-control study of robot-assisted type III radical hysterectomy with pelvic lymph node dissection compared with open radical hysterectomy. Am J Obstet Gynecol. 2008;199:357.e1.
26. Ko EM, Muto MG, Berkowitz RS, Feltmate CM. Robotic versus open radical hysterectomy: a comparative study at a single institution. Gynecol Oncol. 2008;111:425.
27. Geisler JP, Orr CJ, Khurshid N, et al. Robotically assisted laparoscopic radical hysterectomy compared with open radical hysterectomy. Int J Gynecol Cancer. 2010;20:438.
28. Kruijdenberg CB, van den Einden LC, Hendriks JC, et al. Robot-assisted versus total laparoscopic radical hysterectomy in early cervical cancer, a review. Gynecol Oncol. 2011;120:334.

CHAPTER

20

Ovarian Cystectomy

Neelam Suri

INTRODUCTION

Traditionally adnexal masses, more commonly ovarian cysts, have been managed by laparotomy. Subsequently, with the advent of laparoscopy, the standard of care for these cases became laparoscopy which definitely had advantages of shorter hospital stay, faster recovery, minimal loss of blood and fewer complications.

However, laparoscopy has its own disadvantages. Not only does it have a long-learning curve, it also involves putting the surgeon in unnatural posture for long duration. Ergonomically, laparoscopy is a challenge in every case. Moreover, fixed entry point means small movements of instruments and it may actually accentuate the normal human tremors. Lastly, the two-dimensional camera limits the depth perception. Hence, many surgeons would prefer to do complex procedures by the open technique.

Many of the above limitations of laparoscopy are taken care of by the da Vinci robotic system. The use of robotics in gynecological surgery was first approved by the Food and Drug Administrator (FDA) in April 2005. Since then, a list of advancement has been made and, today, most of gynecological surgery, including myomectomy, hysterectomy, oophorectomy, and ovarian cystectomy, resection of endometriosis, sacrocolpopexy and lymphadenectomy, are done with the help of the robot.[1]

Benign and malignant ovarian lesions can both present as adenexal masses. Commonly encountered benign ovarian tumors are ovarian cysts, endometriomas, mature teratoma, serous and mucinous cystadenomas.

Up to recently, laparoscopy has been considered as the approach of choice for evaluating and treating such tumors.[2,3] The indications for managing an adnexal mass by laparoscopy and/or laparotomy are:

- Size >5 cm
- Increasing size
- Suspicious malignancy (size >10 cm, thick septum, vegetations, low resistance index and Doppler flow studies, heterogeneous contents)
- Complicated tumor
- Chronic pelvic pain.

With the advent of da Vinci robot, the surgeon has a choice of using robot for doing the ovarian tumor surgery.[4,5]

Advantages of robot:[6,7]

- Higher degree of magnification of camera
- 3D vision
- Reduced postoperative pain
- Availability of endowrist instruments, which allow 360° rotation
- Reduced hospital stay
- Decreased intraop and postoperative complications
- Faster recovery
- Shorter learning curve for surgeons than that in laparoscopy.

PREOPERATIVE EVALUATION

History and Physical Examination

Every patient with pelvic mass should have a detailed evaluation, starting with a detailed history. Patient should be asked for menstrual irregularities, dysmenorrhea, pelvic pain (pattern and severity), dyspareunia, abdominal protrusion, urinary and bowel disturbance.[8]

A complete general physical examination including evaluation for pallor, thyroid examination, breast examination should be performed for all the patients. Abdominopelvic and rectosigmoid examination should also be performed. Ovarian, uterine or other origin of pelvic masses may be detected by physical examination. Pervaginal examination is done to evaluate the consistency, irregularities, mobility and tenderness of mass. Presence of ascites should also be noted. Mass which is fixed to the surrounding structures in presence of ascites may be suggestive of malignancy.

Investigations

- Complete blood examination like CBC, S. TSH, blood sugar (F/PP), KFT, LFT.
- *Tumor markers:* Serum tumor markers have important role in screening, diagnosis and follow-up of some

gynecologic malignancies. The preoperative evaluation of serum biomarkers should be done before surgery in order to determine malignant disease.

CA-125 is the most valuable marker to predict malignancy. Level of 35 IU/mL or higher is positive, but in some benign conditions (such as pregnancy, endometriosis and leiomyoma), elevated serum level of CA-125 is seen.[9] CA-125 is a specific and sensitive marker (97% and 78%) in postmenopausal women in order to predict cancer.[10] Human epididymis 4 (HE4) is another serum marker which is occasionally checked in combination with CA-125. The major advantage of HE4 is due to its high specificity in borderline and early stage ovarian cancer, but no benefit has been shown from combining CA-125 and HE4 together in routine practice.

Recent data suggests that serial tumor markers are more effective in distinguishing benign from malignant ovarian tumors.

Carcinoembryonic antigen (CEA), alpha-fetoprotein (AFP), lactate dehydrogenase (LDH), inhibin, beta-hCG and mesothelin are some of the other available tumor markers, which may predict the chance of malignant degeneration in ovarian masses.[9,11]

- *Role of ultrasound:* High frequency ultrasound scans are performed as a routine to detect ovarian tumor. Transvaginal sonography gives a greater resolution and provides a more detailed morphological picture than transabdominal sonography.

  Transvaginal Doppler ultrasound is another technique for evaluation of adnexal masses.[12] With tumor angiogenesis, there is increase in the number and tortuosity of vascular supply, but because of absence of muscular intima, the vessels have low impedance flow.

  Low impedance flow in the tumor correlates with higher risk of malignancy.[13] The Pulsatility index (the difference between the peak systolic and the end-diastolic flow velocity divided by mean-flow velocity) lower than 1.0 is indicative of low impedance to blood flow and is indicative of higher risk of malignancy.[12]

  However, preoperative color Doppler study is not a reliable indicator of malignancy because some benign lesions such as hemorrhagic, luteal, dermoid cysts and inflammatory masses may also show low impedance.[12]
- *CT scan and MRI:* These modalities are also used for evaluation of adnexal mass. In patients with a confirmed ovarian tumor by transvaginal sonography, CT scan gives us an additional information about lymphadenopathy, omental disease and metastasis.[13]

  PET-CT is recommended for malignant ovarian tumor. MRI is indicated to assess the adnexal mass, to assess tumor infiltration and provide soft tissue contrast and clear picture of pelvic organs.[8]

  Satoh et al. showed that the best modality to supplement ultrasonography is still open to question and routine CT and MRI after transvaginal sonography has little advantage except in cases of suspected malignant lesion.[14]

SURGICAL APPROACH

Though, at present, laparoscopy is still considered the standard of care in managing the cases of ovarian cyst, but with the advent of robots, it is also being widely used for treating the patients with adnexal masses. Even though robot offers several advantages and its use has also increased but it will still take some years and more studies, for it to become the standard of care in these patients.

The learning curve is shorter than laparoscopy; so many surgeons can use minimally invasive technique to treat their patients.

da Vinci surgery has a special role and infact considered better than laparoscopy in patients with lots of adhesions (due to previous surgeries) and in suspected case of endometriosis.

da Vinci surgery has an important role in surgery for malignant ovarian tumor.

More surgical skill leads to better results and fewer complications of surgery. The surgeon should be experienced and should understand the disease that is being treated.

Informed consent should be taken prior to the surgery. The patient should be explained about the plan of organ conservation or removal as the case may be. Route and type of surgery, complications and possibility of laparotomy should be discussed and documented.

Patients, in whom severe adhesions or malignancy might be detected, should have preoperative bowel preparation. Peglec is commonly used for bowel preparation. All patients should receive antithrombotic stockings and/or sequential compressions devices to prevent deep venous thrombosis.

Position of the Patient

Patient is put in semilithotomy position. In robotic surgery, the legs should be placed in Allen's stirrups (boot-like gel cushioned supports) before docking the robot to allow free movement of robotic arms.Upper extremities are protected with additional cotton wool padding. Take special care for specific pressure points.

Anesthesia

The surgery is routinely done under general anesthesia with tracheal intubation. Foley's catheter is placed to empty the bladder. Orogastric tube is put to empty the stomach contents. With these precautions risks of bladder and bowel injuries are reduced.

Technique

Abdominal skin should be prepared from xiphoid process to mons pubis like an abdominal laparotomy preparation. If the patient has intact uterus, uterine manipulator may be helpful to facilitate adnexal dissection. In case of previous hysterectomy, a vaginally placed sponge on stick is helpful.

Start and boot up the da Vinci system called 'Homing'.

Preparation of camera system, choosing the camera, balancing the contrast settings and gaging with crosshairs (latter essential for a clear 3D image), draping the camera and fall protected positioning is done.[14]

Sterile draping of camera arm is done with special foil and mounting of plates on which endowrist instruments will be mounted later, is also done.

After induction of general anesthesia, pneumoperitoneum is created using a veress needle. The incision is given in supraumbilical area for 12 mm camera port.

- Robotic camera/laparoscopic camera is introduced through the supraumbilical incision to visualize the abdomen from inside and to guide the entry of secondary trocars.
- Length of the trocar to be used depends on the size of adnexal mass and whether the patient is obese or not.
- Long trocars are preferred as the docking of robotic camera becomes easier.
- Incisions are placed in inverted W or M shaped **(Fig. 20.1)**
- Accessory ports are put through 8 mm trocars. (Points 1, 2, 3).
- Points 2 and 3 are placed about 2–3 cm superior to anterior superior iliac spine. Point 1 is about 10 cm away from point 3 as well as from point C.
- One should be careful to keep a distance of at least 10 cm between two points on the same side. It is a standard principle of robotic surgery. The placement of instruments is done in a manner that the robotic arms do not collide and dissection with these instruments becomes easier. The instruments should have full span of mobility.
- Point A (on left side of patient) is the place where (12 mm) trocar is inserted. This is the assistant port from where the assistant can do suction irrigation and manipulation if required. The specimen can be retrieved through this port at the end of the surgery.
- After the camera port is placed, 0° or 30° scope is introduced to visualize the abdomen. The adenexal mass is checked and evaluated.

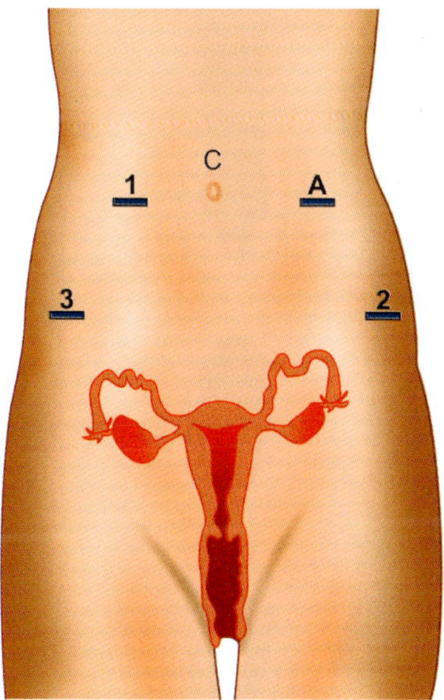

Fig. 20.1: Robotic port placement

- Adhesiolysis is performed when indicated to establish the normal anatomy.
- Adhesiolysis may also be required to be done in case port placement is difficult because of adhesions.
- Any doubts of malignancy should be proved by biopsy and frozen sectioning. If malignancy is found by initial evaluation or by frozen section, management should be continued with involvement of robotic gyneocology surgeon.

Docking

Docking of the robot can be done between the legs (between the legs docking) or from the side (side docking). In our practice, we follow the side docking from bottom right side. This makes the left side free for the assistant to help through assistant port. Also the assistant at vaginal end can easily manipulate the uterus so that the dissection becomes easier for the surgeon sitting at the console. Patient should be put in steep Trendelenburg position before docking the robot. It helps the bowel to move away from the pelvic area where surgery is to be performed.

Instrument Placement

Three robotic arms are used in addition to the camera, though some surgeons use only two arms to cut down the cost. Monopolar scissors is put in Arm no. 1, PK (plasma kinetic forceps) is used with energy in arm no. 2 and bipolar forceps with energy in arm no. 3. Assistant port (A) is used for manipulation, suction irrigation and retrieval of specimen. As a matter of fact, this set of instruments can be used for all robotic gynecological surgeries especially for benign diseases. Though there are other robotic instruments like Prograsp, Harmonic, Maryland, Tenaculum, etc. available, but the choice of instruments depends on the type of surgery and choice of the surgeon.

The first set of instruments is used for dissection till the cyst is completely separated. The second set of instruments which is the large needle driver (with suture cut) and needle driver without suture cut is introduced when the tissues need to be stitched. In case of ovarian cystectomy, the ovarian tissue left after removal of cyst has to be stitched back. So needle drivers are put in arms 1 and 2 instead of scissors and PK forceps. The bipolar forceps can continue to be used along with needle drivers as it helps in stitching.While suturing, bipolar can be used as a grasper and to cauterize the remaining bleeders, if any.

SPECIFIC CONSIDERATIONS

Serous and Mucinous Cystadenomas

Serous Cystadenoma

They are common in women aged between 30 and 40 years. Their diameter is usually less than 15 cm. They are filled with serous fluid. Internal surface is either smooth or has papillary projections in the internal wall.

Mucinous Cystadenomas

They are commonly unilateral. They may reach the size of 30–50 cm or even more in diameter. They are filled with mucinous fluid.

Robotic Ovarian Cystectomy

The incision is made with monopolar scissors on the anti-mesenteric surface of cyst, taking care not to rupture it. With the help of PK forceps in arm 2 and bipolar forceps in arm 3, the cyst wall is dissected from the ovarian parenchyma by stripping technique. Bleeders are cauterized at the base. The whole cyst wall is stripped from the ovarian parenchyma. At the hilum the dissection is carefully done taking care of the hemostasis. The hemostasis is achieved with PK and bipolar forceps **(Figs 20.2 to 20.7)**.

Robotic Salpingo-oophorectomy

This is indicated in large endometriotic cyst and benign ovarian cyst in patients aged above 40 years.

The technique for this surgery is cauterizing the infundibulopelvic ligament with PK forceps or bipolar forceps and cutting with monopolar scissors.

Ovarian pedicle is also coagulated with PK forceps/bipolar forceps and cut with monopolar scissor. Hemostasis is achieved. In cases of oophorectomy, fallopian tube of the same side is also removed.

The specimen is put in the endobag and is retreived later.

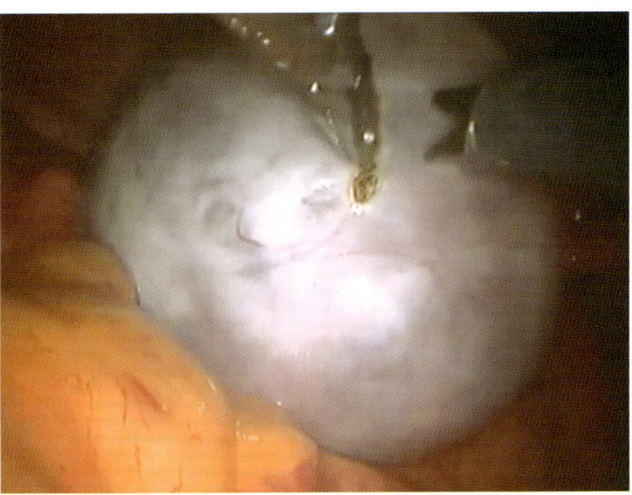

Fig. 20.2: Incision on cyst wall

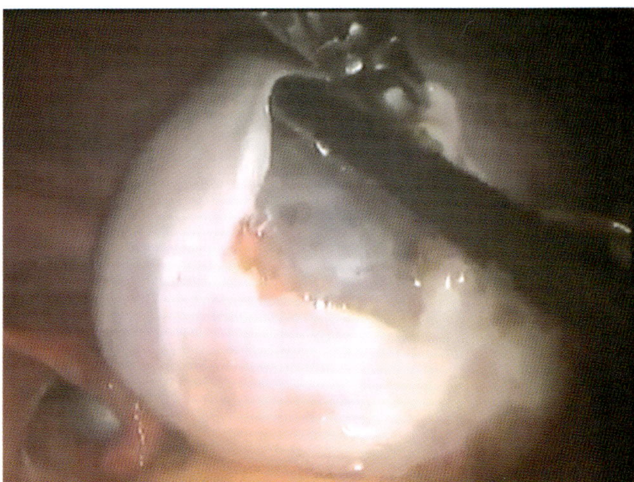

Fig. 20.3: Dissection on cyst wall

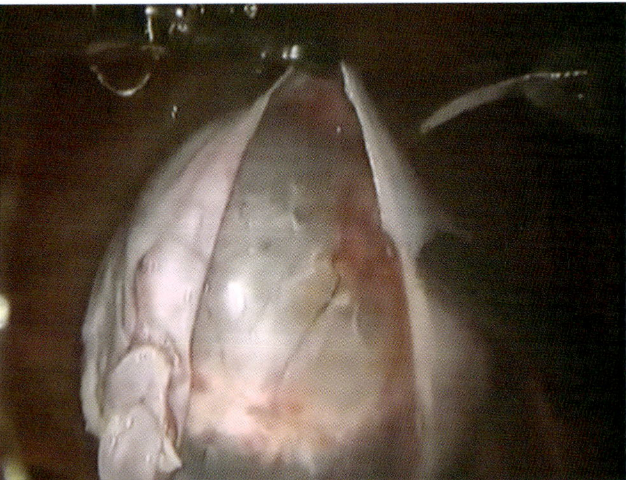

Fig. 20.4: Dissection for removal of ovarian cyst (1)

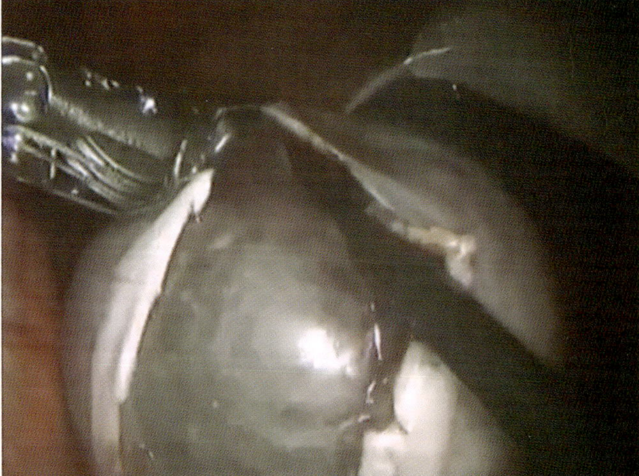

Fig. 20.5: Dissection for removal of ovarian cyst (2) (continued)

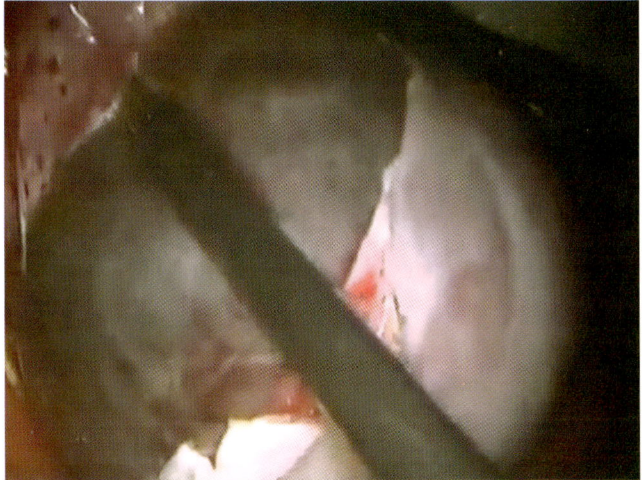

Fig. 20.6: Dissection for removal of ovarian cyst (3)

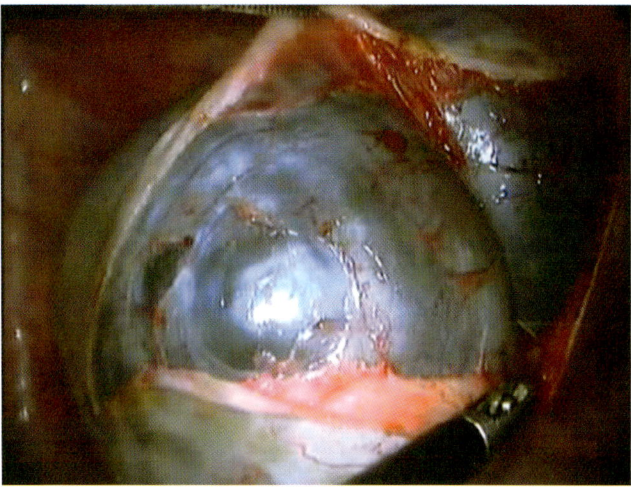

Fig. 20.7: Ovarian cystectomy (4)

Before starting the procedure, it is important to observe the course of the ureter as it crosses the external iliac artery near the bifurcation of the common iliac artery at the pelvic brim.

Endometrioma

It is a frequent benign condition seen mainly in young and infertile women.[15]

Endometriomas are formed due to presence of ectopic endometrium in ovaries. This endometrium undergoes cyclical bleeding every month and thus leads to formation of these chocolate-colored cysts or endometriomas. These are the cause of dysmenorrhea, abnormal uterine bleeding, chronic pelvic pain and infertility. Medical therapies include danazol, GnRh agonist and lately dienogest. These treatment modalities have been compared in some studies.[16,17] About 40–57% decrease in size of endometrioma has been found on medical therapy. But endometriomas equal to or larger than 3 cm are not known to respond well to medical therapy.[18]

The surgical procedures for treatment of endometriomas include:

- Ultrasound-guided or laparoscopic-guided aspiration.
- Aspiration and sclerotherapy.
- Laparoscopic surgery by cystectomy or fenestration and coagulation.
- Robot-assisted excision of endometriomas and endometriotic patches.
- Radical-treatment (oophorectomy or adnexectomy)

Robot-assisted approach is considered the best approach for endometriotic cysts because blood loss during operation, length of hospital stay and need for analgesics is significantly low. Since the magnification of da Vinci camera is very high and provides a 3D vision, so it is easy to excise rather than to just fulgurate the endometriotic spots. Endometriotic patches on vital organs such as bladder and bowel can also be effectively excised without injury to the organ. It is a well-accepted fact that excision of endometriotic tissue is a better approach than simple aspiration or fulguration as the recurrence rate of latter is very high (80–100%).[19]

Although giving GnRh agonist after drainage of endometrioma can reduce the size of cyst up to 50% but it has no effect on prevention of recurrence because of the nature of disease.

Robotic Cystectomy of Endometrioma

This is the first line of choice for treatment of endometriotic cyst. Preoperative assessment and surgical approach remains the same as described earlier. The inner lining of cyst is dissected from the ovary with the help of monopolar scissors and the PK forceps in arms 1 and 2 respectively with the bipolar forceps in arm 3. Because of its adherent nature, it can get ruptured and chocolate-colored fluid can be aspirated.

Although Muzzi et al.[20] reported that in 54% of cases of laparoscopic cystectomy, ovarian tissue was detected with cyst pseudocapsule but chance of getting this by da Vinci technique is much less as the camera magnification is very high. This ovarian tissue does not show any follicular pattern and postcystectomy ovarian response to gonadotropins is comparable to the contralateral ovary.

Along with this, the surgeon should look for all the possible sites of endometriotic patches like pouch of Douglas, uterosacrals, contralateral ovary, bladder, and bowel.

Excision of these patches is recommended to get rid of the disease. da Vinci surgery has made the surgeon's job easier in cases of endometriosis and the results are encouraging.

According to the meta-analysis by Alborzi et al. the excision of cyst in endometrioma is strongly recommended.[16]

Radical Treatment for Endometriomas

This technique includes adnexectomy and ovariectomy. This is seldom required and depends on the degree of endometriosis.

Mature Teratoma

Dermoid cysts are the most common ovarian neoplastic lesion found in adolescents and approximately 70% of benign ovarian tumors in women under the age of 30 years.[21]

They are filled with all tissues deriving from three embryonic layers (ectoderm, mesoderm and endoderm) and filled with hair, teeth, cartilage, semisolid jelly and sebaceous material.[8]

Large demoid cyst (>5 cm in diameter) are under high risk of torsion and symptomatic teratomas need surgical operation.

Robotic surgery has an important role since the dissection of dermoid from the healthy ovarian tissues can be done easily and chances of rupture are also less. Spillage of cyst contents may lead to adhesion formation and peritonitis. So, removal of dermoid in toto and preservation of ovary is the method of choice.

Robotic Dermoid Cystectomy

The instrument choice remains the same. The technique remains the same as described above under the heading of robotic ovarian cystectomy. The surgeon should be careful not to rupture the cyst. The chances of rupture are less because of the wristed robotic instruments. If at all rupture occurs, good peritoneal lavage with ringer lactate should be done.

Retreival of Specimen

The specimen is put in an endobag and retrieved through assistant port which is a 12 mm port. It is done in a similar manner as done in conventional laparoscopic procedures.

Ovarian Torsion

The most common complaint of patients who come to emergency gynecological room in adnexal torsion is acute pelvic pain.

It is defined by Huchon et al. as the twisting by at least one complete turn of the adnexa, ovary or more rarely the tube, around the center line. Its frequency is about 2.5–7.4%.[22]

Early diagnosis of torsion is very important because most of the patients are young and all of them desire future fertility. Sudden onset of pain associated with nausea, vomiting, vagal reflex, leukocytosis peritoneal irritation and fever, are the most common presentations. Doppler imaging is the modality to diagnose, but according to Pena et al, 60% of cases of torsion have normal Doppler, but its positive predictive value is 100%.[23] A certain diagnosis of adnexal torsion is made only by laparoscopy.

The technique of surgery consists of untwisting the adnexa, even when necrosed and resection of cyst and/or ligamentopexy. Robotically assisted surgery is done in the similar manner as described above.

Borderline and Malignant Ovarian Tumors

The preoperative evaluation of an adnexal mass involves the radiological and serum tumor marker evaluation. A high index of suspicion is important and thereby detailed evaluation should be done after inserting the robotic camera.

Approximately, 10% of all ovarian serous tumors are borderline and 50% occur before the age of 40 years.[24]

In case of laparoscopy for evaluation of adnexal mass, high index of suspicion is important. In such cases frozen section of the biopsy from the mass is recommended. If malignant, complete surgical staging should be performed. An early stage ovarian cancer is rarely diagnosed preoperatively and occasionally found incidentally during laparoscopy for benign ovarian tumors.[24]

Robotic surgery is a major breakthrough in such cases as a highly magnified camera allows a complete evaluation and staging.

Advantages of robotic surgery in ovarian cancer includes less traumatic surgery, faster recovery and earlier possibility of chemotherapy administration.Disadvantages include rupture of cyst and spillage of contents, difficulty to remove large ovarian masses, inability to palpate lymph nodes and possibility of trocar metastasis.

Ovarian Tumors in Pregnancy

- The use of laparoscopic and robotic technique is for diagnosis and management of a number of surgical disorders in pregnancy, including the evaluation of adnexal masses.[25]
- The most common pregnancy-associated ovarian tumors are luteomas, benign cystic teratomas and cysts because of ovarian hyperstimulation syndrome (OHSS).
- Generally, pregnant women are young, therefore, malignant ovarian tumors are uncommon during pregnancy. Leiserowitz et al. reported incidence of ovarian masses to be 1% in pregnancy.[26]
- Indications for surgery in pregnancy are suspicion of torsion or rupture, tumor size more than 10 cm, tumor obstructing labor and presence of signs in favor of malignancy, such as nodule, papillary projections or solid component.
- Investigations including high-resolution sonography and color Doppler sonography for better evaluation of adnexal mass. MRI is a helpful diagnostic tool. Tumor markers such as CA125, AFP and beta-hCG are not specific in pregnancy because their levels change in this period. Elective surgery should be avoided in first trimester, because many lesions resolve spontaneously. Sonography should be repeated after 6 weeks to detect persistent cysts.

- General anesthesia is preferred in pregnancy, but one should be careful in view of delayed gastric emptying, esophageal reflux and inferior vena caval and aortic compression.
- Intracervical instruments for mobilization of uterus should be avoided. Tocolytic agents should be used in pre- and postoperative period to avoid abortion.
- Robotic-assisted laparoscopic surgery offers the obstetric patient safe and less invasive alternative to laparotomy or conventional laparoscopy.[27]

SUTURING IN OVARIAN SURGERY

Robotic surgery has a definite advantage over laparoscopy when it comes to suturing. The endowrist manipulation of the needle holders allows suturing to be done easily.

Bipolar and PK forceps are used for hemostasis. Needle drivers are used for stitching the ovarian tissue. When large ovarian tumors are removed, ovarian tissue is restitched. This helps to avoid adhesion formation in a gapped ovary.

Complications of Robotic Ovarian Cystectomy

General

- Cardiopulmonary complications can occur as steep head-down position is required for performing the surgery and usually takes longer operating time.
- Thromboembolic incidents
- Gas embolism
- Incisional hernia at trocar site
- Nerve injury
- Shoulder pain
- Reflux of gastric contents
- Electrosurgical complications
- Hemorrhage
- Gastrointestinal complications
- Bladder injury and injury to ureter
- Infections[28]

Complications Specific to da Vinci Surgery

- Intraoperative malpositioning leading to nerve injury, especially brachial plexus injury.
- Rapid impairment of visibility or disturbed veiw due to blood contamination of endoscope, which is less flexible in handling (undocking from camera arm for cleaning). Thus sufficient cranial trocar placement is suggested and camera too close to surgical field is avoided.
- Confusion of pedals
- Faulty operation of instruments (accidental cutting of thread)
- Collision of robotic arms if trocars are placed too close together
- Trocar dislocation when robotic arms are deflected too much
- System-associated hardware and software failures.

Special Complications

Spillage of Contents

When cystectomy is performed, rupture of cyst may occur. Rupture and spillage of cyst contents is important in mature teratoma, which may create chemical peritonitis and adhesions. In malignant lesion, seedlings of tumor cells may occur.

Chances of rupture and spillage is less in robotic surgery. It is important to use atraumatic grasper and maintain good hemostasis to see the clear planes. Endoscopic bags can be used in the same manner as in laparoscopic surgery. The assistant port (12 mm) is used to introduce endobag. After putting the specimen in endobag, edges of the bag are pulled outside the abdominal wall and clamped. In case of big volume, the cyst contents can be aspirated before pulling the endobag out of the abdominal wall.

If spillage occurs, the patient's position should be changed to reverse. Trendelenburg after undocking the robot and abdominopelvic cavity lavage should be done with several liters of ringer lactate solution.[29]

Adhesions

Adhesion formation is less after robotic surgery than conventional laparotomy.

Many pharmacological agents and mechanical barriers like interceed have been advocated to address this issue.[30]

SUMMARY

- Ovarian reserve should be assessed by hormonal levels/or antral follicle count before surgery in patients with endometriomas, bilateral ovarian cysts or tumors. These levels should be repeated after surgery. Also tumor markers should be checked before operation where there is suspicion of borderline or malignant tumor.
- Transvaginal ultrasound is the best and cheapest modality for imaging the ovarian cysts or adnexal mass. In addition, one may benefit from CT or MRI imaging.
- Bowel preparation is essential in robotic surgery patients with adnexal cyst or mass.
- In patients with benign cysts such as serous, mucinous or dermoid neoplasms, every attempt should be done to avoid rupturing the cyst wall, however, if accidental leakage occurs, pelvic and abdominal cavity should be thoroughly washed. Chances of chemical peritonitis is not high as previously thought.
- Inadverent removal of healthy tissue after endometrioma surgery is much higher than removal of other cysts such as serous, mucinous or dermoid cyst.
- Small endometriomas less than 1 cm in size may effectively be treated by fenestration and coagulation of the inner lining. However, for larger endometriomas, cystectomy is the best technique in terms of chances of recurrence of symptoms and signs, reoperation rate and cumulative pregnancy rate.

- Deep infiltrating endometriosis in ovarian fossa should be excised at the time of cystectomy to avoid recurrence of endometrioma. Covering deperitonealized and operated areas by absorbable barriers significantly reduces the incidence, extent and severity of postsurgical adhesions.
- Extensive cauterization of ovarian tissue can lead to a rise in follicle-stimulating hormone (FSH) levels postoperatively and should be avoided. Fine hemostasis under irrigation with microbipolar and use of sutures to approximate the bed of ovary is the best option to avoid ovarian failure in patients with bilateral endometriomas.
- If there is a large enough area after ovarian cystectomy, reapproximation of ovarian incision in two layers with fine non-reactive sutures with good technique is the best way to avoid adhesion formation.

REFERENCES

1. Advincula AP. World Robotic Gyn Symposium: the dawn of a new age in minimally invasive gynecologic surgery. J Robotic Surg. 2007;1:177-8.
2. Maris V, Ajossa S, Piras B, et al. Treatment of nonendometriotic benign adnexal cyst: a randomized comparison of laparoscopy and laparotomy. Obstet Gynecol. 1995; 86(5):770-4.
3. Yuen PM, Yu KM, Yip SK, et al. A randomized prospective study of laparoscopy and laparotomy in the management of benign ovarian masses. Am J Obstet Gynecol. 1997;177(1):109-14.
4. Liu H, Lu D, Wang L, Shi G, Song H, Clarke J. Robotic surgery for benign gynaecological disease. Cochrane Database of Systemic Reviews, Issue 2. Art. No.: CD008978, 2012.
5. Nezhat C, Saberi NS, Shahmohamady B, Nezhat F. Robotic assisted laparoscopy in gynaecological surgery. Journal of the Society of Laparoendoscopic Surgeons. 2006;10(3):317-20.
6. Pitter MC, Anderson P, Blisset A, Pemberton N. Robotic-assisted gynaecological surgery-establishing training criteria; minimising operative time and blood loss. Int J Med Robot. 2008;4:114-20.
7. Lenihan Jr Jp, Kovanda C, Seshadri-Kreaden U. What is the learning curve for robotic-assisted gynecologic surgery? J Mini Inva Gynec. 2008;15(5):589-94.
8. Malzoni M, Imperato F. Laparoscopic treatment of adnexal masses. In: Mencaglia L, Minelli L, Wattiez A (Eds). Manual Gynaec Laparo Surg, 11th edition. Tuttlingen: Straub Druck + Medien AG. 2009. pp.152-63.
9. Husseinzadeh N. Status of tumor markers in epithelial ovarian cancer—has there been any progress? A review. Gynecol Oncol. 2011;120(1):152-7.
10. Malkasian GD, Knapp RC, Lavin PT, et al. Preoperative evalution of serum CA-125 levels in premenopausal and postmenopausal patients with pelvic masses: discrimination of benign form malignant disease. Am J Obstet Gynecol. 1988:159(2):341-6.
11. Aggarwal P, Kehoe S. Serum tumor markers in gynaecological cancers. Maturitas. 2010;67(1):46-53.
12. Kawai M, Kano T, Kikkawa F, et al. Transvaginal Doppler ultrasound with color flow imaging in the diagnosis of ovarian cancer. Obstet Gynecol. 1997;79(2):163-7.
13. Van Nagell JR, Gershenson DM. Ovarian cancer:etiology, screening and surgery. In: Rock JA, Jones III Hw (Eds). Telinde's Operative Gynecology, 10th edition. Philadelphia: Woters Kluwer/ Lippincott-Williams and Wilkins. 2008. pp.1307-39.
14. Satoh S, Takashima T, Nakano H. Role of imaging modalities in ovarian tumors. Int J Obstet Gynecol. 2002;76(2):195-7.
15. Alborzi S, Momtahan M, Parsanezhad ME, et al. A prospective, randomized study comparing laparoscopic cystectomy versus fenestration and coagulation in patients with endometriomas. Fertil Steril. 2004;82(6):1633-7.
16. Alborzi S, Zarei A, Alborzi S, et al. Management of ovarian endometrioma. Clin Obstet Gynecol. 2006;49(3):480-91.
17. Crikel U, Ochs H, Schneider HP. A randomized comparative trial of triptorelin depot (D-Trp6-LHRH) and danazol in the treatment of endometriosis. Eur J Obstet Gynecol Reprod Biol. 1995;59(1):61-9.
18. Rena N, Thomas S, Rotman C, et al. Decrease in the size of ovarian endometriomas during ovarian suppression in stage IV endometriosis, role of preoperative medical treatment. J Reprod Med. 1996; 41(6):384-92.
19. Saleh A, Tulandi T. Reoperation after laparoscopic treatment of ovarian endometriomas by excision and fenestration. Fertile Steril. 1999;72(2):322-4.
20. Muzii L, Bianchi A, Croce C, et al. Laparoscopic excision of ovarian cysts: is the stripping technique a tissue sparing procedure? Fertile Steril. 2002;77(3):609-14.
21. O'Neill KE, Cooper AR. The approach to ovarian dermoids in adolescents and young women. North Am Soc Pediat Adoles Gynecol. 2011.
22. Bar-On Sh, Mashiach R, Stockheim D, et al. Emergency laparoscopy for suspected ovarian torsion: are we too hasty to operate? Fertile Steril. 2010;93(6):2012-5.
23. Pena JE, Ufberg D, Cooney N, et al. Usefulness of Doppler sonography in the diagnosis of ovarian torsion. Fertile Steril. 2000;73(5):1047-50.
24. Berek JS, Natarajan S. Ovarian and fallopian tube cancer. In: Berek JS (Ed). Berek and Novak's gynaecology, 14th edition. Philadelphia:Lippincott-Williams and Wilkins. 2007. pp.1458-547.
25. Sherard GB III, Hodson CA, Williams HJ, et al. Adnexal masses and pregnancy: A 12-year experience. Am J Obstet Gynecol. 2003;189(2):358-62.
26. Lesiserowitz GS. Managing ovarian masses during pregnancy. Obstet Gynecol Surv. 2006;61(7):463-70.
27. Carter S, Depasquale S, Stallings S. Robotic-assisted laparoscopic ovarian cystectomy during pregnancy. Am J Perinotol Rep. 2011;1:21-24.
28. Soper DE. Gynecologic endoscopy. In: Berek JS (Ed). Berek and Novak's gynecology, 14th edition. Philadelphia-Lippincott-Williams and Wilkins. 2007. pp. 432-500.
29. Mecke H, Savvas V. Laparoscopic surgery of dermoid cysts-intraoperative spillage and complications. Eur J Obstet Gynecol Reprod Biol. 2001;96(1);80-4.
30. Sekiba K.Use of intercede (TC7) absorbable adhesion barrier to reduce postoperative adhesion reformation in infertility and endometriosis surgery. Obster Gynecol.1992;79:518-22.

SECTION 5

Urogynecology

• **Vesicovaginal Fistula Repair**
Nitesh Jain, K Ramesh

CHAPTER

21

Vesicovaginal Fistula Repair

Nitesh Jain, K Ramesh

INTRODUCTION

Vesicovaginal fistula (VVF) is abnormal fistulous tract extending between the bladder and vagina leading to continuous involuntary discharge of urine. In addition to medical symptoms, they affect social and emotional well-being of the women, which needs correction.

Common cause of VVF is obstetric surgery, namely hysterectomy in developed country and prolonged labor in developing country.

Open repair of vesicovaginal fistula is rare in modern era. Minimally invasive treatments for VVF are:

- Laparoscopic repair
- Robotic VVF repair.

Laparoscopic tissue dissection and intracorporeal suturing are technically challenging. Laparoscopic dissection and suturing are difficult in recurrent VVF repair and often suturing by laparoscopic instruments may be difficult for many surgeons. Laparoscopic surgery has a steep learning curve in contrast to short learning curve with robot. These difficulties are overcome by robotic surgical repair.

Using da Vinci robotic system insertion of miniature surgical instruments of the robotic arms though the small incision allow the surgeon to have extremely fine and precise movement and computer-enhanced, stereoscopic camera under the surgeons control allows the surgeon to have three-dimensional view of the surgical area. Robotic surgery overcomes the traditional limitation of the open and laparoscopic surgery by filtering and seamlessly translating the surgeon hand movement into precise micro movement. First robotic repair of vesicovaginal fistula was done in 2005 by Melamud at university of California, United States.

Repair of vesicovaginal fistula can be repaired by vaginal or abdominal approach. Abdominal approach is better for multiple, complex large, supratrigonal or recurrent fistula. Robotic repair can be transperitoneal or extraperitoneal.

HISTORY AND PHYSICAL EXAMINATION

Pervaginal examination by bivalve speculum usually provides a precise assessment of VVF including the location, size and number.

INVESTIGATIONS

Computerized tomography (CT) urogram with cystogram is done to identify the fistula. A tampon is placed pervagina during CT scan may improve the sensitivity for findings the small or occult VVF.

Twelve percent of VVF is associated with ureteric fistula. CT urogram helps to identify the ureteric fistula.

If suspicion for ureteric injury is high then retrograde pyelogram (RGP) may help.

Biopsy is done if malignancy is suspected. Urine culture and sensitivity to exclude any active urine infection.

REPAIR OF VESICOVAGINAL FISTULA

Repair of vesicovaginal fistula is challenging surgery to the surgeon as many of the vesicovaginal fistula are due to complication of previous gynecological surgery. Repair of vesicovaginal fistula is surgical. Rarely small vesicovaginal fistula can be treated by conservative procedure. Best chance of success is the first surgery so appropriate surgery at right time gives the best results.

Repair of VVF can be done by vaginal or abdominal route. Low fistula is generally repaired by vaginal route. Large, complex, recurrent and supratrigonal fistula are treated by abdominal route. Type of approach is also depends on the familiarity and experience of the surgeon. It is better the surgeon choose the route he is familiar and experienced with to get best results.

Timings of Surgery

There has been debate on perfect timing for the repair. Ideal time for surgery is once edema, inflammation in the area settles and infection is treated.

If there is extensive edema and inflammation, it is advisable to wait for 3–6 month, before the elective operation is taken.

Preparation for Surgery

- A preoperative antibiotic is indicated. A broad-spectrum antibiotic along with the anaerobic cover is recommended.

- Urine culture should be sterile.
- Povidone-iodine vaginal douches are given the previous night and on the day of surgery.
- DVT prophylaxis is recommended. TEDS stocking and a prophylactic anticoagulant is advised.
- Estrogen treatment is sometime given before surgery to improve the vascularity of the region.

Position of Patient

Patient is positioned in lithotomy position.

Initially, cystoscopy is done to assess the size, number and position of the fistula. Retropyelogram is done if ureteric injury is suspected. The fistula is cannulated with a guidewire followed by insertion of ureteric catheter. The ureteric catheter is retrieved through the vaginal vault. Occasionally, a Foley's catheter can be used if the fistula is large. Ureteric orifices are cannulated with a ureteric catheter if the fistula is close to the ureteric orifice to avoid damage during repair. Double J stent is placed if needed.

Vaginoscopy is done to inspect if the vaginal vault area is healthy. Vagina is packed with betadine-soaked gauze.

Anesthetic Challenges

Pressure points: All pressure points should be adequately cushioned and protected.

Support of patient: Patient should be support at both shoulders to avoid sliding of patients during steep Trendelenburg position. Chest should strapped but not too tight to compress the chest movement.

Effect of Trendelenburg position: Prolonged surgery in lithotomy position may cause increased venous return and cause alteration in hemodynamics of the patients and add to strain of the heart.

Urine output should be minimized to prevent the soiling of the operative field with urine.

Bowel distension: Any anesthetic agents that cause bowel distension should be avoided and bowel preparation the previous night may reduce the distension.

Cerebral edema and eye edema: Prolonged steep Trendelenburg position can cause cerebral and edema of the eye. Eyes should be adequately protected. Cerebral edema may cause confusion and irritability for the patient in immediate postoperative period.

Procedure

Port Placements

- 12 mm camera port is placed in the supraumbilical region 3–5 cm from the umbilicus depending on the patient.
- Two 8 mm robotic arm port in inserted at the level of the umbilicus, on the right and left pararectal line and the ports should be 10 cm away to avoid clashing of the arm during the procedure.
- Two assistant ports are used.
- 5 mm assistant port is placed lateral to umbilicus.
- A 10 mm port is placed below and lateral to robotic port. This port allows passing and retrieving the sutures.

Robotic instruments required are:

- 0° and 30° lens
- Monopolar-curved scissors
- Maryland bipolar forceps
- Two large needle driver
- Prograsp forceps.

Patient is positioned in steep Trendelenburg position as for prostate surgery. This allows the bowels to be away from operation site. Shoulder should have support not allowing the patient to slide. The chest should be adequately strapped and supported but not too tight to compress the chest. Adequate bowel preparation will be ideal.

Steps of the Surgery

Adhesiolysis

Previous abdominal surgeries in the pelvic area often lead to extensive peritoneal adhesion. Sometimes it may be difficult to insert the post wherein open technique for port insertion is advised. At times laparoscopic release of adhesion is required before further robotic ports are inserted.

Bowel adhesions are released by combination of sharp and blunt dissection. Bowel adhesion should be released to expose the pouch of Douglas. Diathermy should be avoided. Once the adhesions are released to identify the bladder. Movement of the Foley's balloon helps identification of cystostomy site.

Cystostomy

Bladder is divided vertically down to the fistula. Fistulous tract is excised. Scar tissues are excised till healthy tissue. Edges should be healthy with bleeding. Suspicious area of malignancy needs to be biopsied. Vaginal vault is separated from the bladder.

Closure of Fistula

Vaginal vault is closed horizontally with 3/0 Quil (Barbed Monocryl suture) or V-Loc suture. V- LOC suture avoids knotting. Continuous watertight closure with barbed unidirectional suture allows maintaining the tension and helps in watertight closure.

Vascularized Omental Patch

Vascular omental patch is mobilized. Sometimes the omentum is released using laparoscopic instrument before the patient is positioned in the steep lithotomy position. Released omental patch should be able to reach the pelvis if not changing the position of the patient is helpful. Patient is placed back in the horizontal position will and also additionally flexing the hip and knees reduce the distance between the pubis and mesenteric root to achieve tension free anastomosis of omental patch.

Sometimes omental flap is mobilized by dividing the greater epiploe from greater curvature of the stomach and it can also be done laparoscopic method.

Other options are bladder tissue, peritoneum flap or appendices epiploic is used. When omentum is unavailable or cannot be adequately mobilized, the epiploic appendices of the sigmoid colon or a peritoneal flap from the nearest anatomical location is used as tissue for interposition. The interposition tissue is anchored with a suture on the resilient vaginal wall and distally to the end of the vaginal closure line. To prevent laxity on fixation, the interposition tissue is additionally fixed left and right on the peritoneal edges of the cystotomy.

Bladder (Cystostomy Closure)

Bladder closure is done vertically with a barbed unidirectional absorbable monocryl suture. This allows better tissue approximation and tightening. V-Loc suture can also be used. V-Loc suture eliminates the need for tie the knots and saves time. V-Loc is again a unidirectional barbed absorbable monofilament suture allows better tissue tightening and approximation. A vascular omentum is interposed between the bladder and vaginal vault. Bladder is usually closed in single layer. If the cystostomy is long, two separate sutures can be used to begin from both the ends. Watertight closure of the bladder is checked by doing a leak test. 200 mL of saline is instilled into the bladder and should be checked for leak. If minor leaks are present addition sutures are taken.

If retrograde pyelogram shows ureteric injury reimplantation of ureter can be done simultaneously. SPC is usually not required. Drain is kept in pelvis. 20FR Foley's catheter is placed. Vagina is packed with Povidone-iodine soaked gauze and left in place for 24 hours. Port closure-12 mm ports are closed with Vicryl using Carter Thompson. Local infiltration of the port sites reduces the postoperative pain.

Postoperative Care

Antibiotics should be continued for 5 days. Prophylactic anticoagulation should be continued till the patient is fully mobilized. Chest physiotherapy should be started to prevent atelectasis. Povidone-iodine soaked vaginal pack to should be removed after 24 hours. Adequate pain relieve should be given and patient can be mobilized out of bed on the first postoperative day. Catheter removal can be done on 14th postoperative day. Cystogram is not a must. It is advised not to have intercourse for next 6 weeks.

Anticholinergics started to reduce the bladder spasm.

TIPS AND TRICKS

- Lifting the bladder through the suture passed through anterior abdominal wall will allow better vision and helps to identify the ureteric orifice and avoid it during suturing. It also avoids the use of fourth arm and additional port placement.
- Using a V-Loc suture avoids knotting the suture and save operation time.
- Using a barbed Quil allow suture to pass in one direction and allow to maintain adequate tension and watertight closure.
- Monocryl suture cause less irritation of the bladder and allow early absorption.
- Bowel preparation and head-low position allow the intestine away from the operation site.
- Key to successful surgery is providing well vascularized omental patch without tension and good drainage of the bladder during tissue healing.

Principles of good surgical repair are:

- Optimize the tissue condition before surgery-tissue should be free of inflammation, edema, infection or malignancy.
- Complete excision of scar tissue
- Tension free
- Watertight
- Multilayered
- Nonoverlapping suture lines
- Interposition of healthy vascularized tissue between bladder and vaginal suture lines.

Though the cost of robotic surgery repair is more, at present it is likely to come down in future. Definitely robotic repair is indicated in select complex cases for best results.

BIBLIOGRAPHY

1. Kumar S, Kekre NS, Goplakrishnan G. Vesicovaginal Fistula: An update. Indian J Urology. 2007;23(2);187-91.
2. Robotic reconstruction for recurrent supratrigonal vesicovaginal fistula. The Journal of Urology. 2008;180(3):981-5.
3. Sundaram BM, Kalidasan G, Hemal AK. Robotic repair of vesicovaginal fistula: case series of five patients. Urology. 2006;67(5):970-3.
4. Surgery Illustrated-Surgical Atlas Robotic repair of vesicovaginal Fistula (VVF). BJU International. 2012;109:1416-34.

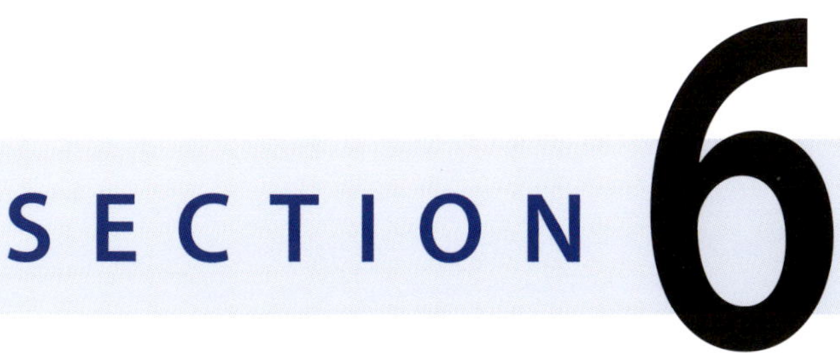

SECTION 6

Pediatric Urology

- **Pediatric Urology: The First Hundred Cases**
  DK Kandpal, SK Chowdhary

CHAPTER

22

Pediatric Urology: The First Hundred Cases

DK Kandpal, SK Chowdhary

INTRODUCTION

The development of minimal access surgery was one of the greatest achievements in the field of medicine in the second half of last century. The absorption of laparoscopic surgery in pediatric patients has remained a very slow process for obvious reasons. The widespread application is still hindered by significant learning curves for pediatric reconstructive procedures. A few studies in pediatric population have confirmed the benefits of minimally invasive surgery (MIS) earlier demonstrated in adult series.[1] However, the limitations of conventional MIS, i.e. two dimensional view, limited degree of movement of the instruments, lack of tactile feedback, poor ergonomic positions of the surgeon and the assistant, lack of training opportunity and steep learning curve continued the delay in extension of this surgical technology to pediatric population for major urological reconstructive procedures.[2]

The surgical robotic systems were designed to overcome many of the drawbacks of conventional laparoscopic surgery as well as enhance the surgical capabilities and skills. The arrival of robotic technology allowed the opportunity for extension of the minimally invasive approach for complex reconstructions in children. The well-known advantages of robotic technology are improved dexterity, three dimensional view, motion scaling, tremor filtration, operator controlled camera and EndoWrist™ instruments that provide seven degrees of freedom of movement. In the Indian context, there was a delay in the arrival and absorption of this revolutionary new way of doing surgery, particularly in the pediatric segment. One of the main reasons for this trend, was for the failure of the evolving health insurance industry in India, to support surgery for congenital malformation depriving the enormous pediatric population from the benefits of private health care revolution and access to modern heath care technology in India.[3]

The da Vinci robotic surgical platform was approved by the United States (US) Food and Drug Administration in 2000. The first robotic minimally invasive case in a child was Nissen fundoplication, reported in 2001.[4] Since then, there were a total of 2393 procedures reported in the following decade.[5] In contrast there were 573,000 procedures performed in adults on the da Vinci system in a single year (2014) alone. The adoption of robotics in pediatric population continues to be slow in the Asian context with very few centers having published their experience yet.[6]

The first pediatric robotic case at Indraprastha Apollo hospital was performed in March 2013, soon after the arrival of this technology in our hospital. Since then, more than a hundred cases have been performed including all complex urological reconstruction in infants and children, without any conversion. At the time of arrival of the robotic platform in our hospital, we had already crossed nearly a thousand laparoscopic procedures in babies which helped us absorb this new way of doing surgery rapidly.[7] The chapter describes the journey of adaptation to a new way of doing surgery and experience of this difficult, but very rewarding journey.

STARTING THE PEDIATRIC ROBOTIC PROGRAM

The pediatric services and volumes constitute a small fraction of the total adult volumes in a large private multispecialty hospital. At this stage, starting an exclusive pediatric robotic program is extremely difficult due to small case load and financial limitations. The financial viability of the robotic operating theater is dependent on all specialities sharing the same theater with the same nurse and operating room technicians helping changing surgical teams so that the supporting staff gains experience rapidly with the sophisticated machinery.

The primary driver to start a robotic program is the reputation of the department as a large tertiary referral center with good numbers of complex reconstructive procedures. Large experience of advanced laparoscopic procedures enables faster assimilation of this new technology. Although there were a few suggestions that laparoscopic skills are not an absolute prerequisite for developing robotic acumen, in our experience, the previous vast exposure to complex laparoscopic reconstructions considerably reduced the learning curve and allowed fast track development of complex robotic pediatric urological reconstructions.

The next step is building a team trained and familiar with the new technology. The chief surgeon and another surgeon with good exposure of laparoscopic work along with dedicated nurses and technicians form the integral part of the team. The safety of the patient is the prime consideration and needs proper communication by the surgeon to the assistants, anesthetist, scrub nurse and technician at all stages. The critical issues for the anesthetist during major robotic reconstructions are prolonged anesthesia in non-physiological position, effects of pneumoperitoneum and hypothermia and restricted access to the patient. In the initial stages the cases need to be selected appropriately for the robotic approach. It maybe a good idea to start with the less complex excisional surgeries rather than reconstructive procedures. Once the surgeon becomes familiar with the technology and the team starts to get together more complex procedures can be undertaken successfully.

Finally, maintenance of the clinical database and video records of the surgery for review and future references will go a long way in improving the skills and promoting research activity. The program as a whole and the individual surgical procedures need a critical review by the team at regular intervals for any course correction.

PYELOPLASTY FOR PELVIURETERIC JUNCTION OBSTRUCTION

The time tested and gold standard treatment for pelvi ureteric junction obstruction is open dismembered pyeloplasty with success rate of 95–100%.[8] One of the first series of laparoscopic pyeloplasty was reported in 1995.[9] The laparoscopic approach was limited to a few centers and never gained wide acceptance due to technical difficulty, long learning curves and concerns regarding risk of complications. Although the technical feasibility of laparoscopic pyeloplasty in infants and children was demonstrated in few studies, it gained limited popularity.[10] Robotic pyeloplasty has the advantage of shorter suturing time, shorter learning curve and magnified 3-D vision, and much less drag and shearing effect on the suture leading to reduced tissue trauma during intracorporeal suturing. Several authors have reported successful outcomes after robotic pyeloplasty **(Table 22.1)**.

We admitted our patients one day prior to surgery and mild bowel preparation was done with lactulose and proctoclysis enema. All the patients underwent preoperative cystoscopy, retrograde pyelography and retrograde DJ stenting. The patients were then placed in position with the affected side raised by 60 degrees for transperitoneal, transmesocolic pyeloplasty. Camera port (12 mm) was placed at the umbilicus or paramedian line at the level of umbilicus on opposite side. Eight or 5 mm working ports were placed with triangulation one below the xiphisternum and other in midclavicular line in the ipsilateral iliac fossa. The assistance port was placed in midline between umbilicus and pubic symphisis.

The pelviureteric junction was exposed on the left by transmesenteric approach and on the right by colonic mobilization. After the exposure of the pelvis and pelviureteric junction, the spatulation was begun on the pelvis first. The scissors were then interchanged to spatulate the ureter laterally. The dismembering of the pelviureteric junction was left to the last preserving the blood supply and allowing the PUJ for traction and excision later on completion of the anastomosis. We used PDS 6-0 or 5-0 suture for the anastomosis. Forty five children underwent robotic pyeloplasty. Two patients were referred for a redo pyeloplasty for failed procedure done earlier. Two patients underwent pyelolithotomy with pyeloplasty. The youngest baby was 4 months and 6 kg in weight. The mean age at the time of surgery was 6.5 years. All underwent cystoscopy, retrograde pyelography and retrograde DJ stenting. The associated renal anomalies were horse shoe kidney, ectopic kidney, malrotated kidney, anterior crossing lower pole vessels and renal calculus with PUJ obstruction. The mean operating time was 160 minutes. There were no conversion to open surgery and no intraoperative misadventures. Mean hospital stay was 3.5 days. DJ stent removal was done at four weeks and they were followed up at 3, 6 months and one year. Ultrasound scan and DTPA scan were done at 6 months. In the last twenty seven months two out of forty five children required a redo pyeloplasty. This was an infant and one of our first cases, who had developed stricture at the anastomotic site and presented with recurrent UTI and persistent dilatation and failure of improvement in drainage. Another has needed redo pyeloplasty after postoperative PUJ dilatation and DJ stenting for 3 months with no improvement. The third complication is in a child with severely limited function and massive pelvis, where although the PUJ is open on flexible URS, the huge pelvis (8 cm) is not draining satisfactorily. Although greater than 90% of young infants and young children operated for pelviureteric junction by the robotic approach have had an

Table 22.1: Robotic assisted pediatric pyeloplasty: complications and outcomes

Author	n	Mean age (years)	Operating time (minutes)	Hospital stay (days)	Complications (%)	Follow-up (months)	Success (%)
Lee et al. 2006	33	7.9	219	2.3	3	10	94
Olsen et al. 2007	67	7.9	146	2	17.9	12.1	94
Sorenson et al. 2011	33	9.2	326	2.2	15	17	97
Minnillo et al. 2011	155	10.5	198.5	1.9	11	31.7	96
Barbosa et al. 2013	58	7.2	NA	NA	1.7	33	76.9
Our series (unpublished), 2015	45	6.5	160	3.5	6.0	20	94

Table 22.2: Comparative table of open and robotic pyeloplasty in children

Author	n	Mean age (years)	Operative time (minutes)	Hospital stay (days)	Complications (%)	Follow-up (months)	Success (%)
Lee et al. 2006							
Open	33	7.6	181	3.5	0	20	100
Robotic	33	7.9	219	2.3	3	10	94
Sorenson et al. 2011							
Open	33	8.2	236	NA	9	19	97
Robotic	33	9.2	326	2.2	15	17	97
Barbosa et al. 2013							
Open	154	1.2	NA	NA	4.3	31	67.9
Robotic	58	7.2	NA	NA	1.7	33	76.9
Our series (unpublished), 2015							
Open	280	2.5	110	4.5	1.7	48	98.3
Robotic	45	5	180	3.5	6	20	94

excellent outcome in our experience with desired regression in pelvic drainage and dilatation, there is need for caution and close follow-up. Several authors from the western world, have demonstrated that the success rate of transperitoneal and retroperitoneal robotic pyeloplasty are similar to open pyeloplasty **(Table 22.2)**.

URETERIC REIMPLANTATION FOR REFLUXING/OBSTRUCTED/ECTOPIC URETERS, RETROCAVAL URETER

We have adopted the extravesical approach as described by Lich-Gregoir for treatment of vesicoureteric reflux. For grade I-III and symptomatic or deteriorating upper tract with unilateral or bilateral VUR we prefer endoscopic treatment by Deflux™ injection. In a case with grade IV-V, bilateral VUR, our preferred approach remains the open transtrigonal Cohen's reimplantation. Those patients with a unilateral grade IV-V VUR, obstructed ureters or ectopic ureters are ideal candidates for the robotic extravesical reimplantation. In patients with obstructed giant megaureters (>10 mm) especially in infants with poor renal function a side to side ureteroneocystostomy was done without disconnecting the ureter from the bladder.

Ectopic ureters with functioning moieties/kidneys presenting with incontinence can be managed very elegantly by the robotic approach. Ectopic ureters opening into the bladder neck, posterior urethra, vagina or the vestibule can be disconnected and reimplanted into the bladder by minimally invasive approach using robotic assistance. A variety of procedures on the lower ureters like trans uretero-ureterostomy, ipsilateral ureteroureterostomy and correction of retrocaval ureter have been shown to be safe and feasible by robotic approach.

The patient were placed in lithotomy position and camera port was placed at the umbilicus and pneumoperitoneum created. In smaller children the camera port was placed between umbilicus and xiphisternum to create more working space and to avoid the robotic arms colliding with each other. Two 8 mm ports were placed at the level of umbilicus in the anterior axillary line. The robot was docked from the foot end. The posterior bladder wall was exposed by a stay suture taken from the dome of the bladder. The lower ureter was mobilized and the detrusor was spilt till the mucosa is visible. The ureter was placed in this tunnel and overwrapped by the detrusor. A cystogram was done at the end of the procedure to check for VUR. For obstructed megaureters, a refluxing side to side reimplant was done with a DJ stent *in situ*. The catheter was left for 3–5 days and DJ stent removed after 4 weeks.

Twelve children underwent a unilateral extravesical ureteric reimplantation for unilateral high grade VUR. The age range was from 2 to 12 years. The mean operating time was 90 minutes with a range of 70 to 100 minutes. Most of the children were discharged the next day. None of the patients had a recurrence of the reflux during the mean follow-up of nine months. As compared to open procedure there was no hematuria, clot retention or dysuria in any of the patients. Ten other children with primary obstructed megaureters and two with postureteric reimplantation obstruction underwent a refluxing reimplantation. A side to side neo ureterocystostomy was done across a stent without disconnecting the ureter from the bladder. The urethral catheter was removed after 3–5 days. At this stage, now we are able to discharge children after robotic ureteric reimplant within 24 hours. This is going to translate to huge saving on health care spending in the long run. The extravesical robotic ureteric reimplantation has been shown to be an efficacious and safe procedure in children **(Table 22.3)**.

Robotic approach for lower ureteric surgery in cases of ectopic ureters, retrocaval ureter etc. provides excellent opportunity for a minimally invasive repair. Reimplantation of ectopic ureters and trans ureteroureterostomy were done in three patients with good results.

Table 22.3: Extravesical robotic ureteric reimplantation for vesicoureteric reflux in children: complications and outcomes

Author	*n*	*Mean age (years)*	*Operative time (minutes)*	*Hospital stay (days)*	*Complications (%)*	*Follow-up (months)*	*Success (%)*
Casale et al. 2008	41	3.1	139	1	None	3–6	97.6
Kasturi et al. 2012	150	3.5	108	1	None	3–24	99.3
Hayashi et al. 2014	15	11	268	7.4	Recurrence 1	3–4	93.3
Akhavan et al. 2014	78	7.2	NA	2	Ileus 2 Obstruction 1 Ureter injury 1	14	92.4
Our series, 2015	12	6	90	3	None	16	100

PARTIAL NEPHRECTOMY/HEMI-NEPHROURETERECTOMY/NEPHRO-URETERECTOMY FOR COMPLEX RENAL ANOMALIES

Preoperative preparation was done as per protocol for pyeloplasty. Cystoscopy, RGP, DJ stenting of the functioning moiety was done to protect and identify the normal ureter. The patient was positioned in the same way as for pyeloplasty. The camera port was placed at the level of umbilicus in opposite paramedian line and working ports just below the xiphisternum and ipsilateral midclavicular line below the umbilicus. The kidney was exposed by mobilizing and reflecting the colon along the line of Toldt. The dissection was started at the renal hilum and affected pole vessels identified, ligated and divided. The dissection of the plane between upper and the lower pole was particularly difficult in patients with history of recurrent upper urinary tract infection. After the heminephrectomy was completed, patient was placed in lithotomy position and ports rearranged for the pelvic part of the surgery. The position of the camera and the working ports was swapped for surgery in the pelvis. The dissection of lower ureteric end was completed and ureteric stump was ligated with either suture or hemoclip close to the bladder wall. The specimen was delivered through the camera port.

Thirteen patients underwent heminephroureterectomy for symptomatic nonfunctioning pole/kidney. The magnified and three dimensional view allowed precise dissection without any risk of injury to the vessels or ureter of functioning moiety. One patient developed perinephric collection after heminephroureterectomy which resolved on conservative management.

AUGMENTATION CYSTOPLASTY WITH URETERIC REIMPLANTATION

Augmentation cystoplasty is the gold standard for neuropathic bladder refractory to medical management. Laparoscopic augmentation was reported by a few authors but never gained acceptance due to technical problems in intracorporeal suturing in limited space of a child's pelvis. The full potential of the robotic technology is realized in complex reconstructions like these. Gundeti et al. reported their experience of six patients with robotic augmentation ileocystoplasty in 2011.[11] They demonstrated the safety and feasibility of this approach.

We have our own experience of robotic augmentation cystoplasty and bilateral ureteric reimplantation in four children with a median follow-up of 15 months. The age range was from two years to fifteen years. All four cases were completed by the minimally invasive robotic approach with intracorporeal suturing without the use of staplers. The mean operative time was 330 minutes (300–360 minutes). The morphine requirement was significantly less in the robotic group as compared to the open group. The bladder capacity increased from a preoperative mean of 83 mL to postoperative mean of 163 mL at three month after surgery. All are on clean intermittent catheterization through the native urethra with a dry interval of more than 4 hours. The peak detrusor pressure decreased from a mean of 60 cm of water to 20 cm of water postoperatively at one month. There was no anastomotic leak or any postoperative major morbidity. The Hospital stay was 8–14 days. The follow up ranges from six months to twenty months with a median period of 15 months **(Table 22.4)**.

The robotic augmentation cystoplasty will reduce the total hospital stay and eventually cut down the cost of treatment with superior cosmetic and overall long-term results. The immediate postoperative period and the early results are very encouraging **(Table 22.5)**. The robotic assistance allows the minimally invasive approach to replicate the open procedure step by step and thus reproduce the excellent results of the open surgery. These cases were selected very carefully and none of these required a bladder neck procedure. In future as our experience increases bladder neck procedure can be added to the augmentation cystoplasty, wherever indicated in more complex patients.

In our experience of first 100 consecutive cases there were no robotic malfunction or instrument failures. FDA's MAUDE (manufacturer and user facility device experience) database has reported 565 robotic instrument failures in a two year period between 2009 and 2010.[12] The age range of our patients was from 4 months to 16 years, twelve patients were less than one year of age. None of the patients required conversion to open surgery. The smallest child operated by us was 4 months old and 6 kg in weight, who underwent robotic pyeloplasty. In neonates and smaller children there are technical difficulties of using robotic technology due to space constraints which

Table 22.4: Comparative chart of robotic augmentation ileocystoplasty

Author	n	*Mean age*	*Medical management*	*Bowel prep*	*Surgery*	*Technique of ileocystoplasty*	*Postoperative urodynamics*	*Follow-up in months (range)*
Gundeti et al. 2010	6*	10 years	CIC4/6 AntiCh 6/6	None	Augmentation ileocystoplasty 6/6 Mitrofanoff 5/6 Bladder neck reconstruction none Ureteric reimplant none	Bladder bivalved in coronal plane Detubularized ileal loop sutured directly to bladder	Not recorded	18 (14–22)
Current, 2015	4	9.5 years	CIC 4/4 AntiCh 4/4 Botox 2/4	All	Augmentation ileocystoplasty 4/4 Ureteric reimplant 3/4 Mitrofanoff none Bladder neck reconstruction none	Bladder bivalved in sagittal plane Detubularized Ileal loop made into a U plate duplicating open technique	Done in all	15 (6–20)

*conversion to open 1

Table 22.5: Comparison of open and robotic ileocystoplasty, n = 4

	Open ileocystoplasty	*Robotic ileocystoplasty*	*p*
Mean operative time	240 minutes	330 minutes	<0.05
Mean morphine requirement	42 mg	12 mg	<0.05
Mean hospital stay	16 days	10 days	<0.05
Mean percentage increase in bladder capacity	175%	177%	Not significant

result in internal cluttering of instruments and external collision of robotic arms. Miniaturization of the robot and dedicated instruments with smaller articulating length will allow the pediatric robotic urology to take off in true sense. Until then, the indications and application of robots at our center will be limited to infants greater than 6 kilograms or 6 months.

CONCLUSION

Robotic technology is an innovation which will take the minimally invasive surgery to another orbit. Robotics will decrease the steep learning curve for advanced laparoscopic procedures. The conventional laparoscopic surgery will continue to have its important place and laparoscopy and robotics will remain complimentary to each other. With further evolution of this technology the robotics has the potential to become an essential armamentarium of the pediatric urologist.

REFERENCES

1. Chowdhary SK, Kandpal DK. Minimal access surgery in children: a 5 year study. Indian Pediatr. 2012;49:971-4.
2. Esposito C, Valla JS, Yeung CK. Current indications for laparoscopy and retroperitoneoscopy in pediatric urology. Surg Endosc. 2004;18:1559-64.
3. Nerli R, Reddy M, Chowdhary SK. The Asian Continent: is it ready for the new technology? An Indian perspective. In: Gundeti MS (Ed). Pediatric robotic & reconstructive urology: a comprehensive guide. West Sussex, England: Wiley Blackwell. 2012. pp. 305-12.
4. Meininger DD, Byhahn C, Heller K, Gutt CN, Westphal K. Totally endoscopic Nissen fundoplication with a robotic system in a child. Surg Endosc. 2001;15:1360-1.
5. Cundy TP, Shetty K, Clark J, Chang TP, Sriskandarajah K, Gattas NE, Najmaldin A, Yang GZ, Darzi A. The first decade of robotic surgery in children. J Pediatr Surg. 2013;48:858-65.
6. Chowdhary SK, Kandpal DK, Agarwal D, Sibal A, Srivastava RN. Robotic augmentation ileocystoplasty with bilateral ureteric reimplantation in a young child with neuropathic bladder. J Indian Assoc Pediatr Surg. 2014,19:162-5.
7. Chowdhary SK, Kandpal DK, Agarwal D, Balan S, Jerath N, Sibal A, Broor SL. Endoscopic esophageal substitution for pure esophageal atresia and wide gap esophageal atresia: a report of five cases with minimum follow-up of twelve months. J Pediatr Surg. 2015.
8. O' Reilly PH, Brooman PJ, Mak S, Jones M, Pickup C, Atkinson C, Pollard AJ. The long-term results of Anderson-Hynes pyeloplasty. BJU Int. 2001;87:287-9.
9. Peters CA, Schlussel RN, Retik AB. Pediatric laparoscopic dismembered pyeloplasty. J Urol. 1995;153:1962-5.
10. Tan HL. Laparoscopic Anderson-Hynes dismembered pyeloplasty in children. J Urol. 2008;180:1689-92.
11. Gundeti MS, Acharya SS, Zagaja GP, Shalhav AL. Paediatric robotic-assisted laparoscopic augmentation ileocystoplasty and Mitrifanoff appendicovesicostomy (RALIMA): feasibility of and initial experience with the University of Chicago technique. BJU Int. 2011;107:962-9.
12. Friedman DC, Lendvay TS, Hannaford B. Instrument failures for the da Vinci surgical system: a Food and drug administration MAUDE database study. Surg Endosc. 2013;27:1503-8.

SECTION 7

Adult Urology

- **Radical Prostatectomy**
  Hariharan Palayapalayam Ganapathi, Kenneth J Palmer, Gabriel Ogaya-Pines, Travis Rogers, Vipul R Patel
- **Role of Pelvic Lymphadenectomy in Robot-assisted Radical Prostatectomy**
  Varun Mittal, NP Gupta
- **Radical Cystoprostatectomy**
  Sudhir Rawal
- **Partial Nephrectomy**
  Ajit Saxena
- **Donor Nephrectomy**
  Vinay Mahendra, Jaydip Bhadra Roy, Tridibes Mondal
- **Adrenalectomy**
  Sohrab Arora, Gagan Gautam
- **Urolithiasis: Expanding the Horizons of Robotic Surgery**
  Siddharth Yadav, Prabhjot Singh, Prem Nath Dogra
- **Pyeloplasty**
  Manu Gupta
- **Ureteric Reimplantation**
  Vipin Tyagi

CHAPTER

23

Radical Prostatectomy

Hariharan Palayapalayam Ganapathi, Kenneth J Palmer, Gabriel Ogaya-Pines, Travis Rogers, Vipul R Patel

INTRODUCTION

Radical prostatectomy is one of the surgical treatments for clinically localized prostate cancer. Since introduced in 2000 robotic assistance has significantly changed the surgical management of clinically localized prostate cancer.[1] Within a decade, robot assisted laparoscopic radical prostatectomy (RALP) is being utilized worldwide. In the USA, more than 80% of radical prostatectomies are performed with robot assistance.[2] Several technical modifications evolved with the principle of achieving trifecta. Our group introduced the concept of pentafecta with key components of local tumor control with negative surgical margins, less perioperative morbidity while preserving continence and sexual function.[3]

Currently, RALP is performed with the da Vinci® system (Intuitive Surgical, Sunnyvale, CA). RALP has attracted the attention of urologists to take advantage of its immersive three-dimensional (3-D) vision, 7° of freedom of movement truly mimicking the movements made during standard open surgery, tremor filtration, motion scaling, and superior ergonomics compared to standard laparoscopy. These advantages favor shorter learning curve for complex laparoscopic skills such as intracorporeal suturing and knot tying.

Multiple RALP series demonstrated safety, efficiency, and reproducibility of the procedure. Meta-analysis across multiple high volume centers demonstrated clear advantages in perioperative morbidity and functional outcomes.[3-6]

Our technique is based upon a fusion of the open approach as described by Walsh and the standard laparoscopic approach. However, after having performed more than 9,000 cases (single surgeon series—VP), our technique has evolved significantly, including several refinements to further improve surgical outcomes and reduce patient morbidity. In the present manuscript, we perform a detailed description of our surgical technique of RALP and provide practical recommendations based on available reports and personal experience. We herein describe the surgical technique we currently perform at our institution.

Preoperative Preparation

One hour prior to incision, the patient receives 1 g IV Cefazolin (first-generation cephalosporin). Prior to induction of anesthesia, sequential compression devices are placed on the lower extremities and the patient receives 5,000 units of subcutaneous heparin. At this point the patient is positioned in low lithotomy, ensuring that thighs are not overextended to avoid neuropraxia. All pressure points including shoulders, elbows and wrists are carefully and thoroughly padded **(Fig. 23.1)**. The patient is placed within a bean bag which is fixed to the table aided by adhesive tape. Abdominal hair is trimmed and the patient is prepped and draped in a sterile fashion. An orogastric tube is inserted before insufflation along with an 18-French Foley catheter with 15 cc sterile water in the balloon.

Intra-abdominal Access and Trocar Placement

Most published RALP series follow the same basic principles with only subtle modifications. Positioning of the patient in extended lithotomy and steep Trendelenburg is the standard. Likewise, most series utilize the transperitoneal approach as it provides a larger working space, particularly important during lymph-node dissection and urethrovesical anastomosis.[5-7] A six-trocar transperitoneal approach is utilized in all cases. Access to the abdominal cavity is obtained via a 1 cm supra-umbilical incision using a Veress needle insufflating up to 15 mm Hg **(Fig. 23.2)**. **Figures 23.3 and 23.4** indicate our port placement.

Step 1: Incision of the peritoneum and entry into the space of Retzius.

Instruments

- *Right arm (Xi Arm #4):* Monopolar scissors (Da Vinci Si setting: 25W or Xi setting: 2)
- *Left arm (Xi Arm #2):* Bipolar forceps (Da Vinci Si setting: 25 W or Xi setting: 2)
- *Fourth arm (Xi Arm #1):* Prograsp forceps
- *Camera port (Xi Arm #3):* Telescope 0° lens
- *Assistant:* Microfrance grasper and suction.

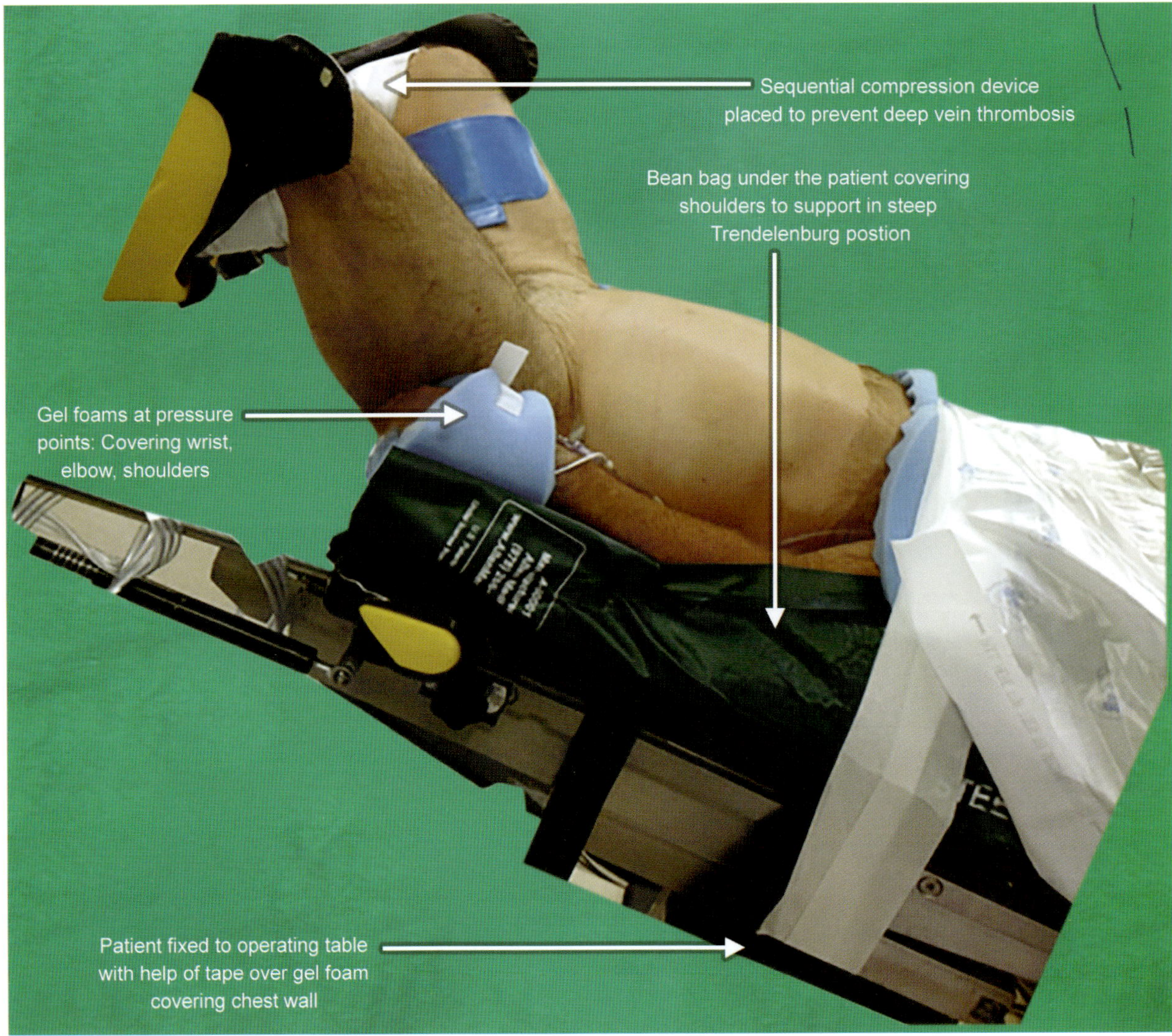

Fig. 23.1: Patient positioning for robot assisted laparoscopic radical prostatectomy

A transverse peritoneal incision is made through the median umbilical ligament and extended on both sides in an inverted U fashion to the level of the vasa deferens laterally. The fourth arm provides countertraction for this step. The peritoneum is dissected down to the pubic tubercle, which is the anatomical landmark used to follow the pubic rami lateral and horizontally so as to not produce inadvertent injury to epigastric vessels above the rami. It is important to dissect the peritoneum all the way up to the base of the vasa for optimum release of the bladder to allow a tension-free vesicourethral anastomosis.

Step 2: Incision of the endopelvic fascia (EPF) and identification of the dorsal venous complex.

Instruments

- *Right arm (Xi Arm #4): Monopolar scissors (Da Vinci Si setting: 25W, Xi setting: 2)*
- *Left arm (Xi Arm #2): Bipolar forceps (Da Vinci Si setting: 25 W, Xi setting: 2)*
- *Fourth arm (Xi Arm #1): Prograsp forceps*
- *Camera port (Xi Arm #3): Telescope 0° lens*
- *Assistant: Microfrance grasper and suction.*

The important landmarks are bladder neck, base of the prostate, levator ani muscles, and apex of the prostate. After defatting the prostate, the fourth arm is used to retract it contralaterally so as to provide adequate exposure and tension on the EPF. The EPF is opened (with sharp dissection) toward the base of the prostate and then followed toward the apex of the prostate to identify the notch between dorsal venous complex (DVC) and urethra where the DVC ligation and suspension stitch will be placed. This step is performed using cold scissors and taking extra caution in identifying any accessory pudendal arteries that may travel along the EPF. Proceeding from the base to the apex, the fibers of the levator ani are dissected off the prostate with the round edge of the scissors until the DVC and urethra are visualized **(Fig. 23.5)**. Use caution when dissecting and cutting the puboprosatic ligaments because if carried out too medially it will definitely

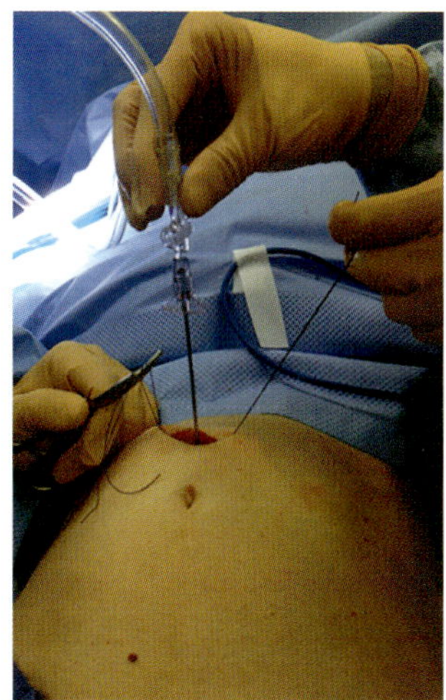
Fig. 23.2: Supraumbilical incision, support stiches in the rectus sheath and Veress needle insufflation

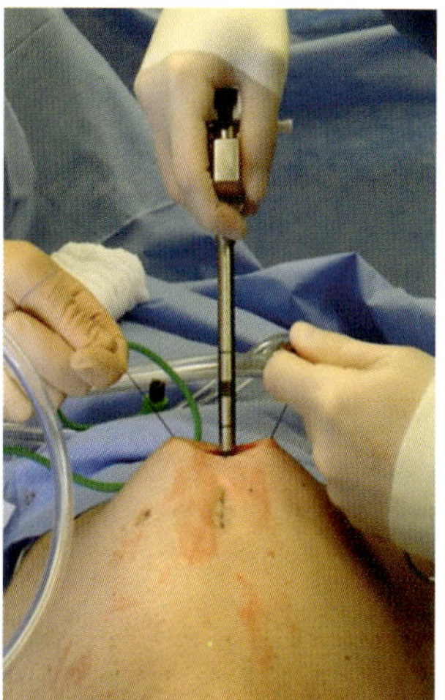
Fig. 23.3: Camera port placement (da Vinci Xi 8 mm trocar)

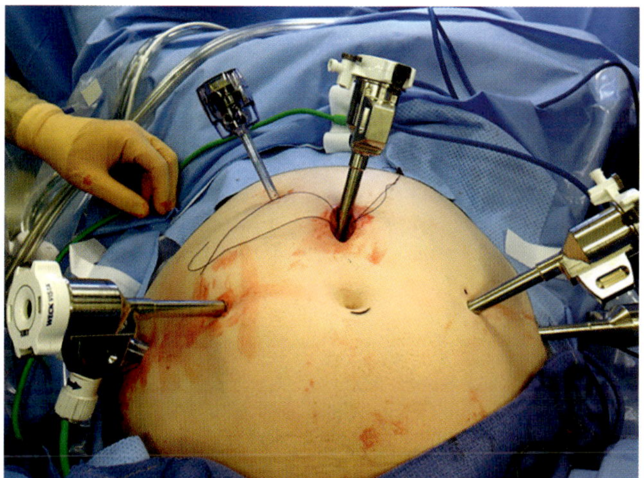
Fig. 23.4: Ports in place for da Vinci Xi surgical robot assisted radical prostatectomy

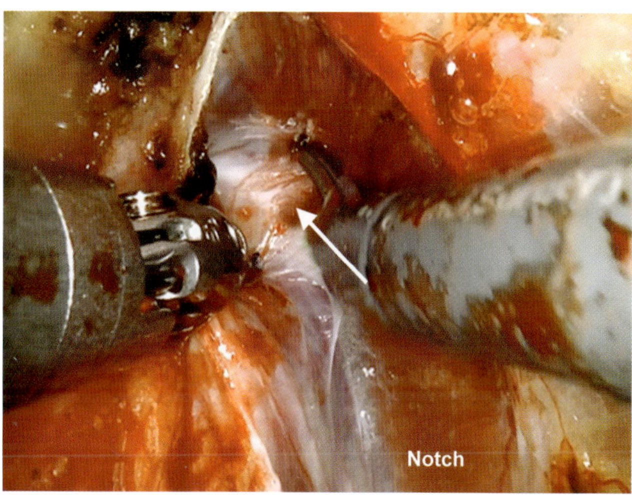

Fig. 23.5: Incision of endopelvic fascia and identification of notch between dorsal venous complex and urethra

lead to injury of the DVC and unnecessary bleeding. Full dissection of the apex is best performed at the end of the procedure.

Step 3: Ligation of the DVC.

Instruments

- *Right arm (Xi Arm #4):* Large robotic needle driver
- *Left arm (Xi Arm #2):* Large robotic needle driver
- *Camera port (Xi Arm #3):* Telescope 0° lens
- *Fourth arm (Xi Arm #1):* Prograsp forceps
- *Assistant:* Laparoscopic scissors and needle driver.

We use 12 inch length Caprosyn 1 on a large CT1 needle. The needle is held two-third back at a 45° angle and placed in the notch between the urethra and DVC. The needle is pushed straight across at 90° and then the wrist is turned to curve around the apex of the prostate **(Fig. 23.6)**. At this point we prefer to use the slip knot to tie as it prevents the suture from loosening as it is tied. A second suture is then placed to suspend the urethra to the pubic bone and secondarily ligate the DVC. The DVC is encircled and then stabilized against the pubic bone along with the urethra **(Fig. 23.7)**.

Step 4: Anterior bladder neck (BN) dissection.

Instruments

- *Right arm (Xi Arm #4):* Monopolar scissors (Da Vinci Si setting: 25W, Xi setting: 2)
- *Left arm (Xi Arm #2):* Bipolar forceps (Da Vinci Si setting: 25 W, Xi setting: 2)
- *Fourth arm (Xi Arm #1):* Prograsp forceps
- *Assistant:* Microfrance grasper and suction
- *Camera port (Xi Arm #3):* Telescope 30° lens directed downward.

The scope is changed to a 30° down-facing lens for the BN dissection. Although some authors use 0° scope throughout

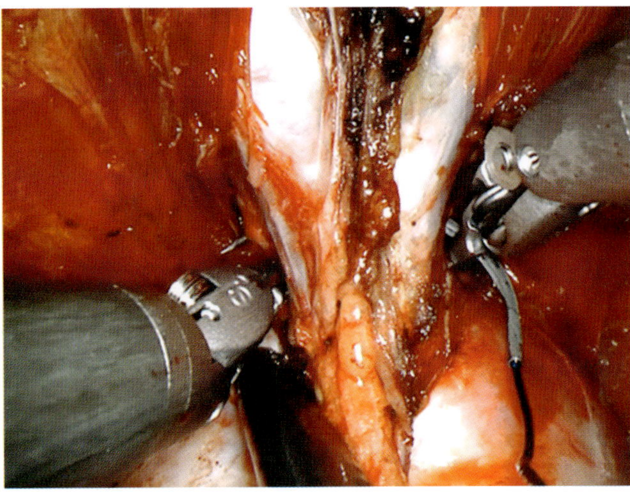

Fig. 23.6: Ligation of dorsal venous complex

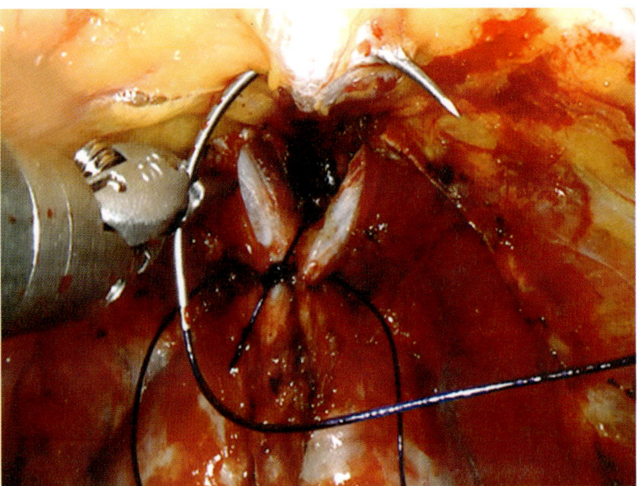

Fig. 23.7: Anterior suspension stitch

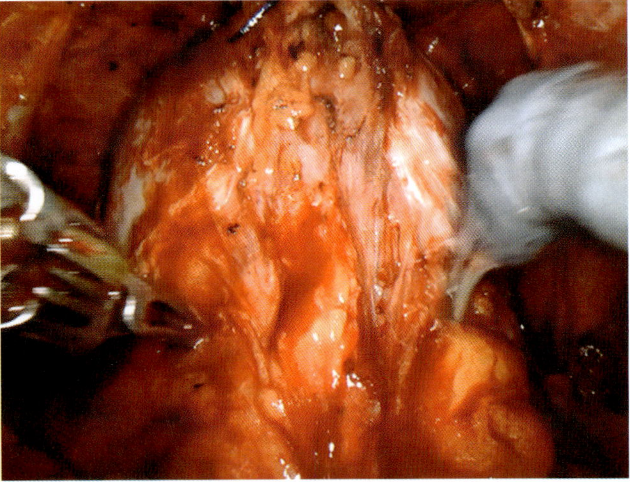

Fig. 23.8: Identifying anterior bladder neck by fat line and pinching with robotic arms

the case, we believe that this angled lens is optimal to see inferiorly and to visualize the correct planes. Key points here to correctly identify the BN is identifying where the bladder fat ends on the prostate in the form of an inverted "U" **(Fig. 23.8)**; another trick is to pull on the Foley catheter and visualize the balloon as it reaches the base of the prostate. However, although useful, this can be misleading in patients with prior transurethral resection of the prostate (TURP) or in the presence of median or anterior lobes. The robotic arms also provide a moderate amount of visual feedback to facilitate localization of the boundaries (double-pinch maneuver). This step is begun by cauterizing the superficial veins that are located in the midline with the bipolar forceps. Then the bladder is dissected off the prostate in the midline using a continuous sweeping motion of the monopolar scissors and traction with the bipolar forceps while visualizing the bladder fibers. The key is to stay in the midline to avoid lateral venous sinuses until the anterior bladder neck is opened and the Foley catheter visualized. Once the anterior urethra is divided, the Foley catheter is retracted out of the bladder using the fourth arm, in an upward manner to expose the posterior bladder neck.

Step 5: Posterior bladder neck.

Instruments

- *Right arm (Xi Arm #4):* Monopolar scissors (Da Vinci Si setting: 25W, Xi setting: 2)
- *Left arm (Xi Arm #2):* Bipolar forceps (Da Vinci Si setting: 25 W, Xi setting: 2)
- *Fourth arm (Xi Arm #1):* Prograsp forceps
- *Assistant:* Microfrance grasper and suction
- *Camera port (Xi Arm #3):* Telescope 30° lens directed downward.

The posterior BN dissection is generally considered to be the most challenging step of the operation for the novice robotic surgeon. The difficulty is in appreciating the posterior tissue plane between the bladder and prostate and the direction and depth of dissection necessary to locate the seminal vesicles. After incising of the anterior BN, any remaining peripheral bladder attachments should be divided to flatten out the area of the posterior bladder neck and allow precise visualization and dissection of the posterior plane. The full thickness of the posterior bladder neck should be incised at the precise junction between the prostate and the bladder. The lip of the posterior BN is then grasped with the fourth arm and retracted upward. The bipolar forceps is then used for traction thus visualizing the correct plane between prostate and bladder. The dissection is directed posteriorly and slightly cephalad (toward the bladder) to expose the seminal vesicles. It is important to avoid dissecting caudally (toward the prostate) as there is a possibility of entering the prostate and missing the seminal vesicles completely.

Step 6: Seminal vesicle (SV) dissection.

Instruments

- *Right arm (Xi Arm #4):* Monopolar scissors (Da Vinci Si setting: 25W, Xi setting: 2)
- *Left arm (Xi Arm #2):* Bipolar forceps (Da Vinci Si setting: 25 W, Xi setting: 2)
- *Fourth arm (Xi Arm #1):* Prograsp forceps
- *Assistant:* Microfrance grasper and suction
- *Camera port (Xi Arm #3):* Telescope 30° lens directed downward.

Once the posterior BN dissection is complete, the vasa and SVs can be identified. The thin fascial layer over the SVs and vasa should be opened to free the structures for retraction. The fourth arm is used to retract the left vas superiorly and laterally. Dissection continues on the medial side of the vas due to the inexistence of vessels in this area, until the tip of the left SV is reached. When this occurs it is grasped and retracted with the fourth arm elevating it away from the neurovascular structures that lie beneath (hypogastric plexus). The vas is then clipped with a 10 mm hem-o-lock followed by clipping of the vessels of the tip of the SV. Then the SV is dissected completely to the base. This procedure is carried out similarly on the right side.

Step 7: Denonvilliers' fascia and posterior dissection.

Instruments

- *Right arm (Xi Arm #4):* Monopolar scissors (Da Vinci Si setting: 25W, Xi setting: 2)
- *Left arm (Xi Arm #2):* Bipolar forceps (Da Vinci Si setting: 25 W, Xi setting: 2)
- *Fourth arm (Xi Arm #1):* Prograsp forceps
- *Assistant:* Microfrance grasper and suction
- *Camera port (Xi Arm #3):* Telescope 30° lens directed downward.

Once the SVs have been dissected completely to the base, the right SV is handed over to the assistant for upward traction; the left SV is retracted using the fourth arm. Downward traction of the undersurface of the prostate with the bipolar forceps is applied and blunt dissection using the monopolar scissors on the base of the SVs correctly identifies Denonvilliers' fascia (visualized as a bright pearly white plane **(Fig. 23.9)**. Denonvilliers' fascia is then entered and dissected laterally and caudally until reaching the apex of the prostate.

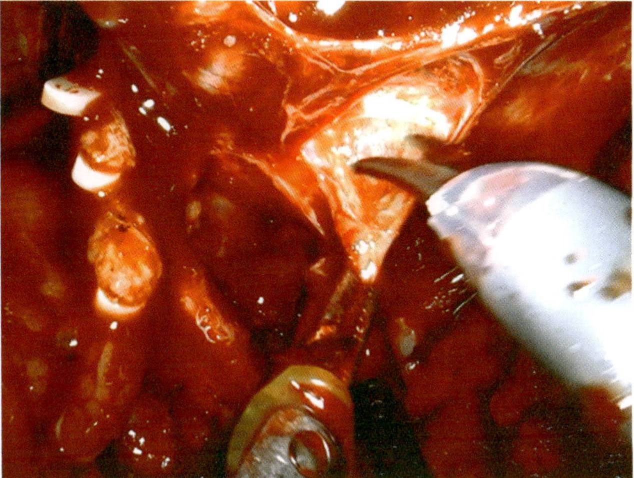

Fig. 23.9: Incision of Denonvilliers fascia

Step 8: Neurovascular bundle (NVB) preservation.

Instruments

- *Right arm (Xi Arm #4):* Monopolar scissors (Da Vinci Si setting: 25W, Xi setting: 2)
- *Left arm (Xi Arm #2):* Bipolar forceps (Da Vinci Si setting: 25 W, Xi setting: 2)
- *Fourth arm (Xi Arm #1):* Prograsp forceps
- *Assistant:* Microfrance grasper and suction
- *Camera port (Xi Arm #3):* Telescope 30° lens directed upward then downward.

Athermal early retrograde release: Our approach to nerve-sparing portion is unique as we perform it in a retrograde fashion, mirroring the open approach. It is based upon the philosophy of minimal traction, athermal, and early release of the neurovascular bundle with precise identification at the mid-prostate prior to ligating the prostatic pedicle.

Prior to performing this portion, it is essential to fully dissect the posterior plane up to the apex and laterally to the bundles. Prior DVC ligation is also key as this decompresses large periprostatic veins that can potentially be a frustrating source of bleeding. Posteriorly at mid prostate level plane between neurovascular bundle and prostatic capsule created by athermal blunt dissection using bipolar forceps. Camera rotation of 180° to look upward (instant toggling of endoscope from 30 down to up) helps to better visualize and dissect at this step. This feature is available in the Da Vinci Xi surgical system using touch screen control panel in the console. For release of the left NVB, the assistant grasps the prostate and rotates it contralaterally (to the right). When dissecting the right NVB the fourth arm is used instead of the assistant to rotate and elevate the prostate, grasping the SVs and border of the prostate in an alternating manner.

With the prostate rotated laterally, the lateral pelvic fascia is incised and peeled like an onion until the neurovascular bundle is identified. Once this is accomplished, early release of the neurovascular bundle can then be performed. The levator fascia is elevated with the bipolar forceps and incised along the lateral aspect of the prostate. At the level of the apex and mid-portion of the prostate, the avascular plane between the neurovascular bundle and prostatic fascia is developed with caution, using the bipolar forceps to maintain the neurovascular steady and the monopolar scissors used to peel the prostate off the bundle. The importance of the assistant in this step cannot be stressed enough as they are in charge of maintaining a bloodless operating field for clear visualization of the bundle as well as contralateral traction. Once the posterior plane is reached, the retrograde dissection begins toward the prostatic pedicle and then toward the apex of the prostate. No thermal energy is used during dissection of the bundle or ligation of the pedicle. The path of the bundle

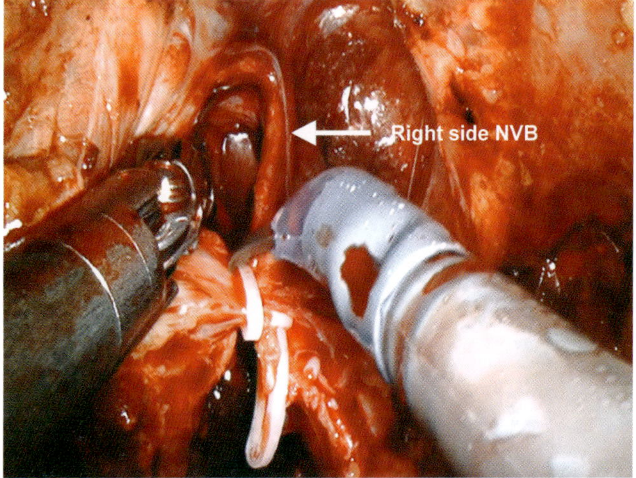

Fig. 23.10: Preservation of neurovascular bundle (NVB)—right side

Fig. 23.11: Transection of urethra with adequate stump length

has now been clearly delineated and focus can now turn to controlling the prostatic vascular pedicle. The pedicle is controlled with hem-o-lock clips placed above the level of the already released bundle **(Fig. 23.10)**. This technique allows complete neurovascular bundle sparing without the use of any thermal energy, trauma, or inadvertent damage.

Step 9: Apical dissection.

Instruments

- *Right arm (Xi Arm #4):* Monopolar scissors (Da Vinci Si setting: 25W, Xi setting: 2)
- *Left arm (Xi Arm #2):* Bipolar forceps (Da Vinci Si setting: 25 W, Xi setting: 2)
- *Fourth arm (Xi Arm #1):* Prograsp forceps
- *Assistant:* Microfrance grasper and suction
- *Camera port (Xi Arm #3):* Telescope 30° lens directed downward.

The landmarks are the ligated DVC, urethra, apex of the prostate, and NVB. Again, it is essential to have securely ligated DVC to prevent bleeding, which may interfere with the apical dissection and division of the urethra under direct vision. Cold scissors are used to carefully divide the DVC and create a long urethral stump facilitating the anastomosis. Complete dissection of the apex and urethra is facilitated by the 10X magnification that the robot provides. Once the urethra has been identified, the bipolar forceps is used to create a plane on the posterior surface of the urethra separating it from the musculofascial plate before incising with cold scissors. The rhabdosphincter is then incised with caution, avoiding any posterior lip that the prostate may have at this location **(Fig. 23.11)**.

Step 10: Bladder neck reconstruction, posterior reconstruction and urethrovesical anastomosis.

Instruments

- *Right and left arms (Xi Arm #2 & 4):* Large robotic needle drivers
- *Camera port (Xi Arm #3):* Telescope 30° lens directed downward.

Before starting the bladder neck reconstruction it is essential to check the position of ureteral orifices and their distance from the edge of the bladder neck. Bilateral plication over the lateral aspect of the bladder is then performed using sutures of 2-0 Quill Monoderm® 8 cm long in VP 2000Q needle (16 cm double armed suture cut in to equal half). The suture begins laterally and runs medially until the bladder neck size matches that of membranous urethra.

Prior to performing the vesicourethral anastomosis, we perform a modified reconstruction of the pelvic floor, re-attaching Denonvilliers' fascia to the rhabdosphincter. For this step, we use a 2-0 Quill® variable loop suture 20 cm length (Quill knotless tissue closure device). We proceed to identify the free edge of Denonvilliers' fascia, which is approximated to the posterior aspect of the rhabdosphincter and posterior median raphe running one of the arms of the suture and tied. A second layer is then run with the second arm of the suture, approximating the posterior bladder neck to the posterior lip of the urethra **(Fig. 23.12)**.

A continuous modified van Velthoven vesicourethral anastomosis is then performed. Single 2-0 Quill Monoderm® loop double armed suture of 16 cm long on VP 2000Q needles are used for the anastomosis. The posterior urethral anastomosis is performed first with one arm of the suture starting at the 5 o'clock position until reaching the 10 o'clock position in a clockwise fashion. This is followed by completion of the anterior anastomosis with the second arm of the suture in a counterclockwise fashion and then tying both sutures on the urethral stump. The key to performing an efficient rapid watertight anastomosis is to use both hands when suturing; that is, the left hand feeds the suture to the right and so forth. Having a long urethral stump, normal-sized bladder neck, clear operative field, and exerting perineal pressure (in some instances) contribute to this also. Once the anastomosis is completed, a new 18 Fr Foley catheter is placed and saline solution is used to irrigate and eliminate any clots and also to confirm a watertight anastomosis. A Jackson–Pratt drain is placed at the pelvic rim and then all trocars are removed under direct vision.

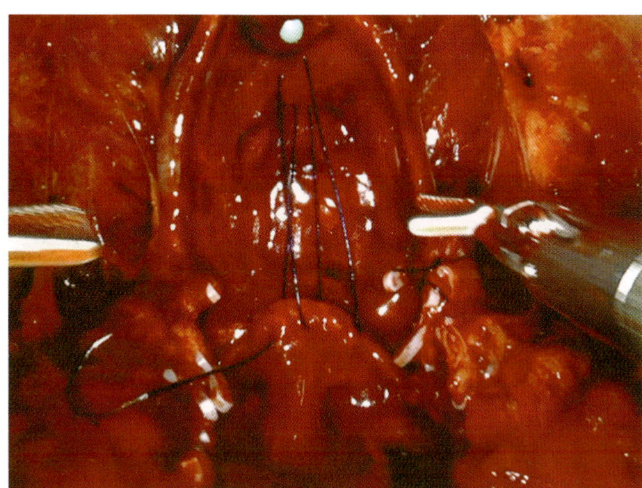

Fig. 23.12: First layer of the posterior reconstruction—Denonvilliers fascia sutured with the rhabdosphincter

CONCLUSION

Fifteen years after the first RALP was performed, multiple large series are currently mature enough to demonstrate outcomes with at least comparable data to most experienced open centers.

It is clear that the evolution of minimally invasive surgery from standard laparoscopy to robotics has given the surgeon a great advantage over the later, regarding magnification.

However, these advantages provided rely solely on the expertise of the surgeon, team, and the manner in which he applies his surgical knowledge. As with any foray into new technology and surgical procedures, the development of technical modifications and surgical refinements are inevitable with increasing experience, explaining the role of surgical volume in ultimately improving the outcomes. During our learning experience, we developed several technical modifications that currently allow us to perform the procedure with shorter operative time, improved oncological and functional outcomes, and low overall complication rates.

REFERENCES

1. Brawley OW. Prostate cancer epidemiology in the United States. World J Urol. 2012;30:195-200.
2. Cooperberg MR, Broering JM, Carroll PR. Time trends and local variation in primary treatment of localized prostate cancer. J Clin Oncol. 2010;28:1117-23.
3. Patel VR, Sivaraman A, Coelho RF, et al. Pentafecta: a new concept for reporting outcomes of robot-assisted laparoscopic radical prostatectomy. Eur Urol. 2011;59:702-7.
4. Ficarra V, Novara G, Rosen RC, et al. Systematic review and meta-analysis of studies reporting urinary continence recovery after robot-assisted radical prostatectomy. Eur Urol. 2012;62:405-17.
5. Ficarra V, Novara G, Ahlering TE, et al. Systematic review and meta-analysis of studies reporting potency rates after robot-assisted radical prostatectomy. Eur Urol. 2012;62:418-30.
6. Novara G, Ficarra V, Rosen RC, et al. Systematic review and meta-analysis of perioperative outcomes and complications after robot-assisted radical prostatectomy. Eur Urol. 2012;62:431-52.
7. Patel VR, Tully AS, Holmes R, et al. Robotic radical prostatectomy in the community setting—the learning curve and beyond: initial 200 cases. J Urol. 2005;174:269-72.

CHAPTER

24 Role of Pelvic Lymphadenectomy in Robot-assisted Radical Prostatectomy

Varun Mittal, NP Gupta

INTRODUCTION

Lymph node invasion in carcinoma prostate is an important factor for overall long-term survival of the patient. The role of pelvic lymphadenectomy (PLND) in prostate cancer (PCa) is now being increasingly defined. The central role of a PLND is to determine the loco-regional extent of cancer, and to help evaluate the need for adjuvant therapy and the risk of cancer progression and recurrence. Recent contemporary literature also suggests that PLND is therapeutic and promotes a cancer specific survival benefit. Due to the low sensitivity of available preoperative imaging modalities pelvic lymph node dissection, as a staging modality, remains an important component of radical prostatectomy (RP). Computed tomography (CT) and magnetic resonance imaging (MRI) are able to detect approximately only 40% of cases with low volume nodal involvement.[1] Emerging technologies as 68Ga-PSMA positron emission tomography-computerised tomography (PET-CT), C11-Acetate PET-CT, 18F-Choline PET-CT, lymphonanotropic MRI (LN-MRI), scan, have shown some potential but still have questionable sensitivity and specificity especially as primary staging modality.[2] Thus, as of now, PLND remains the most reliable technique for the detection of nodal spread in PCa. Several questions have been raised regarding the PLND during robot-assisted radical prostatectomy (RARP) as:

- Imaging for N staging in cancer prostate?
- Is it necessary in all patients or what are its current indications?
- What is the optimal anatomic extent of dissection?
- Is there any survival benefit?
- Complications associated with it?
- Technical advancements as robotic and its current status? The present chapter focuses on all the above issues.

LYMPHATIC DRAINAGE OF PROSTATE

Anatomic studies have been performed to define the periprostatic subcapsular lymphatic network that drains the prostate. From the prostatic acini, large intraprostatic trunks are formed. These penetrate the prostatic capsule and form the periprostatic lymphatic plexus. This plexus yields lymphatic vessels which follow the vascular network of the prostatovesical arteries.[1] This network is composed of the ascending, lateral and posterior groups draining into the external iliac or obturator, internal iliac and presacral lymph nodes respectively **(Fig. 24.1)**.

IMAGING FOR LYMPH NODE INVOLVEMENT

Low sensitivity of the standard radiological investigations used for primary diagnosis and staging of prostate cancer in detecting metastatic involvement of pelvic lymph nodes has led to PLND being the most reliable tool for staging N status in PCa. Multiple novel techniques are emerging to improve the sensitivity, specificity and predictive value of nodal involvement in cancer prostate.

Computed Tomography Scan

It is a widely used tool for initial evaluation of the nodal involvement. According to the accepted size criteria, any node with a short-axis diameter greater than 1 cm and any rounded node larger than 8 mm is concerning for malignancy. However, as nodal evaluation on CT relies solely on nodal size rather than on nodal function and physiology, this method is limited in its accuracy, as small nodes may harbour micrometastases and enlarged lymph nodes may be reactive in nature and therefore not regarded as the staging investigation of choice.[3,4]

Positron Emission Tomography Scan

18F-Fluorodeoxyglucose (FDG) has a low sensitivity and accuracy in staging prostate cancer, likely due to, low rates of accumulation of the tracer in the prostate cancer cells.[2] Also the FDG is eliminated by kidneys, the excreted FDG activity accumulating in the ureters and bladder may limit the evaluation of adjacent structures such as the prostate and pelvic lymph nodes.

C11-Choline acetate is a preferred tracer for prostate and bladder cancer as it lacks the urinary radioactivity seen with 18F-FDG. Choline is one of the components of

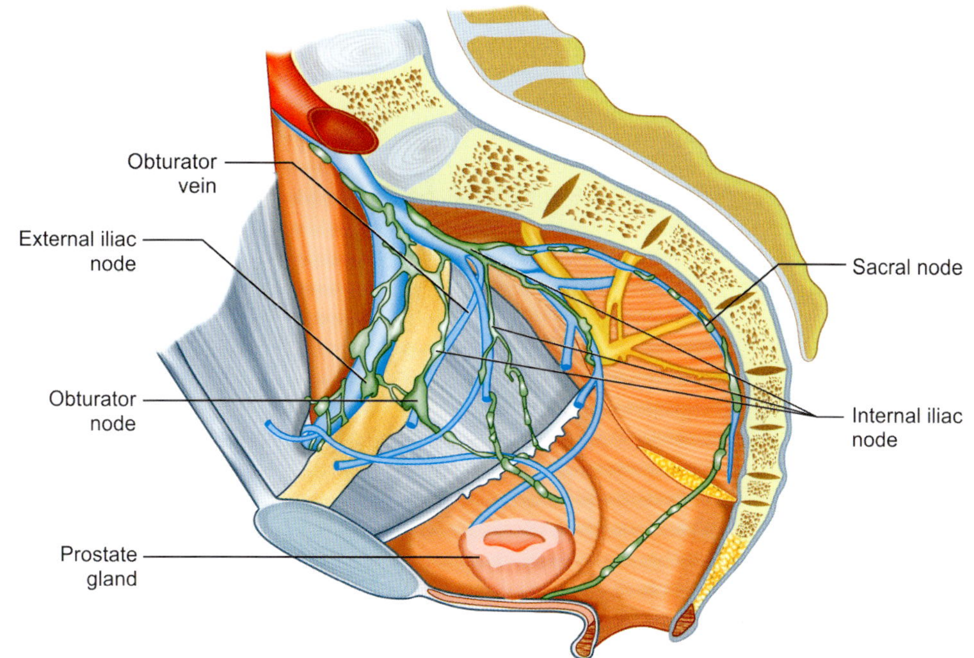

Fig. 24.1: Lymphatic drainage of prostate

phosphatidylcholine, an essential element of phospholipids in the cell membrane. Malignant tumors show a high proliferation and increased metabolism of cell membrane components that will lead to an increased uptake of choline. Sensitivity for staging metastatic lymph node disease in patients with prostate cancer is of 80%, a specificity of 96%, and an accuracy 93%. It can also detect solitary extra regional lymph node metastases. Limitation of choline is its short half-life and requiring a cyclotron to be in close proximity to the hospital.[5]

In recent years, a new PET compound (anti-3-(18)F-FACBC or (18) F-fluciclovine has been tested for the detection of prostate cancer relapse. It accumulates in metabolically active cells and therefore can be detected on PET-CT. Sensitivity and specificity is approximately 45% and 96%, respectively. Positive and negative predictive values are 82% and 92%, respectively.[6] Nanni C et al. evaluated 28 consecutive patients with biochemical relapse after radical prostatectomy with anti-3-18F-FACBC PET/CT and 11C-choline PET/CT to evaluate the site of disease recurrence and concluded that the detection rate of anti-3-18F- Choline PET-CT is greater in comparison with 11C-choline, with approximately 20% of additional patients and approximately 60% additional lesions detected.[7] Choline acetate and 18F-FACBC PET imaging have been hampered by decreased specificity in differentiating malignant from benign hyperplastic prostatic lesions. Also (11)C-choline and (18)F-fluoromethylcholine have poor sensitivity at low PSA levels.

Prostate specific membrane antigen (PSMA) is a promising, well-characterized biomarker specific for prostate cancer, which has also been associated with prostate tumor aggressiveness. Several 18F-PSMA–targeted agents are being developed to stage the cancer prostate, as 18F-DCFBC and 68Ga-PSMA and 18F-DCFPyL. These are being evaluated as imaging modalities for primary diagnosis, risk stratification and staging of prostate cancer.[8]

Single-photon Emission Computed Tomographic Imaging (SPECT)

In addition to changes in metabolism, malignant cells express tumor-specific antigens. SPECT imaging uses radioactive-labeled antibodies against such antigens e.g Indium-111 capromab pendetide (ProstaScint) is a radioactively labelled monoclonal antibody directed against the intracellular portion of the prostate-specific membrane antigen (PSMA), a glycoprotein that is expressed by the prostate epithelium and is upregulated in metastatic prostate cancer.[9] Recent literature on PSMA scan provides its sensitivity of 62%, specificity of 72%, positive predictive value of 62%, and negative predictive value of 72%.[10] Improves selection of candidates for definitive local therapy in men with clinically localized prostate carcinoma and significant risk of lymph node involvement. It has also been evaluated for its use in evaluation of the risk of lymph node metastases prior to pelvic lymph node dissection in high risk cases.

Lymphotropic Nanoparticle-enhanced Magnetic Resonance Imaging (LN-MRI)

LN-MRI is a novel tool for lymph node staging in genitourinary malignancies. This examination uses ultra small superparamagnetic iron oxide particles. The iron oxide particles are small enough to pass across capillary walls, drain via the lymphatic circulation, and localize in the lymph nodes where they allow for detailed characterization of these nodes independent of typically accepted size criterion of conventional MRI or CT.[11,12] Once delivered to the lymph node, the nanoparticles are phagocytosed by macrophages of the reticuloendothelial system (RES), resulting in nanoparticle accumulation within the nodes. Such accumulation results in shortening of T2 and subsequent signal loss in T2 weighted images. As metastatic lymph nodes lack normally functioning RES, their signal intensity remains intermediate to high on the T2-weighted sequences secondary to lack of USPIO accumulation. Harisinghani and colleagues reported 100% per-patient sensitivity, 95.7% per-patient specificity, and 97.5 per-patient accuracy of the LN-MRI in detection of nodal involvement with PCa. This result was a significant improvement over conventional MRI relying on size with per-patient sensitivity, specificity, and accuracy of 45.4%, 78.7%, and 65%, respectively.[13] In addition, LN-MRI was demonstrated to have high sensitivity, specificity, and accuracy of 96.4%, 99.3%, and 98.9%, respectively, for detection of metastases in lymph nodes with short axis of 5-10 mm.[13] Such nodal metastases would commonly be overlooked based on the size criteria of conventional MRI. LN-MRI is also useful tool for detecting lymph node metastases outside the routine lymph node dissection area.

Diffusion-weighted Magnetic Resonance Imaging

Diffusion-weighted MRI (DW-MRI) relies on Brownian motion of water molecules in the tissues, and is highly influenced by the cellular environment of water. Thus, the findings on DW-MRI can reflect biological abnormalities of the underlying tissues.[14] Apparent diffusion coefficient (ADC) values, derived from DW-MRI, are often used as a quantitative parameter to describe the microscopic water diffusibility. DW-MRI has proved to be crucial for detection of primary PCa, increasing sensitivity and specificity of routine MRI.[15,16] Although malignant nodes theoretically expected to show impeded diffusion, resulting in low ADC values, because most primary malignant tumors show impeded diffusion caused by high cellularity, its role in the detection of nodal metastases is still under investigation. Hence DW-MRI cannot be recommended for routine clinical use in nodal staging of high risk prostate cancer patients before initial treatment.

Sentinel Lymph Node Imaging

The lymphatic drainage pattern of a cancer determines the extent of lymph node dissection, allowing for less extensive surgery when appropriate and thus potentially decreasing the morbidity. Preoperative visualization of lymphatic drainage via lymphoscintigraphy involves injection of a radiopharmaceutical agent into the organ of interest followed by planar imaging and/or SPECT as well as intraoperative visualization with gamma probe. The feasibility and accuracy of sentinel node lymphadenectomy in PCa has been demonstrated in few series.[17] An advantage of sentinel node lymphadenectomy is the fact that sentinel nodes outside of the routinely dissected area and possibly outside the ePLND region can also be localized and removed increasing the LNY and probably adds to therapeutic benefit and may also prolong recurrence free interval. With the combination of SPECT and CT, the nodal tracer uptake detected by SPECT can be fused with CT, providing the surgeon with better information on the anatomic location of the sentinel node. Out of the 46 patients of PCa examined by Vermeeren et al. 23 revealed additional sentinel nodes on SPECT-CT which were not seen on planar imaging in 29 (63%). 35% of all patients had uncommon location of sentinel nodes outside the pelvic area, and 56% of these were seen only on SPECT/CT. In addition, of the 15 patients with positive sentinel nodes, 7 (47%) were present exclusively in the nodes detected by SPECT/CT only.[17]

INDICATIONS OF PELVIC LYMPHADENECTOMY

In the era of prostate specific antigen (PSA) screening, downward stage migration has been noted in PCa. The incidence of nodal involvement in presumed clinically localized PCa patients with standard PLND (obturator/external iliac lymph nodes) has decreased from 20 to 40% in the 1980s to 4% to 6% in the most recent contemporary series.[18-22] Mayo series revealed a marked decline in the incidence of positive lymph nodes at the time of radical prostatectomy (RP), from 9.1% between 1988 and 1993 to 1.8% between 1998 and 2001.[23] This stage migration has been held responsible for overall decline in the performance of PLND in the United States over the past few decades. It has been demonstrated that there is a trend towards omitting PLND for low-risk and intermediate-risk PCa.[18,19]

To determine who should undergo a PLND, the benefits must be weighed against the risks and applied only to those who are at a risk of metastatic disease. A number of nomograms have been developed to stratify patients at risk for lymph nodal involvement. Currently PLND during RARP is omitted at many centers in patients with low risk PCa (preoperative PSA <10 ng/mL, a biopsy Gleason score (GS) <7, clinical stage cT1/cT2a) or when the likelihood of lymph node metastases is less than 2% and 5% based on the Partin or Kattan and Briganti nomograms respectively.[24,25] Although these tools provide guidance during clinical decision making, but they have several drawbacks as these are based on the earlier studies with variable patient selection criteria and staging procedures, inconsistent surgical technique and extent of lymph node dissection, variable gleason scoring and histopathology reports.

To overcome this Briganti et al. published a nomogram predicting the probability of lymph node invasion among patients undergoing open retropubic radical prostatectomy (RRP) and an extended PLND (ePLND) and has been externally validated both RRP and RARP series and has shown the highest accuracy as compared to other similar prognostic tools.[26,27]

The incidence and predictive factors for lymph node involvement has been studied in some series. Recently Batra et al. have analysed 100 out of total 452 patients who underwent combined RARP and ePLND Lymph node positivity rates and lymph node density were analyzed on the basis of preoperative prostate specific antigen (PSA), Gleason score, clinical stage, D'Amico risk category and magnetic resonance imaging (MRI) findings. Seventeen patients (17%) had positive lymph nodes (median of 1, range 1-6). Median lymph node density in these patients was 10%. On multivariate analysis, clinical stage >T2a was the only significant factor impacting lymph node positivity. They concluded that a higher clinical stage predisposes to an increased incidence of lymph node metastases.[28]

Many series have demonstrated the low likelihood of lymph node involvement in patients with low risk prostate cancer. Narayan et al. performed retrospective analysis on 932 patients to determine subset of patients in whom PLND could be avoided and concluded that it was unnecessary in patients with GS ≤ 6 and preoperative PSA ≤10 ng/mL.[29] Bluestein et al. concluded the same after they found low risk of only 1–2% of lymph node involvement in low risk patients.[30] These series may underestimate risk of lymph node involvement at a given PSA and GS as they are based on PLND that did not include the internal iliac lymph nodes.[31] Lymph node yield of PLND in these series ranged from 6–9 and hence carried a risk of understaging at a given PSA and GS. Schumacher and colleagues analyzed patients with a PSA ≤10 ng/mL who underwent RRP and PLND. Lymph node involvement was found in 11% of men. In patients with GS ≤6, only 3% had positive lymph nodes, while 25% of men with pathologic GS 7 or higher had positive nodes. Biopsy specimens have been found to understage, undergrade or upgrade the tumor in 30–40% of cases.[32,33] Grossfeld et al. analyzed record of PCa patients who underwent RRP and found undergrading of primary and secondary Gleason patterns in 13 and 29% of patients, respectively, whereas understaging in 24% of these.[33] According to the latest update of Partin tables, lymphadenectomy may be omitted in men with Gleason 3 + 3 disease, unless they have a PSA > 10 ng/mL AND a clinical stage ≥ T2b. Even in Gleason 3 + 4 disease, PLND can be avoided in men with cT1c disease, unless PSA >10 ng/mL.[34]

To summarize, although it may be permissible to desist from performing PLND in low-risk patients with a PSA <10 ng/mL and a biopsy GS ≤6, there is still an inherent risk of biopsy related understaging or undergrading. An ePLND should be performed in all patients in intermediate and high risk category requiring a prostatectomy and men with a PSA level >10 ng/mL as well as those with a PSA level ≤10 ng/mL but a Gleason score ≥7.

EXTENT OF PELVIC LYMPHADENECTOMY

From the existing contemporary literature, standardized universal definitions for PLND prostate cancer are still controversial. The most guidelines recommend an extended template dissection which includes the dissection and removal of lymphatic tissue from the level of the external iliac vein to the obturator nerve, extending proximally to the common iliac artery bifurcation and distally to the proximal femoral canal to include the node of Cloquet **(Figs 24.2A and B)**.

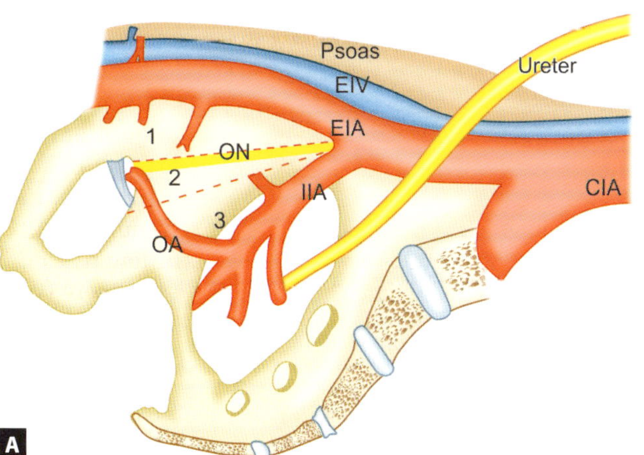

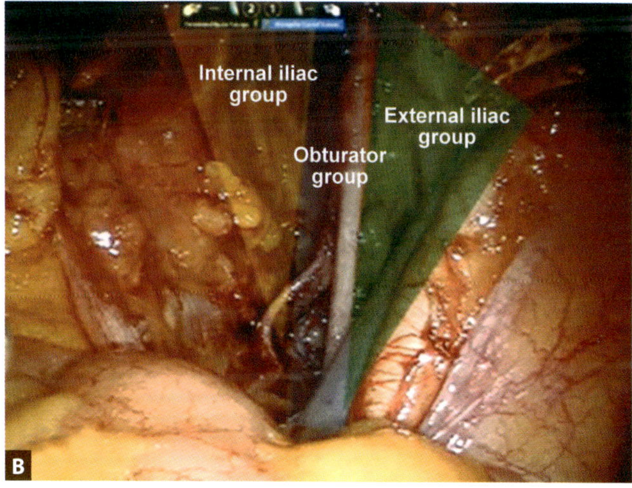

Figs 24.2A and B: (A) ePLND (right side) including the external iliac (zone 1), obturator (zone 2), hypogastric (internal iliac) (zone 3) group of lymph nodes; (B) Intraoperative picture of robotic ePLND (right side) showing the important landmarks and zones of dissection

Abbreviations: CIA, common iliac artery; EIV, external iliac vein; EIA, external iliac artery; IIA, internal iliac artery; OA, obturator artery; ON, obturator node

An ePLND is the extension of standard resection to include the lymphatic tissue surrounding the internal iliac vein and presacral region.[35,36] Superextended templates including the pre-sacral and common iliac groups have also been described, but their role in prostate cancer treatment is yet to be established.[7,23]

SURVIVAL BENEFIT WITH PELVIC LYMPHADENECTOMY

While the role of PLND in improving PCa staging is well established, there is evolving evidence of a therapeutic benefit as well. Previously, high rates of local recurrence were seen even in the presence of organ confined primary tumors and this was probably related to left out nodal disease and hence lymphadenectomy was suggested. Presently, although there are as yet no randomized trials in cancer prostate that have demonstrated differences in survival with or without lymphadenectomy, but there is strong evidence supporting lymphadenectomy. In addition, various prognostic factors have been characterized only through PLND which may improve risk stratification and better direct the adjuvant treatment. These factors represent the volume of metastatic disease and its biological aggressiveness and include the number and volume of positive lymph nodes, extranodal extention, lymph node density, and molecular occult metastases.

There are many contemporary series which have which tried to stratify the lymph node positive patients as per the number and volume of involved lymph nodes. Golimbu et al in 1987 analyzed 42 patients of PCa with a mean follow-up of 5 years and observed higher survival rates in patients with low tumor bulk and a single lymph node metastasis.[37] In 1988, Catalona et al. in their small series of 12 patients confirmed a 75% and 58% recurrence free survival advantage at 5 and 7 years respectively with treatment of lymph node in lymph node positive disease.[38] Similarly, Pound et al. in their series, confirmed a 68% 10-year metastasis-free survival rate in patients with lymph node micro-metastasis even without adjuvant therapy.[39]

Recently, Boorjian and colleagues retrospectively reviewed a large series of patients from the Mayo Clinic with positive lymph nodes with or without adjuvant hormonal therapy and demonstrated that in comparison to patients with single lymph node metastasis, patients with two or more lymph node metastases has two fold risk of systemic progression as well as prostate cancer death.[40]

In addition to number of lymph nodes removed as a factor in survival, Griebling et al. found that the 5-year overall survival rate for patients with extracapsular nodal extension was 55%, compared with 71% for those with histologically confined prostatic nodal metastases.[41]

In terms of the lymph node density, an advantage in PSA progression-free survival was reported in men with <15% as compared to those with ≥15% involved nodes. In addition, a <15% density in patients conferred a 5-year PSA progression-free survival rate of 43% following an extended PLND, compared with only 10% after a limited PLND. Daneshmand et al. reported 72% 10 year recurrence free survival rate with ≤ 20% LND as compared to 47% in patients with >20% LND.[42]

There is evidence from contemporary literature regarding the survival advantage with lymphadenectomy in men without lymph node involvement. Based on the analysis of the Surveillance, Epidemiology, and End Results program database in 1923 patients, Josyln and colleagues also concluded that an extended PLND reduced the long-term risk for prostate cancer-related death, even in patients with negative nodes, compared with those who had no PLND.[43] A group from the Memorial Sloan-Kettering Cancer Center observed that, in men without nodal involvement, a higher number of nodes removed correlated significantly with freedom from biochemical recurrence and survival rates. The benefit of removing negative nodes is perhaps related to the presence of occult lymph node metastases.[44,45]

Role of molecular markers for predicting nodal micrometastasis in PCa is being explored. Miyake et al. Ferrari et al. and Pagliarulo et al. has highlighted the role of molecular markers of micro-metastasis for PCa using real-time reverse transcriptase polymerase chain reaction and immunostaining on lymph nodes. In these series the mere presence as well as the level of these markers was significantly associated with a higher rate of cancer recurrence and shorter survival.[46-48]

The presence of lymph node metastasis in men diagnosed with clinically localized prostate cancer is a poor prognostic finding and hence has important implications on the initiation of adjuvant therapy. Even removing all the positive lymph nodes with PLND during RARP may not be curative. Survival benefit of adjuvant therapy in pN1 disease in addition to PLND is still questionable. Messing et al. demonstrated, in their study, that early adjuvant androgen-deprivation therapy (ADT) following RP in men with node-positive disease is associated with longer survival.[49] The indications, timing and duration of ADT in pN1 disease are dubious. Abdollah F et al. evaluated 1107 patients with pN1 PCa treated with RP, PLND and ADT between 1988 and 2010 and concluded that some patients with pN1 PCa have favorable cancer specific mortality (CSM) free rates at 10 years. They have developed and internally validated the nomogram to accurately predict CSM free rate in these patients and guide adjuvant therapy.[50] Touijer et al. analyzed 369 men with pN1 disease from 1988 to 2010 and found favorable outcomes as per overall survival , cancer-specific survival, freedom from biochemical recurrence and distant metastasis, in patients with GS <8 and low nodal metastatic burden. The above series has raised the concern for need of risk subclassification of pN1disease.[51]

COMPLICATIONS ASSOCIATED WITH PELVIC LYMPHADENECTOMY

With increased understanding of the anatomy and technical advancements in surgical techniques there are only a few complications associated with PLND. Lymphocele, adjacent structures as ureter, nerve and vessel injuries are the most common.

Lymphocele

A lymphocele is defined as a collection of lymphatic fluid without distinct epithelial lining, resulting from the transaction of afferent lymphatic channels, and is the most frequent postoperative complication related to PLND.[52] Although the incidence of lymphocele ranges from 27 to 61%, only a few become symptomatic.[53] It has to be noted, however, that because routine imaging is not performed after prostatectomy, the incidence of subclinical lymphoceles might be higher than expected. A greater rate has been suggested for patients undergoing extraperitoneal PLND as in RRP.[54] The low rate of lymphoceles in the RARP literature may be due to increasing technical experience as well as the transperitoneal nature of RALP, which allows for easier egress of the lymphatic fluid, thus preventing collection formation. The reported incidence of symptoms related to lymphoceles are fever in 47%, abdominal pain in 40%, lower swelling in 37%, genital swelling in 25%, groin pain in 22%, abdominal swelling in 9%, and back and flank pain in 6% and 5%, respectively. In addition, compression of the pelvic veins by the lymphocele increases the risk of thromboembolic events.[55] Physical examination may reveal a fluctuant mass in the lower abdomen and the diagnosis may be confirmed by radiological imaging. On ultrasound imaging, lymphoceles appear as anechoic cystic structures that may contain thin septations and debris. On CT scan, lymphoceles are seen as thin-walled hypodense lesions with negative HU values. A finding of a thickened wall with regional enhancement suggests the presence of infection. Suggested factors mounting the risk of lymphocele after PLND are excessive use of diathermy, the presence of metastatic lymph nodes, the long term use of steroids or diuretics, prior radiation therapy, and subcutaneous heparin. Linear relationship has been proposed with number of lymph nodes retrieved and lymphocele. Treatment of lymphoceles varies depending on the degree of symptoms. Small asymptomatic lymphoceles are typically observed but, for larger symptomatic collections, initial management involves percutaneous aspiration. Fluid obtained by percutaneous aspiration is evaluated for bacterial culture and analysis of creatinine to exclude urine leak. The collections requiring repeated aspirations may require placement of a percutaneous drain. Sclerosing agents such as 96% ethanol, 10% povidone-iodine, and tetracycline have been used via percutaneous drain with variable success.[56] Surgical options include marsupialization into the peritoneal cavity, which may be performed using an open or laparoscopic approach.[57] Open external drainage is generally reserved primarily for loculated, infected lymphoceles that fail to respond to percutaneous drainage and antibiotic therapy.

Ureteral Injury

Injury to the ureter occurs in <1% of cases. Most common site of injury is near the crossing over the iliac vessels to enter the pelvis, by inadvertent clip placement or aggressive dissection.[54]

Nerve Injury

The close anatomic relationship between the pelvic lymph node chains and pelvic nerves puts these nerves at risk for injury during PLND. The reported incidence of nerve injuries after PLND is approximately 3.2%.[55,56] It encompasses neuroparexia, axontomesis, or neurontomesis.

- Obturator nerve injuries are the most frequent type of nerve injury associated with PLND.[58] This is reported in 0–1.8% cases. The obturator nerve is an important landmark during PLNDs. the obturator nerve is used as the inferior extent of dissection. It may be injured by excessive traction, cautery, clip, or inadvertent transaction. Clinically, the Howship-Romberg sign has been shown to be suggestive of injury to the obturator nerve. It is represented by pain down the medial thigh into the knee, and occasionally into the hip, and is exacerbated by extension and abduction or inward thigh rotation.
- Genitofemoral nerve is a mixed nerve with a preponderance of sensory fibers. The nerve commonly lies adjacent to the common iliac vessels, in the groove between the vessels and the medial aspect of the psoas muscle. Injury occurs infrequently during an extended PLND, when it may occur where the nerve courses lateral to the iliac artery during dissection of the common and external iliac lymph nodes. Injury may present with neuropraxia of the medial aspect of the ipsilateral groin and thigh. Typically, these paresthesias are self-limiting.[56]
- Femoral nerve injuries result from direct compression injury from the placement of self-retaining retractors and indirect compression from retracting the psoas muscle laterally while pressing on the nerve against the pelvic sidewall and is therefore does not happen in RARP. Femoral neuropathy is managed by physical therapy to prevent muscle wasting. Femoral nerve compression almost invariably resolves spontaneously; however, the time to resolution remains variable. Chronic neurogenic pain may be treated with nonnarcotic analgesics. Drugs such as carbamazepine and amitriptyline are useful adjuncts to analgesics.

ROBOT-ASSISTED PELVIC LYMPHADENECTOMY: CURRENT STATUS

In the era of minimal invasive urology, robot-assisted radical prostatectomy has become the preferred approach over the open radical prostatectomy by virtue of better perioperative outcomes. The feasibility of PLND during RARP is now well established, with several large series demonstrating comparable yield and perioperative outcomes to the RRP.

Earlier because of the technical limitations of the robotic arm pitch in accessing the pelvic sidewall and undersurface of the iliac bifurcation, uro-oncologists questioned the adequacy of robotic PLND. Yates J et al. in 2009 compared the lymph node yield between open and robot-assisted lymphadenectomy and found that robot-assisted laparoscopic PLND yielded fewer lymph nodes compared to open PLND at the time of radical prostatectomy for organ confined disease. The mean number of lymph nodes obtained via open PLND was 7.3 while the mean number obtained via robotic PLND was 3.3.[58] On the contrary Zorn KC et al. in the same year, 2009 described their standard template pelvic lymphadenectomy (PLND) technique during robot-assisted radical prostatectomy and evaluated the nodal yield and perioperative outcomes. They confirmed the feasibility and low complication rate of robotic standard-template PLND with lymph node yields comparable to those with open PLND.[59] Truesdale MD et al. in 2010 conducted a retrospective study in patients who underwent pelvic lymphadenectomy during open and found only a borderline significant difference in LNY between ORP and RARP (7.49 vs 6.35 nodes, respectively, P = 0.06). They concluded that there are no significant differences in LNY during RARP and RRP for intermediate and high-risk men and an experienced surgeon in RARP can achieve equivalent LNY as RRP. The extent of pelvic lymphadenectomy during RARP has been defined and evidence demonstrates that ePLND yields a greater number of positive nodes.[60] Yee DS et al. in 2010 performed ePLND in 32 patients of cancer prostate undergoing RARP. They concluded that ePLND produces a high lymph node yield and may result in improved pathologic staging. It has been shown in multiple retrospective analyses that an adequate ePLND principally can be performed with the open, laparoscopic or robot-assisted technique.[61] Ploussard G et al. in 2014 reviewed the literature on ePLND during RARP and observed that it can be performed effectively and safely. The overall number of nodes removed, the likelihood of node positivity, and the types and rates of complications of PLND are similar to pure laparoscopic and open retropubic procedures.[62]

The concerns have been raised about the technical issues while doing robot assisted PLND and technique has improved over the time. Mattei A et al. in 2013 described a monoblock technique of ePLND during RARP and found that robot-assisted monoblock ePLND technique is simple to perform, offers a good overview of the operative field during the entire procedure, permits complete and radical removal of the lymphatic tissue contained in the ePLND template, and avoids spreading of fatty and lymphatic tissue within the abdominal cavity.[63] Recently Williams SB et al. described a novel, step-by-step approach to robot-assisted extended pelvic lymph node dissection (ePLND) at the time of robot-assisted radical prostatectomy (RARP).[64]

The indications to perform the PLND remain the same for both. With the technical advancement in robotics and more and more application in urology the now PLND is being performed with robot assistance during RARP.

REFERENCES

1. Bader P, Burkhard FC, Markwalder R, Studer UE. Disease progression and survival of patients with positive lymph nodes after radical prostatectomy. Is there a chance of cure? J Urol. 2003;169:849-54.
2. Spermon JR, De Geus-Oei LF, Kiemeney LA, et al. The role of 18fluoro-2-deoxyglucose positron emission tomography in initial staging and re-staging after chemotherapy for testicular germ cell tumors. BJU Int. 2002;89:549-56.
3. Tiguert R, Gheiler EL, Tefilli MV, et al. Lymph node size does not correlate with the presence of prostate cancer metastasis. Urology. 1999;53:367-71.
4. Saksena MA, Kim JY, Harisinghani MG. Nodal staging in genitourinary cancers. Abdom Imaging. 2006;31:644-51.
5. de Jong IJ, Pruim J, Elsinga PH, et al. 11C-choline positron emission tomography for the evaluation after treatment of localized prostate cancer. Eur Urol. 2003;44:32-8.
6. Beheshti M, Imamovic L, Broinger G, et al. 18F choline PET/CT in the preoperative staging of prostate cancer in patients with intermediate or high risk of extracapsular disease: a prospective study of 130 patients. Radiology. 2010;254:925-33.
7. Nanni C, Schiavina R, Brunocilla E, Boschi S, Borghesi M, Zanoni L. 18F-Fluciclovine PET/CT for the Detection of Prostate Cancer Relapse: A Comparison to 11C-Choline PET/CT. Clin Nucl Med. 2015;40:386-91.
8. Rowe SP, Gage KL, Faraj SF, Macura KJ, Cornish TC, Gonzalez-Roibon N. ^{18}F-DCFBC PET/CT for PSMA-Based Detection and Characterization of Primary Prostate Cancer. J Nucl Med. 2015;56:1003-10.
9. Pouliot F, Johnson M, Wu L. Non-invasive molecular imaging of prostate cancer lymph node metastasis. Trends Mol Med. 2009;15: 254-62.
10. Rosenthal SA, Haseman MK, Polascik TJ. Utility of capromab pendetide (ProstaScint) imaging in the management of prostate cancer. Tech Urol. 2001;7:27-37.
11. Feldman AS, McDougal WS, Harisinghani MG. The potential of nanoparticle-enhanced imaging. Seminars and Original Investigations. Urol Oncol. 2008;26:65-73.
12. Weissleder R, Elizondo G, Wittenberg J, et al. Ultrasmall superparamagnetic iron oxide: an intravenous contrast agent for assessing lymph nodes with MR imaging. Radiology. 1990;175:494-8.
13. Harisinghani MG, Barenztsz J, Hahn PF, et al. Noninvasive detection of clinically occult lymph-node metastases in prostate cancer. N Engl J Med. 2003;348:2491-9.
14. Petralia G, Thoeny HC. DW-MRI of the urogenital tract: applications in oncology. Cancer Imaging. 2010;10:S112-23.
15. Haider MA, van der Kwast TH, Tanguay J, et al. Combined T2-weighted and diffusion-weighted MRI for localization of prostate cancer. AJR Am J Roentgenol. 2007;189:323-8.
16. Yoshimitsu K, Kiyoshima K, Irie H, et al. Usefulness of apparent diffusion coefficient map in diagnosing prostate carcinoma: correlation with stepwise histopathology. J Magn Reson Imaging. 2008;27:132-9.
17. Vermeeren L, Valde´s Olmos RA, Meinhardt W, et al. Value of SPECT/CT for detection and anatomic localization of sentinel lymph nodes before laparoscopic sentinel node lymphadenectomy in prostate carcinoma. J Nucl Med. 2009;50:865-70.

18. Gil-Vernet JM. Prostate cancer: anatomical and surgical considerations. Br J Urol. 1996;78:1618.
19. Weingartner K, Ramaswamy A, Bittinger A, Gerharz EW, Vöge D, Riedmiller H. Anatomical basis for pelvic lymphadenectomy in prostate cancer: results of an autopsy study and implications for the clinic. J Urol. 1996;156:1969-71.
20. Schuessler WW, Pharand D, Vancaillie TG. Laparoscopic standard pelvic node dissection for carcinoma of the prostate: is it accurate? J Urol. 1993;150:898-901.
21. Sivalingam S, Oxley J, Probert JL, Stolzenburg JU, Schwaibold H. Role of pelvic lymphadenectomy in prostate cancer management. Urology. 2007;69:203-9.
22. Heidenreich A, Varga Z, Von Knobloch R. Extended pelvic lymphadenectomy in patients undergoing radical prostatectomy: high incidence of lymph node metastasis. J Urol. 2002;167:1681-6.
23. Heidenreich A, Ohlmann CH, Polyakov S. Anatomical extent of pelvic lymphadenectomy in patients undergoing radical prostatectomy. Eur Urol. 2007;52:29-37.
24. Kattan MW, Eastham JA, Stapleton AM, Wheeler TM, Scardino PT. A preoperative nomogram for disease recurrence following radical prostatectomy for prostate cancer. J Natl Cancer Inst. 1998;90:766-71.
25. Cagiannos I, Karakiewicz P, Eastham JA, Ohori M, Rabbani F, Gerigk C, et al. A preoperative nomogram identifying decreased risk of positive pelvic lymph nodes in patients with prostate cancer. J Urol. 2003;170:1798-803.
26. Briganti A, Chun FK, Salonia A, Zanni G, Scattoni V, Valiquette L, et al. Validation of a nomogram predicting the probability of lymph node invasion among patients undergoing radical prostatectomy and an extended pelvic lymphadenectomy. Eur Urol. 2006;49:1019-26.
27. Briganti A, Chun FK, Salonia A, Gallina A, Farina E, Da Pozzo LF, et al. Validation of a nomogram predicting the probability of lymph node invasion based on the extent of pelvic lymphadenectomy in patients with clinically localized prostate cancer. BJU Int. 2006;98:788-93.
28. Batra V, Gautam G, Jaipuria J, Suryavanshi M, Khera R, Ahlawat R. Predictive factors for lymph node positivity in patients undergoing extended pelvic lymphadenectomy during robot assisted radical prostatectomy. Indian J Urol. 2015;31:217-22.
29. Narayan P, Fournier G, Gajendran V, Leidich R, Lo R,Wolf Jr JS, et al. Utility of preoperative serum prostate-specific antigen concentration and biopsy Gleason score in predicting risk of pelvic lymph node metastases in prostate cancer. Urology. 1994;44:519-24.
30. Bluestein DL, Bostwick DG, Bergstralh EJ, Oesterling JE. Eliminating the need for bilateral pelvic lymphadenectomy in select patients with prostate cancer. J Urol. 1994;151:1315-20.
31. Heidenreich A, Ohlmann CH, Polyakov S. Anatomical extent of pelvic lymphadenectomy in patients undergoing radical prostatectomy. Eur Urol. 2007;52:29-37.
32. Grossfeld GD, Chang JJ, Broering JM, Li YP, Lubeck DP, Flanders SC et al. Under staging and under grading in a contemporary series of patients undergoing radical prostatectomy: results from the cancer of the prostate strategic urologic research endeavor database. J Urol. 2001;165:851-6.
33. Bhatta-Dhar N, Reuther AM, Zippe C, Klein EA. No difference in six-year biochemical failure rates with or without pelvic lymph node dissection during radical prostatectomy in low-risk patients with localized prostate cancer. Urology. 2004;63: 528-31.
34. Eifler JB, Feng Z, Lin BM, Partin MT, Humphreys EB, Han M, et al. An updated prostate cancer staging nomogram (Partin tables) based on cases from 2006 to 2011. BJU Int. 2013;111:229.
35. Mohler JL, Kantoff PW, Armstrong AJ, Bahnson RR, Cohen M, D'Amico AV, et al. Prostate cancer, version 1.2014. J Natl Compr Canc Netw. 2013;11:14719.
36. Heidenreich A, Bellmunt J, Bolla M, Joniau S, Masone M, MatveevfV, et al. EAU guidelines on prostate cancer, I: Screening, diagnosis, and treatment of clinically localized disease. Eur Urol. 2011;59:6171.
37. Golimbu M, Provet J, Al-Askari S, et al. Radical prostatectomy for stage D1 prostate cancer. Prognostic variables and results of treatment. Urology. 1987;30:427-35.
38. Catalona WJ, Miller DR, Kavoussi LR. Intermediate-term survival results in clinically understaged prostate cancer patients following radical prostatectomy. J Urol. 1988;140:540-43.
39. Pound CR, Partin AW, Eisenberger MA, et al. Natural history of progression after PSA elevation following radical prostatectomy. JAMA. 1999;281:1591-7
40. Boorjian SA, Thompson RH, Siddiqui S, et al. Long-term outcome after radical prostatectomy for patients with lymph node positive prostate cancer in the prostate specific antigen era. J Urol. 2007;178: 864-70; discussion 870-1.
41. Griebling TL, Ozkutlu D, See WA, et al. Prognostic implications of extracapsular extension of lymph node metastases in prostate cancer. Mod Pathol. 1997;10:804-9.
42. Daneshmand S, Quek ML, Stein JP, et al. Prognosis of patients with lymph node positive prostate cancer following radical prostatectomy: Long-term results. J Urol. 2004;172:2252-5.
43. Joslyn SA, Konety BR. Impact of extent of lymphadenectomy on survival after radical prostatectomy for prostate cancer. Urology. 2006;68:121-5.
44. Masterson TA, Bianco FJ Jr, Vickers AJ, et al. The association between total and positive lymph node counts, and disease progression in clinically localized prostate cancer. J Urol. 2006;175:1320 -4; discussion 1324-5.
45. Herr HW, Bochner BH, Dalbagni G, et al. Impact of the number of lymph nodes retrieved on the outcome in patients with muscle invasive bladder cancer. J Urol. 2001;167:1295-8.
46. Miyake H, Hara I, Kurahashi T, et al. Quantitative detection of micrometastases in pelvic lymph nodes in patients with clinically localized prostate cancer by real-time reverse transcriptase-PCR. Clin Cancer Res. 2007;13:1192-7.
47. Ferrari AC, Stone NN, Kurek R, et al. Molecular load of pathologically occult metastases in pelvic lymph nodes is an independent prognostic marker of biochemical failure after localized prostate cancer treatment. J Clin Oncol. 2006;24:3081-8.
48. Pagliarulo V, Hawes D, Brands FH, et al. Detection of occult lymph node metastases in locally advanced node-negative prostate cancer. J Clin Oncol. 2006;24:2735-42.
49. Messing EM, Manola J, Yao J, et al. Immediate versus deferred androgen deprivation treatment in patients with node-positive prostate cancer after radical prostatectomy and pelvic lymphadenectomy. Lancet Oncol. 2006;7:472-9.
50. Abdollah F, Karnes RJ, Suardi N, Cozzarini C, Gandaglia G, Fossati N, et al. Predicting survival of patients with node-positive prostate cancer following multimodal treatment. Eur Urol. 2014;65:554-62.
51. Touijer KA, Mazzola CR, Sjoberg DD, Scardino PT, Eastham JA. Long-term outcomes of patients with lymph node metastasis treated with radical prostatectomy without adjuvant androgen-deprivation therapy. Eur Urol. 2014;65:20-5.

52. Patel A. Complications of Urologic Surgery: Prevention and Management, 3rd edition. Philadelphia: Saunders; 2001. pp.370-85.
53. Solberg A, Angelsen A, Bergan U, et al. Frequency of lymphoceles after open and laparoscopic pelvic lymph node dissection in patients with prostate cancer. Scand J Urol Nephrol. 2003;37(3):218-21.
54. Musch M, Klevecka V, Roggenbuck U, et al. Complications of pelvic lymphadenectomy in 1,380 patients undergoing radical retropubic prostatectomy between 1993 and 2006. J Urol. 2008;179(3):923-8.
55. Heinzer H, Hammerer P, Graefen M, et al. Thromboembolic complication rate after radical retropubic prostatectomy. Impact of routine ultrasonography for the detection of pelvic lymphoceles and hematomas. Eur Urol. 1998;33:86-90.
56. Patel A. Complications of Urologic Surgery: Prevention and Management, 3rd edition. Philadelphia: Saunders; 2001. pp.370-85.
57. Fallick ML, Long JP. Laparoscopic marsupialization of lymphocele after laparoscopic lymph node dissection. J Endourol. 1996;10: 533-4.
58. Yates J, Haleblian G, Stein B, Miller B, Renzulli J, Pareek G. The impact of robotic surgery on pelvic lymph node dissection during radical prostatectomy for localized prostate cancer: the Brown University early robotic experience. Can J Urol. 2009;16: 4842-6.
59. Zorn KC, Katz MH, Bernstein A, Shikanov SA, Brendler CB, Zagaja GP, et al. Pelvic lymphadenectomy during robot-assisted radical prostatectomy: Assessing nodal yield, perioperative outcomes, and complications. Urology. 2009;74:296-302.
60. Truesdale MD, Lee DJ, Cheetham PJ, Hruby GW, Turk AT, Badani KK. Assessment of lymph node yield after pelvic lymph node dissection in men with prostate cancer: a comparison between robot-assisted radical prostatectomy and open radical prostatectomy in the modern era. J Endourol. 2010;24:1055-60.
61. Yee DS, Katz DJ, Godoy G, Nogueira L, Chong KT, Kaag M, et al. Extended pelvic lymph node dissection in robotic-assisted radical prostatectomy: surgical technique and initial experience. Urology. 2010;75:1199-204.
62. Ploussard G, Briganti A, de la Taille A, Haese A, Heidenreich A, Menon M, et al. Pelvic lymph node dissection during robot-assisted radical prostatectomy: efficacy, limitations, and complications-a systematic review of the literature. Eur Urol. 2014;65:7-16.
63. Mattei A, Di Pierro GB, Grande P, Beutler J, Danuser H. Standardized and simplified extended pelvic lymph node dissection during robot-assisted radical prostatectomy: the monoblock technique. Urology. 2013;81:446-50.
64. Williams SB, Bozkurt Y, Achim M, Achim G, Davis JW. Sequencing robot-assisted extended pelvic lymph node dissection prior to radical prostatectomy: a step-by-step guide to exposure and efficiency. BJU Int. 2016;117:192-8.

CHAPTER

25

Radical Cystoprostatectomy

Sudhir Rawal

INTRODUCTION

Robotic radical cystectomy is fast becoming the preferred surgical procedure for removing an invasive bladder cancer. The cancerous bladder is removed by urologic surgeon who uses a combination of high-definition three-dimensional magnifications, miniature instruments with the help of robotic technology for perfection of procedure.

Robotic radical cystectomy involves removal of urinary bladder, seminal vesicles, prostate and surrounding tissues like fat peritoneal attachments in males. In females, there is removal of urethra, cervix, uterus, anterior vaginal wall, and many a times the ovaries are also removed. Concurrently, the pelvic lymph node dissection is also performed.

In this robotic procedure, the da Vinci Surgical System is used in which the surgeon's movements are imitated by robotic arms where the precision gets amplified. Robotic radical cystectomy provides bladder cancer patients the prospect of a highly effective surgery and better postsurgical recovery **(Fig. 25.1)**. This robotic surgical procedure allows the surgeon to make smaller incisions by which vital delicate nerves and muscle tissues are spared. The patient experiences a hospital stay of shorter duration, less complications, and quick recovery time.

The robotic radical cystectomy usually requires a urinary diversion with reconstruction for the removed bladder. The robotic da Vinci Surgical System helps the surgeon with a better visualization plane and improvised surgical dexterity at the time of removal of bladder and reconstructive procedures.

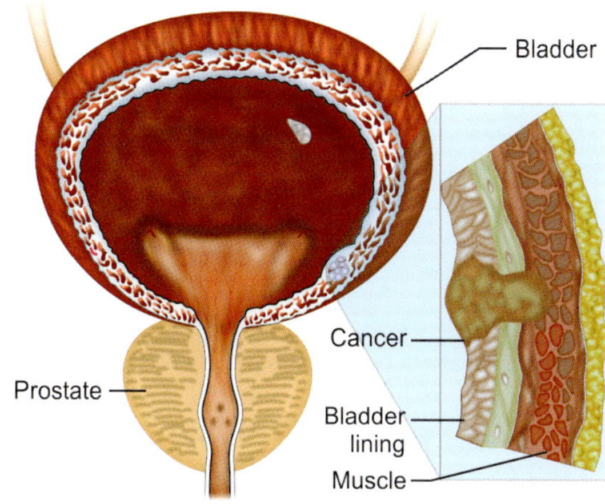

Fig. 25.1: Urinary bladder cancer

PATIENT SELECTION

Earlier robotic radical cystectomy was conducted in patients with history of minimal prior pelvic or abdominal surgeries who could tolerate pneumo peritoneum. However, currently the experienced surgeons are conducting Robotic radical cystectomy in more complex cases. It can be chosen for patients with locally advanced disease, a high body mass index (BMI), or an higher American Society of Anaesthesiologists (ASA) score.

Robotic radical cystectomy is mostly avoided in patients with decreased pulmonary compliance who may not tolerate the Trendelenburg position. It is also avoided in patients who had previous extensive abdominal surgeries and patients with bulky tumor.

PREOPERATIVE PREPARATION

Bowel preparation with antibiotic coverage is to be started one day before the procedure. The second-generation cephalosporin is preferred antimicrobial agent prior to incision as antibiotic prophylaxis. For nearly 24 hours prior to surgery, the patient is asked to have a clear liquid diet. Usually, patient is advised not to eat anything starting at midnight the night before the surgery.

Preoperative evaluation includes stratification of cardiovascular risks, serum laboratory studies, and three-dimensional imaging (CT/MRI). This will help to precisely correlate relationship of the mass of tumor to adjacent organs and lymph nodes.

Before surgery, the patient must be carefully counseled on all options available, the risks and benefits involved and probable outcomes based on surgeon's individual experience. All elements of informed consent need to be covered before the surgical procedure.

Patients' needs to be advised to stop smoking well in advance of surgery, be active, and maintain good diet. Platelet inhibitors are required to be stopped well in advance of surgery.

The set of specific instructions with details of expected steps of the hospitalization, discharge, and postoperative period needs to be given to each patient.

Each patient is different, so few medications like Aspirin, Ibuprofen, Advil are stopped prior to surgery as these drugs can increase the risk of bleeding during surgery. The clinician may be consulted to be sure whether it is safe to discontinue the medications or switch to an alternative medicine, specifically if the patient has a serious condition which may need to be taken into consideration.

Technique

OT Setup and Equipment

Robotic procedure works on the da Vinci Surgical System where a robotic arm imitates the surgeon's movements by which it increases their precision. The instruments, sutures, and pledgets are to be carefully prepared prior to the start of tumor removal.

For a surgeon the user interface consists of the display system, master arms, footswitch, and panel control/touchpad.

Display system: A three dimensional stereoscopic high-definition display with up to 10X magnification for the surgeon in the console is provided by the current systems. For the rest of the operating room team additional two dimensional displays are available.

Master arms: The master controls receive the inputs from the surgeon's finger and thumb and translate these movements in real time to the robotic arms and Endo Wrist instruments.

Control/touchpad: An integrated surgeon interface helps surgeon for selecting desired video, audio, and system settings. This includes changing between two dimensional and three dimensional displays, motion scaling adjustments, and selecting camera perspectives. Unique user settings could be stored in a surgeon's user profile, and the surgeon can benefit from the available ergonomic settings to minimize fatigue.

Footswitch panel: The camera movements, changing between different types of energy and deployment of diathermy are controlled with clutch mechanisms and foot switches.

Patient Positioning

The patient is kept in modest Trendelenburg position following induction of anesthesia and the robotic camera is usually placed near the umbilicus. Sufficient padding is applied around the shoulder and pressure points and the arms are tucked in. A urethral catheter and a nasogastric tube are usually inserted **(Fig. 25.2)**.

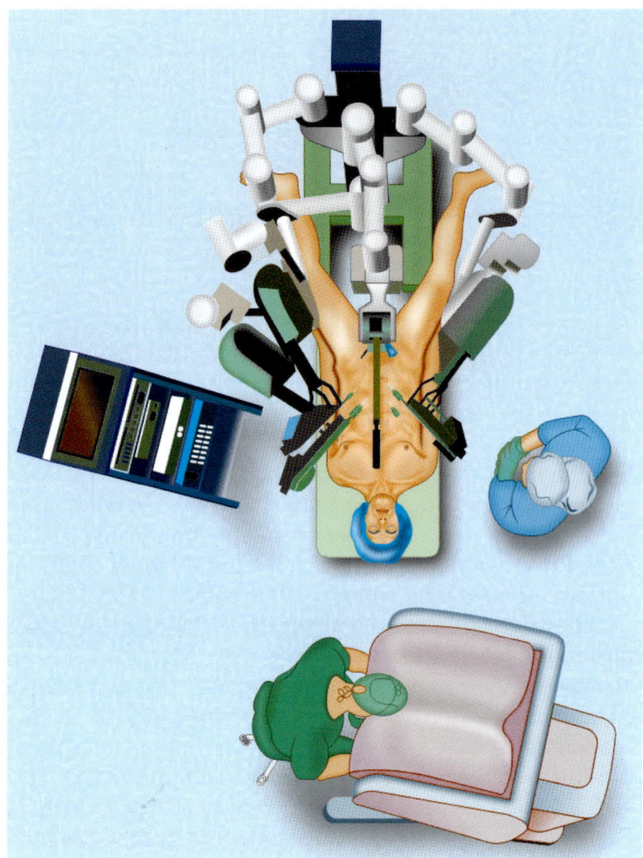

Fig. 25.2: Patient positioning where operating table is maintained in a modest Trendelenburg position

Port Placement

For successful surgery appropriate port placement is vital **(Fig. 25.3)**. Usually, six ports technique is used where the camera port is placed 5 cm above the umbilicus in midline. Pneumoperitoneum around 10 and 12 mm Hg is desirable during the surgery, but during port placement pressure around 18 mm Hg is considered advantageous. Two robotic ports are positioned on the left and right sides, lateral to the rectus sheath at the level of umbilicus.

Usually, the left port is inserted around 8 cm from midline and the right port is kept around 10–11 cm from the midline which gives more space for the assistant's port. The third robotic instrument port is inserted 2 cm above and medial to the left anterior superior iliac spine by a 15 mm port. Two assistant ports are then placed on either side of the right robotic instrument port.

ROBOTIC RADICAL CYSTECTOMY

Initially, the ureters are identified there after the covering peritoneum is opened with care. The ureters are then dissected out towards the urinary bladder, with the periureteral tissue

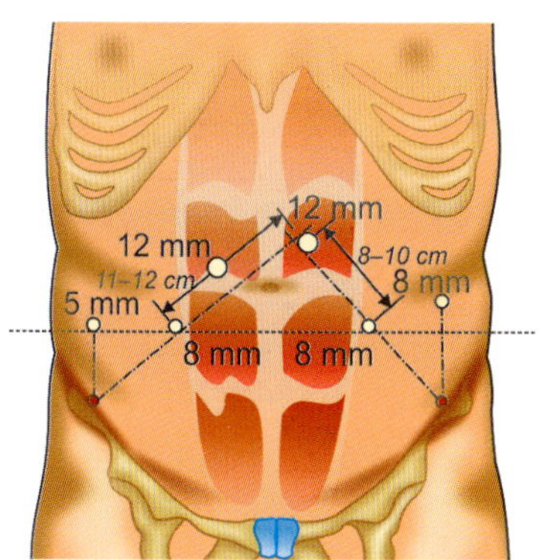

Fig. 25.3: Preferred locations of port placements

holding them are maintained adequately. They are divided close to ureterovesical junction with the help of two Hem-o-Lok clips. Usually, a stay suture is kept on the two proximal clips for easy identification and manipulation of ureters during construction of the urinary diversion.

The levels of the vas deferens are usually identified before posterior dissection. Peritoneum is retracted by an assistant. To expose the seminal vesicle and vas deferens an incision is done in peritoneum, with the help of tips of the scissors above the seminal vesicles.

Further dissection is to be carried out behind the seminal vesicles to exposes the Denonvilliers fascia. After opening the Denonvilliers fascia, a surgical plane gets developed between the rectum and the Denonvilliers fascia which is attached to the prostate. Retroprostatic dissection proceeds anterior to the perirectal fat to avoid any rectal injury. The erectile nerves are usually situated in close proximity laterally to the seminal vesicles. In the cases of nerve sparing situation, the seminal vesicles are divided close to the prostate by which undue damage is avoided.

Identification of the medial umbilical ligaments is done near the abdominal inguinal ring. Incision of the peritoneum is done lateral to the ligaments which is extended till the medial region of external iliac artery towards the space of Retzius. The space between lateral wall of the urinary bladder and the pelvic sidewall is created by using the combined sharp and blunt dissection till the end pelvic fascia.

At this point of dissection the umbilical ligaments and urachus are left intact to ensure that the bladder does not fall down into the operating field. Then the endopelvic fascia is opened following which the lateral surface of the prostate is separated from the levator ani muscle, prostatic apex, and the dorsal vein complex (DVC) are isolated. Due care is taken to avoid any injury to obturator nerve.

For opening of the space medial to external iliac vessels the vas deferens has to be divided and the lateral dissection is continued. Using the fourth arm, the bladder is retracted towards umbilicus. Good retraction helps in identification of the lateral pedicles for division. Division of superior vesicle artery can be done at its origin. Division of the inferior vesicle artery and vesicoprostatic artery is done. To preserve the neurovascular bundles (NVBs) division of the pedicles can be stopped at the upper lateral aspect of prostate around the level of seminal vesicles. The neurovascular bundles on posterior lateral aspect of the prostate are easily transacted in this fashion all the way down to the apex of the prostate.

The median umbilical ligaments and the urachus can be coagulated with bipolar cautery and cut. By staying in the correct plane and following the areolar tissue the urinary bladder is then taken down. The dorsal vein complex (DVC) is divided with cold scissors following which a continuous hemostatic suture with a V-Loc suture can be placed. Maximum sparing of urethra is to be performed and to avoid spilling tumor cells; a suture or Hem-o-Lok clip can be placed on the prostatic apex prior to cutting. When the specimen is totally freed, it can be immediately placed in an endocatch retrieval bag.

Reconstruction Procedures

At present, two main procedures are ilial conduit and Neobladder.

Very few centers are doing it robotically. The use of staplers has made these procedures possible robotically and we should see more centers taking it up. Cost is a big constraint at present.

POSTOPERATIVE CARE

With proper preoperative planning, meticulously done surgery, proper patient selection, and attention to detail, robotic procedures can be performed with minimal morbidity and excellent outcomes for most patients.

Following the robotic surgery the patient spends some time in recovery room or postanesthesia care unit. Then the patient is allowed to move to a designated hospital ward or bed once the patient regains consciousness or awareness and the vital signs are found under control or within normal limits.

Pain after robotic surgery: Majority of patients feel pain of mild intensity post robotic surgery in the initial days near the incision location which is managed by either oral or injectable analgesics. Few patients may experience some transient discomfort in shoulder for few days due to the residual carbon dioxide gas used for the abdominal distension during the robotic procedure.

Nauseating sensation: There may be urge to vomit after the surgical procedure due to general anesthesia (GA). This sensation is temporary and easily controlled by antiemetic agents as necessary.

Catheterization of urinary bladder: Many times the urethral catheter is kept to drain the urinary bladder during the operation. This is done to measure the output of urine on the initial days after operation. The urethral catheter is taken out as soon as the patient starts moving and walks with comfort mostly on the same day or one day following the surgery. Many a times the patient may find his or her urine being blood-tinged for some time after the operation when the urethral catheter is not removed.

Food and diet: Based on tolerability the food pattern of patient is slowly changed from liquid diet to solid diet. Many times patients do not feel hungry and eat properly for nearly seven days after the operation. The gastrointestinal tract may be operating slowly due to the effects of surgical procedure and general anesthesia (GA). Due to this kind of causes, the patient is advised to take smaller quantity of liquids orally till the patient starts passing gas and natural desire to eat food comes back. During this time, interval fluids administered by intravenous route maintains the hydration till the patient start taking oral food adequately.

Weakness or fatigue: Usually the patients feel tired and fatigued after operation which subsides in a few days.

Ambulation: Patient is advised initially to make effort to walk which can be supervised by an attendant. This will help in prevention of blood clot formation in deep veins of leg also expedites the recovery of gastrointestinal tract motility.

TECHNICAL TIPS AND TRICKS

Posterior Dissection (Non-organ Sparing Technique) in Female Patient

Following an incision of inverted U shape the dissection of the posterior aspect of cul-de sac is performed. The same incision may be continued bilaterally for few centimeters above the common iliac vessels as per surgeon's preference. By using the fourth arm of robot the uterus is tilted to anteversion position. The infundibulopelvic suspensory ligaments and the ovarian pedicle are clipped and divided following their identification. The clipping and division of uterine artery is done after it's identified. The uterus and adenexa can be retracted by the fourth arm of Robert following proper homeostasis. The uterus is put under tension by proximal retraction following which the junction between the uterus and vagina. Sometimes the vagina gets identified by putting a sponge inside the vagina. The anterior wall of vagina is removed with specimen after incision. The autonomic nerves which are found near the lateral wall of vagina needs to be preserved to retain better sexual function.

Posterior Dissection (Organ-sparing Technique) in Female Patient

The uterus is preserved by vaginal sparing dissection when the tumor invasion is minimal and uterus is not affected. While preserving the uterus the uterine and ovarian pedicles are protected and preserved along with suspensory ligament. By placing a sponge inside vagina a space is created between uterus and urinary bladder. Near to cervix the anterior wall of vagina is opened to create a plane. Then the dissection continues behind the urinary bladder till its neck.

The vascular pedicles are identified after dissection near lateral aspect of urinary bladder where umbilical ligaments situated. Clipping and division of superior vesicle pedicle and round ligament is done. Robotic fourth arm draws back the urinary bladder. The vascular pedicles are identified, clipped and divided as per surgeon's preference. The external iliac blood vessels and rectum are not injured in this process. Sometimes the surgeon dissects the individual branches originating from the anterior trunk of internal iliac artery and then clips and divides them if required.

COMPLICATIONS

While the benefits of the robotic surgery can be significant, it is important for any surgeon performing these procedures to be well versed about the associated likely complications.

Cardiopulmonary Complications

Sinus tachycardia is commonly observed as arrhythmia. However, the bradyarrhythmias may develop independently or in combination with tachycardia during the robotic procedure. Conditions which may lead to arrhythmias are CO_2 insufflation, increased vagal tone due to traction on pelvic or peritoneal structures, hypercapnia, Trendelenburg position, anesthetic drugs (especially halothane in combination with spontaneous ventilation), patient anxiety, intubation, and gas embolism. To treat and manage hypercapnia the ventilator rate and tidal volume can be adjusted. It has been observed that use of positive end expiratory pressure (PEEP) and lowering of abdominal pressure also helps control of hypercapnia.

Vascular Injury

The injuries to blood vessels are prevented by using blunt trocars in magnified surgical field and performing the procedure slowly. The chance of injury to abdominal wall veins and arteries is more. The injury needs to be quickly identified and managed by ligation or clipping of vessels. During robotic surgery blood may be found dripping near ports where vessels may be injured. A big figure of eight suturing helps in compression of blood vessel.

Postoperative Ileus (POI)

After operation, the recovery of gastrointestinal motility may be delayed this can result in pain abdomen with distension. This may also be associated with vomiting and nauseating sensation. Robotic surgeries prevent or reduce the intensity of postoperative ileus. By not performing any bowel preparation before surgery the POI can be avoided. Mostly the treatment of POI is conservative in nature. In rare instances, gastric decompression can be advised.

Deep Vein Thrombosis (DVT)

Pain and tenderness in calves with swelling are considered as features of deep vein thrombosis. Sometimes patient develops pulmonary embolism as a complication. Treatment includes immediate anticoagulation. The inferior vena cava filter can be advised for the patients whom anticoagulation therapy contraindicated. Deep vein thrombosis can be avoided by using standard measures such as pneumatic sequential compression devices and/or mini dose of heparin and postoperative early ambulation. The robotic approach can be of particular advantage in this regard by allowing early ambulation.

Complications of Urinary Diversion and Urine Leak

These complications include problems like bowel leak, urine leak and ureteroenteric strictures. In addition, patients with urinary diversions may have electrolyte and acid base abnormalities related to urine reabsorption. The commonly seen disturbance is hyperchloremic, metabolic acidosis due to the use of ileum. Many times it is mild not requiring any treatment, but systemic alkalinization may be required if bone resorption or fatigue is associated with it.

EVIDENCE

In 2009, more than five hundred robotic-assisted radical cystectomy (RARC) had been reported to the International Robotic Cystectomy Consortium (IRCC) from fifteen institutions worldwide.

Many centers now have developed techniques for robotic-assisted radical cystectomy with a complete intracorporeal urinary diversion.

Ng et al. in a prospective study of 187 patients undergoing Open Radical Cystectomy (n=104) or robotic-assisted radical cystectomy (n=83) showed a significant lower complication rate in robotic-assisted radical cystectomy, 59% vs 41%.

Nix et al. in a prospective randomized study of robotic-assisted radical cystectomy (RARC) versus open radical cystectomy (ORC) in 41 patients, reported a 33% versus 50% overall complication rate, respectively but not statistically significant.

SUMMARY

Robotic radical cystectomy is a minimally invasive method for the treatment of invasive bladder cancer. The miniaturization, higher range of motion, better vision and mechanical precision offer significant benefits for robotic radical cystectomy patients. This includes less blood loss, less chance of requiring blood transfusions, less postoperative pain and need for any postoperative analgesics, early recovery and return of normal activities and less scarring.

By offering the surgeon a high definition three dimensional view, the da Vinci surgical robot is able to distinguish the vital muscles and delicate nerves surrounding the operative field, providing opportunity to preserve them. The EndoWrist instruments offer surgeons the dexterity not available to them when using conventional instruments. By taking advantage of the da Vinci robot, surgeons can dissect and reconstruct the urinary bladder with relative ease.

BIBLIOGRAPHY

1. Beecken WD, Wolfram M, Engl T, et al. Robotic-assisted laparoscopic radical cystectomy and intra-abdominal formation of an orthotopicilealneobladder. EurUrol. 2003;44:37-9.
2. Beecken WD, Wolfram M, Engl T, et al. Robotic-assisted laparoscopic radical cystectomy and intra-abdominal formation of an orthotopicilealneobladder. Eur Urol. 2003;44:337-9.
3. Collins JW, Tyritzis S, Nyberg T, et al. Robot-assisted radical cystectomy: description of an evolved approach to radical cystectomy. Eur Urol. 2013;64:654-63.
4. Hellenthal NJ, Hussain A, Andrews PE, et al. Surgical margin status after robot assisted radical cystectomy: results from the International Robotic Cystectomy Consortium. J Urol. 2010;184:87-91.
5. Hellenthal NJ, Hussain A, Andrews PE, et al. Surgical margin status after robot assisted radical cystectomy: results from the International Robotic Cystectomy Consortium. J Urol. 2010;184:87-91.
6. Kyle A. Richards, A. Karim Kader, and Ashok K. Hemal. Robotic Radical Cystectomy: Where are We Today, Where will We be Tomorrow? The Scientific World Journal. 2010;10:2215-27. doi:10.1100/tsw.2010.217
7. Luchey AM, Agarwal G, Poch MA. Robotic-assisted Radical Cystectomy. Cancer Control. 2015;22(3).
8. Ng CK, Kauffman EC, Lee MM, et al. A comparison of postoperative complications in open versus robotic cystectomy. Eur Urol. 2010;57:274-81.
9. Nix J, Smith A, Kurpad R, Nielsen ME, Wallen EM, Pruthi RS. Prospective randomized controlled trial of robotic versus open radical cystectomy for bladder cancer: perioperative and pathologic results. Eur Urol. 2010;57:196-201.
10. Smith AB, Raynor MC and Pruthi RS. Peri- and postoperative outcomes of robot-assisted radical cystectomy (RARC). BJU International. 2011;108:969-75. doi: 10.1111/j. 1464-410X.2011.10456.x

CHAPTER

26

Partial Nephrectomy

Ajit Saxena

INTRODUCTION

Partial nephrectomy is a standard surgical procedure for management of small renal masses. To reduce the perioperative morbidity involved with open approach, robotic platforms are being introduced. Robotic partial nephrectomy procedure is being carried out in many patients with Renal cancer or benign renal tumor. In this technique, the tumor is removed but it keeps the rest of the parts of kidney intact as such. By this suitable approach it is observed that there is better postoperative kidney function in patients. The procedure is minimally invasive in nature. Hence there is less trauma and faster recovery time.

Robotic kidney surgery offers significant advantages like minimal trauma, less scarring and faster recovery than open surgery. This robotic surgery technique involves small incisions and avoids cutting through muscle or bony structures. During Robotic Partial Nephrectomy blood supply to the kidney is cut off for a shorter time. Therefore patients undergoing robotic surgery also have decreased loss of blood during surgery and quicker recovery time. Usually the recovery time in robotic method needs 2 weeks, as opposed to 6–8 weeks for the open procedure for partial nephrectomy.

In robotic partial nephrectomy procedure the surgeon gets three dimensional view of field of operation. This robotic procedures permits wider range of motion of the surgical instruments which makes it easier to perform any complex surgical maneuvers required in this procedure.

PATIENT SELECTION

In recent years the understanding of renal cell carcinoma has evolved and the role of partial nephrectomy has expanded more. Partial nephrectomy was earlier done only in patients with a solitary kidney, bilateral masses, or poor renal function. Recently, partial nephrectomy became the standard of care among patients with renal masses smaller than 4 cm. There are many surgeons who argue that partial nephrectomy is current standard of care regardless of tumor size, when it is technically feasible. While checking feasibility for partial nephrectomy, the ability to safely remove all tumor completely becomes the primary consideration. The position of the tumor within the kidney with respect to the blood vessels and collecting system are most important factors when partial nephrectomy is being considered.

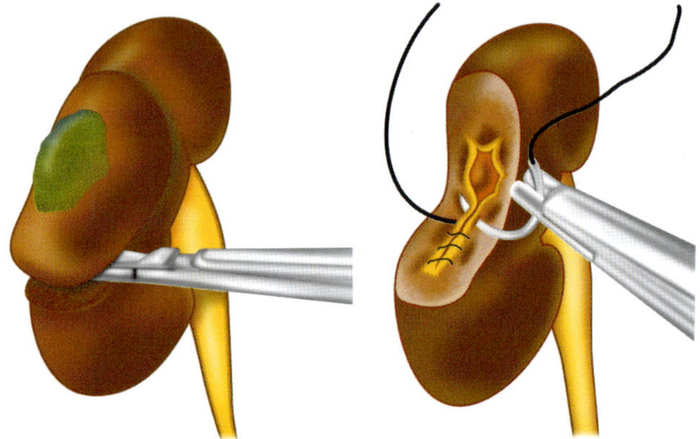

Fig. 26.1: Removal of part of a kidney or a lump from a kidney by partial nephrectomy (robotic)
Source: http://www.laparoscopy-endourology.com/main/for-patients/robotic-surgery/robotic-partial-nephrectomy/

However, the larger tumors and those closer to hilar vessels decrease the ability to successfully perform robotic partial nephrectomy. But, larger central tumors may also be removed robotically based on the location of the tumor and experience of the surgical team **(Fig. 26.1)**.

Other medical conditions like severe heart or lung disease may make the robotic approach less suitable.

In general indications are bilateral synchronous or metachronous tumors, tumor in a solitary functioning kidney, or renal tumors due to manifestation of syndromes such as von Hippel-Lindau (VHL) disease or Birt-Hogg-Dubé (BHD) syndrome, due to its multifocality and bilaterality.

PREOPERATIVE PREPARATION

The preoperative screening of robot-assisted procedure is similar to nephrectomy/partial nephrectomy. Evaluations depend on anesthesia risk and tumor stage, its size, and location. Any patient found suitable for an open partial nephrectomy is also suitable for a robot-assisted partial nephrectomy.

Evaluations required preoperatively include identification of cardiovascular risks, blood or serum laboratory investigations, and 3-dimensional imaging investigations (CT or MRI) to accurately identify the relationship of the mass to the renal vasculature and collecting system. The renal vessels and presence of any aberrant vasculature are to be identified and may be further examined with MRI. Perioperative antibiotics can be administered as per standard nephrectomy procedure.

Before surgery the patient must be carefully counselled on all options available, the risks and benefits involved and probable outcomes based on surgeon's individual experience. All elements of informed consent needs to be covered before the surgical procedure.

Full bowel preparation may not be required routinely for robotic partial nephrectomy. However to decompress the bowel and facilitate colon mobilization patient can be requested to drink magnesium citrate the night before surgery.

Patients needs to be advised to stop smoking well in advance of surgery, be active, and maintain good diet. Platelet inhibitors are required to be stopped well in advance of surgery.

The set of specific instructions with details of expected steps of the hospitalization, patient discharge, and then postoperative duration needs to be explained to each patient. Ideally the specific details about likelihood of drain placement, type of incision closure, recommendations for postoperative activity are to be provided.

An emphasis on the team approach to surgery is required for any Robotic partial nephrectomy. The operating room nursing staff and primary assistant and play vital role in the success of the procedure. For tasks such as application of hilar clamp, introducing the sutures and clips, and provision of suction and countertraction during the tumor excision are critical responsibilities of the assistant.

Many surgeons prefer administration of a second-generation cephalosporin antimicrobial prior to incision as antibiotic prophylaxis.

Robotic partial nephrectomy procedure is performed under general anaesthesia. A urinary catheter is always inserted and stays in place until the patient is mobile after the operation.

TECHNIQUE

OT Setup and Equipment

The instruments, sutures, and pledgets should be carefully prepared prior to commencing the tumor excision. It is advised that the surgeon has to ideally discuss the procedural steps in detail with the bedside assistant, scrub nurse, and any other operating room personals involved in the case.

The Robotic Console of da Vinci Surgical Robot

For a surgeon the user interface consists of the display system, master arms, footswitch, and panel control/touchpad.

Display System

A three dimensional stereoscopic high definition display of nearly 10X magnification for the surgeon in the console is provided by the current systems. For the rest of the operating room team additional 2-dimensional displays are available.

To facilitate training the Si model has dual console capabilities, with a second console with three dimensional vision and ability to take proper control of instruments.

Master Arms

Inputs to the master controls provided from the surgeon's finger and thumb and the operator's movements are translated in real time to the robotic arms and the EndoWrist instruments. Some of the basic force feedback is also given to the surgeon. Motion-scaling settings permit the scaling of hand-to-instrument movement ratios adequately.

Control/Touchpad

The integrated surgeon interface allows control of the audio, video, and system settings for the console surgeon in charge. This usually includes toggling between two dimensional and three dimensional displays, adjustment of motion scaling, and choosing the camera perspectives. Unique user settings could be stored in the surgeon's user profile, and the surgeon would benefit from the available ergonomic settings which can minimize fatigue. The newer Si model has features of a programmable touchpad.

Foot Switch Panel

Camera movement, swapping between different varieties of energy and deployment of diathermy is controlled with the help of a clutch mechanism and the foot switches.

Robotic Arms

Usually the da Vinci system comprises of 2 or 3 arms for mounting surgical instruments, and a separate camera arm is dedicated for the camera exclusively. The robotic arms are preferably mounted on a mobile platform that is draped and properly secured in place alongside the patient once the patient is appropriately positioned. The robotic arms have to be mounted to 8 mm trocars inserted through the abdominal wall of patient.

Surgeon within the console can be easily control the arms. However instrument exchanges, required suctioning, and suture delivery had to be done by the assisting surgeon near the bedside, alongside the robotic arms.

The robotic console, the robotic arms and the other instruments used are depicted in **Figure 26.2**.

Port placement and installation of the robot is a very important aspect of the robotic procedure. It is important to

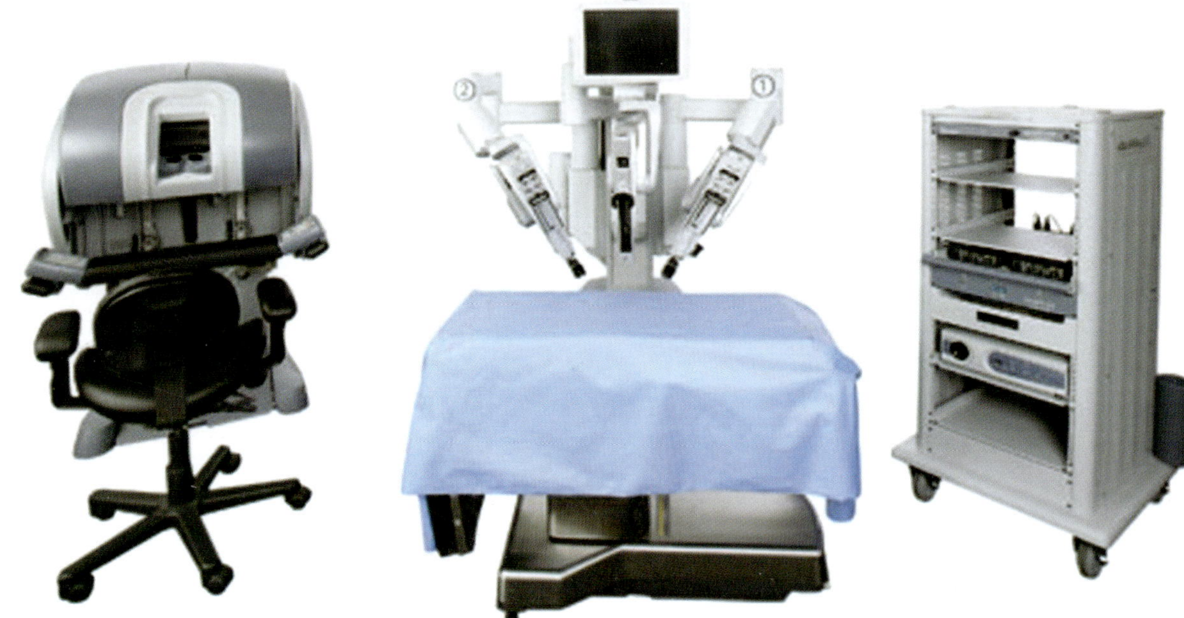

Fig. 26.2: The da Vinci Si robotic surgery system
Source: http://chennaiurologyclinic.in/uro-oncology.html

keep in mind the timing of docking the robot, as table rotation would not be feasible once the robot is docked.

Patient Positioning

Following general anesthesia administration, a nasogastric tube is placed, and a Foley catheter is inserted. The patient has to be placed in modified lateral position with a gel roll behind the buttock and another gel roll behind the shoulder.

Table flexion permits more working space for the robotic instruments and avoids clashing of the robotic arms during the surgical procedure and most surgeons prefer flank position for the patient where the table is moderately flexed.

An axillary roll has to be kept to avoid injury of brachial plexus and all other pressure points need to be padded and protected accordingly. The upper arm may be moved and secured above the down arm or positioned along the patient's hip as upper arm adducted position, as demonstrated in **Figures 26.3A and B**.

Patient positioning in the upside arm adducted (UAA) position maximizes access to the abdomen while avoiding robotic interference with the patient's arm.

Port Placement and Docking

Precise port placement is essential. The diagram below shows the placement of the ports for the instruments.

The port for camera is placed nearly 8–10 cm below the costal margin on an axis of 90° to costal margin. The simple rule of thumb is that the port for camera is placed one average male hand's breadth away from the costal margin and perpendicular to it.

For the novice surgeon, it is useful to use an approach that minimizes the likelihood of disorientation, and many surgeons feel that positioning the operative arms on the long axis of the torso avoids this risk which will in result provide better vision in the caudal direction unhampered.

The abdomen insufflation is done via Veress needle placement before the camera port insertion, or direct port placement can be done in a decompressed abdomen. However placement under direct vision approach can be used without prior insufflation .

While using the 'S' or 'Si' systems, generally the robotic and camera ports should be at least 8 cm apart to minimize clashing. Surgeons who use the 'standard' Da Vinci system may prefer to perform initial abdominal entry, as well as kidney preparation and dissection, before the robot docking for partial nephrectomy owing to the lesser availability of operative field with the earlier model of robot.

It is advised to select a port size adequate to accept a CT-1 needle, clip, and bulldog clamp appliers and mini-laparotomy pad, if required. Many surgeons use a 15-mm port for one of the assist ports and a 12-mm or 15-mm port for the secondary assist port **(Fig. 26.4)**.

Usually the robot is docked from behind of the patient. Adequate care is taken to minimize the potential arm clashing during the extensive side movement necessary for renal mobilization. A 30° down lens can be used. When operating on the right side, an additional 5 mm port could be introduced in the subxiphoid region, if necessary, to allow a blunt grasper to be placed beneath the liver edge and which is secured to the body wall in order to retract the liver superiorly for getting better upper pole access.

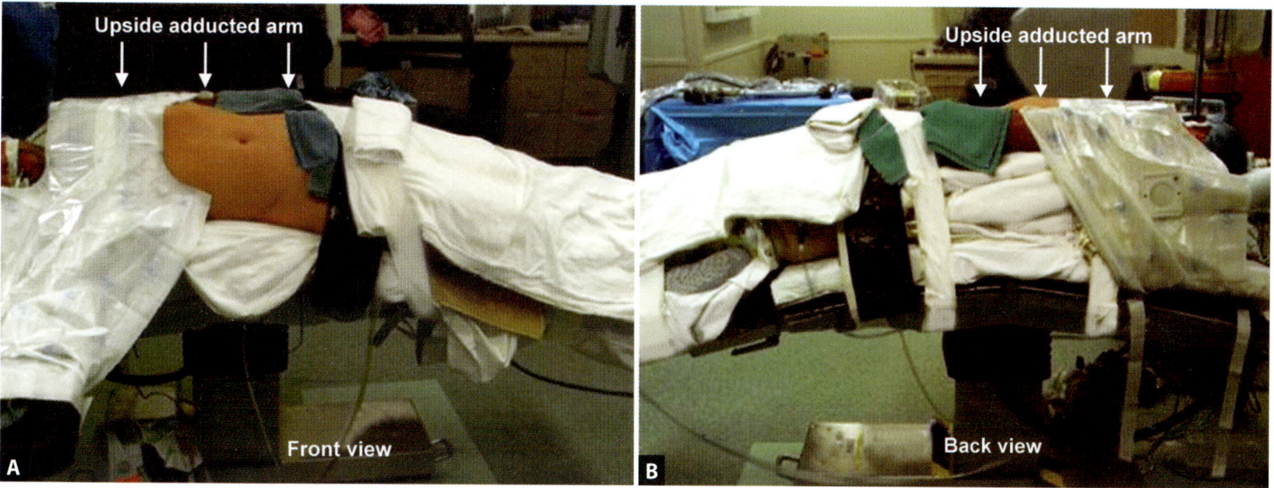

Figs 26.3A and B: (A) Front view of positioning in the upside arm adducted (UAA) position; (B) Back view of positioning in the upside arm adducted (UAA) position. Positioning in the upside arm adducted (UAA) position. This position maximizes access to the abdomen while avoiding robotic interference with the patient's arm.
Source: http://emedicine.medscape.com/article/2036677-technique#c2

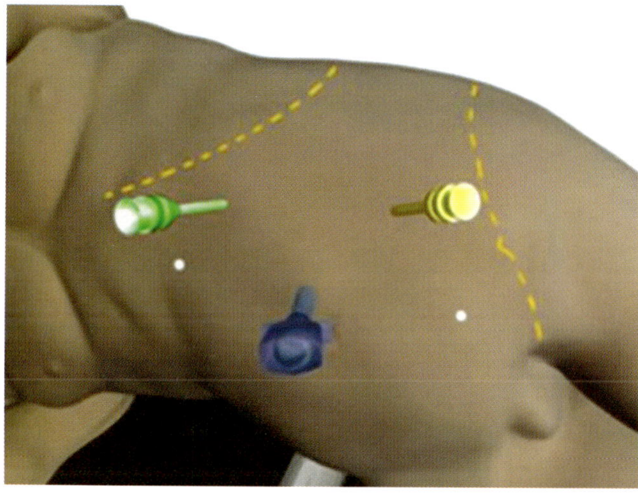

Fig. 26.4: Trocar configuration for laparoscopic and robotic partial nephrectomy
(*Courtesy:* Intuitive Surgical Inc, Sunnyvale, CA)
Source: http://urology.ufl.edu/patient-care/robotic-laparoscopic-urologic-surgery/procedures/laparoscopic-and-robotic-partial-nephrectomy/

ROBOTIC PARTIAL NEPHRECTOMY (RPN)

The operative time could vary from one patient to other; usually the average operating time observed is approximately 3–4 hours.

During robotic partial nephrectomy many small keyhole (<1 cm) incisions are made in the abdomen, which allow the surgeon to insert trocars.

The abdomen is filled with carbon dioxide gas to create a larger working space for the surgeon to accomplish the operation. After finishing the operation the gas is evacuated from the abdomen. The da Vinci S Surgical Robotic System is assembled to the trocars prior to start of the operation with the help of robotic technique.

The operating surgeon seats a few feet away from the operating console. The robotic instrumentation with highly precise motion scaling is controlled by the surgeon in real time. The surgeon controls two or three multi-jointed robotic instruments to accomplish the tasks of dissection, cutting, cauterization and suturing.

In addition, the robotic surgeon visualizes three dimensional, high definition image of the anatomy of kidney. The kidney which is affected has to be dissected and exposed. The tumor is then located and visualized in real time within the kidney. The blood supply to affected kidney is temporarily clamped to decrease blood loss during excision of the tumor. The tumor and its surrounding fat and a rim of healthy kidney are removed along with any visible surrounding lymph nodes. The tumor is excised from the affected kidney and removed later intact at the end of the operation. The defect in kidney is then closed with the help of sutures and surgical glue and the blood supply to the kidney restored later. A small drain is usually left at the end of the procedure exiting from one of the keyhole incisions. A summary of the steps involved is given in **Table 26.1**.

Table 26.1: Individual steps in robotic partial nephrectomy
• Removal of fat overlying renal mass
• Demarcation of renal mass margin
• Excision of renal mass
• Cauterization and sutured closure of renal defect
• Remove clamp from artery
• Place drain

Source: http://urology.ufl.edu/patient-care/robotic-laparoscopic-urologic-surgery/procedures/laparoscopic-and-robotic-partial-nephrectomy/

POSTOPERATIVE CARE

In most of the patients robotic partial nephrectomy can be performed with minimal morbidity and patients have excellent outcome with proper preoperative planning, meticulous surgical technique and attention to detail. The placement of a closed suction drain is considered essential after operation.

Small bleeding vessels can be tamponaded easily. The surgeon had to tie the sutures properly without any risks for tear of the kidney capsule with help of Gore-Tex, specifically when the arterial clamp is taken out in transverse resections during larger tumor removal.

Post-surgery discharge the patients are advised to visit again in 4–6 weeks for serum creatinine estimation and intravenous pyelography. In the absence of any obstruction, the patient would undergo CT scan every 6 months for 2 years and then every yearly for the next 5 years, following which, the frequency of scanning is reduced to every 2 years. Chest radiography and evaluation of serum calcium, liver function tests, serum alkaline phosphatase, and serum creatinine are done yearly for first 5 years and then biannually. Sometimes a surgeon may advice the frequency of postoperative evaluation as per the initial tumor stage, with less rigorous structured follow-up for any of the low-stage, smaller size tumors.

After a period of recovery in the Recovery Room, patient is transported to hospital room once the patient gains awareness and the vital signs are found stable.

Postoperative pain: Although most patients in the first few days after surgery may have mild pain at incision sites, this can be controlled by use of intravenous pain medication, patient-controlled anesthesia pump, or oral pain medication. Few patients may experience some minor transient shoulder pain (1-2 days) related to the carbon dioxide gas used to inflate the abdomen during the robotic surgery.

Nausea: Nausea may be reported following operation especially for those surgeries that need general anesthesia. This is mostly transient in nature and can be controlled by medication which is administered on as needed basis.

Urinary catheter: Urinary bladder is catheterized (e.g. Foley catheter) to drain urine at the time of surgery. This is in efforts to monitor the urine output over the first day or so following surgery. This is generally removed once patient postoperatively starts moving comfortably. It is not uncommon to have blood-tinged urine for a few days after the surgery while the catheter is in place.

Flank drain: A small clear tube or drain is placed during surgery exiting out of the side of the flank. The drain output would appear blood tinged but should be minimal. The drain helps in identifying any excess bleeding or any urine leak from the partial nephrectomy site. The drain is typically removed on the day patient gets discharged from the hospital.

Diet: Patient diet is advanced slowly following surgery from liquid diet to solid diet as tolerated. Mostly the appetite will be poor for up to a week following surgery. In addition, the intestinal function may be sluggish due to surgery and general anesthesia. It is for these two reasons that the patient is recommend taking only small amounts of liquids by mouth at any one time until the patient begins to pass flatus and the appetite returns. In the meantime, the intravenous catheter provides the necessary hydration to body as oral intake improves over a period.

Fatigue: Fatigue is commonly seen following surgery and usually subsides in a few weeks following surgery.

Ambulation: On the evening of surgery it is advised to get out of bed and begin walking with the supervision of a nurse or family member to help prevent blood clots from forming in the legs. In the days that follow surgery, patients are advised to walk nearly 6 different times a day in the ward. This serves to further reduce the change of deep vein thrombosis and helps in return of bowel functions.

Hospital stay: The duration of hospital stay after robotic partial nephrectomy is generally 1–2 days.

TECHNICAL TIPS AND TRICKS

Renal Access

The lateral attachments of the colon are carefully taken down with the help of a monopolar scissor in right robotic hand and a bipolar grasper in the left hand, due care is taken to avoid exposure of the bowel to electrocautery. Few surgeons prefer the Maryland bipolar grasper in their left hand.

The assistant would provide traction to bowel in a downward direction with the help of tip of suction irrigator when the surgeon gives upward counter traction to maximize exposure of the intervening structures. Colon is reflected medially to enter the anterior pararenal space, care has to be taken to identify and then selectively transect the ligamentous attachments to the upper-quadrant structures and minimize risk of any traction injury to the spleen or liver. Lateral body wall attachments of the kidney are mostly left intact, and Gerota fascia is not entered usually.

Hilar Access

After colon is safely released and reflected, careful identification and dissection of renal vasculature is done.

Preoperatively adequate planning and understanding of the anatomy would be obtained through appropriate scan or imaging studies which helps to note all arterial and venous variations and any duplication.

By direct approach access to the vessels of the hilum is obtained, in difficulty the identification of the ureter, inferior great vessel and gonadal vein on the appropriate side helps and surgeon can proceed with careful progression superiorly to the hilum. Due care is taken to identify and preserve any of the accessory lower-pole vessels. The duodenum is usually kocherized towards the right side. By using lateral traction on the kidney to stretch the hilar attachments, the vessels are dissected and made free from all surrounding tissue to allow easy and unhindered placement of occlusive vascular 'bulldog' clamps temporarily. Complete circumferential freedom of the blood vessels is critical to the effectiveness of vascular control. Inclusion of any excess tissue in the clamp could prevent complete occlusion and which may worsen both bleeding and visualization during tumor resection procedure.

Renal Mobilization

After the hilum is adequately freed, attention is given to acquiring access to the renal tumor before the clamping procedure. Better access in the region of the tumor is of importance hence it is recommend that nearly 2–3 cm surrounding the margins of the proposed resection is to be freed of perirenal fat and made accessible to the operating surgeon. For the posterior or upper pole tumors, complete freedom of the kidney may be required to allow the kidney to be turned into a favorable orientation. Gerota fascia is then entered and the plane on the renal capsule developed with focus on dividing the perirenal fat in an orientation that will permit reconstruction of the fat over the tumor resection bed at the concluding phase of the case.

The kidney could be repositioned into the optimal orientation for resection as adequate renal freedom has been obtained.

Identification of the Tumor

For tumor masses of exophytic nature the tumor is generally identified visually during careful dissection of Gerota fascia. Care is taken to avoid any inadvertent tumor entry and, to isolate the perirenal fat over the tumor and leave it attached mostly as an island.

Tumor Resection

While making preparations for resection of tumor, approximately 12.5 g of mannitol is intravenously administered 10 minutes before clamping. Once ready the bulldog clamps are applied to the renal vessels.

Attempts are done to lower the blood pressure is to be undertaken to decrease the bleeding. Some evidences suggest that the deleterious effects of warm ischemia are somewhat decreased by clamping only the arterial inflow without the vein clamping.

The time is noted after vascular clamps are placed and focus is rapidly turned to tumor resection procedure. After the capsule is cut and the adjacent normal parenchyma is rapidly entered. Maintaining an appropriate orientation of resection angle is of critical importance to ensure negative margins. Initially, it is useful to direct the scissor tips away from the mass.

After reaching appropriate depth, the scissors can be turned 'tips up' in order to prevent unnecessary diving into the kidney, the Da Vinci monopolar scissors are 1 cm long can assist in assessing depth adequately.

Entry into the collecting system would be noted and the tumor resection is completed in less than 5 minutes usually.

Renorrhaphy

When the tumor mass gets excised, it is set safely aside in a retrievable location and repair procedure immediately starts. Robotic instruments are exchanged for needle drivers and many surgeons mostly prefer to repair the tumor bed with the help of 6-in, 3-0 V-Lok suture starting outside the resection bed and repair violations in collecting system. The V-Lok suture is cut after running repair of the tumor bed gets completed. This step may not be required in uncomplicated small resections.

COMPLICATIONS

Most complications can be managed conservatively. The least morbidity occurs in which most tumors are smaller and peripherally located.

Hemorrhage

Commonly observed intraoperative complication is excessive bleeding. In this aspect, attention to detail, perfect dissection, and ligation of intra-parenchymal vessels are important. Easy access for renal hilum, is provided by identifying and isolating the renal artery early. Postoperative hemorrhage may be self resolving and could be confined to the retroperitoneum or may present as gross hematuria, decreased hematocrit, or flank ecchymosis. Treatment is mostly expectant which consists of volume resuscitation, serial hematocrits evaluation, and bedrest. In unusual case embolization is an option, if bleeding persists after conservative management and it may require multiple transfusions. Reexploration is considered as last resort for intractable severe bleeding.

Urinary Fistula

Risk factors for development of urinary fistula include central location of mass, larger size of tumor, and increased complexity of nephron sparing surgical procedure. A small amount of urinary leakage may be common which usually stops spontaneously. Any persistent drainage observed through the drain suggests larger leak, which can be still managed expectantly. In the absence of any ureteral obstruction, most of the leaks seal as more of tissue healing occurs. If a urinoma develops following the removal of flank drain, percutaneous drainage by catheter is indicated to prevent any abscess formation.

Renal Insufficiency

In most of the cases renal insufficiency following surgery could be result of transient ischemia during surgery which may spontaneously subside. Intraoperative measures to reduce the complication requires few preventive measures like hydration preoperatively, correction of electrolyte abnormalities, use of mannitol, maintaining minimum duration of arterial clamp time, and use of surface hypothermia in many cases.

Other Complications

Other complications can include infections or those caused by anesthesia (e.g. atelectasis or pneumonia). Appropriate antibiotic treatment and postoperatively use of incentive spirometry could decrease these incidences.

EVIDENCE

Robotic partial nephrectomy is a suitable option for patients and surgeons who desire a minimally invasive alternative for the performance of nephron-sparing surgery which has now become the norm for the management of small renal masses. Numerous evidences have shown favorable outcomes for robotic partial nephrectomy. Robotic partial nephrectomy is a safe and feasible alternative for minimally invasive nephron-sparing surgery with a shorter learning curve. Robotic partial nephrectomy extends the benefits of minimally invasive nephron-sparing surgery to a wider section of surgeons and patients and may be an acceptable alternative for small renal masses.[1]

SUMMARY

Robotic partial nephrectomy helps in achievement of similar oncologic outcomes, less blood loss, minimal effects on renal function, and an excellent safety profile.

The robot offers many advantages over conventional surgeries. The binocular camera helps the surgeon in depth perception to easily operate in three dimensions. Another advantage is that the 'wrist' of robotic arms has seven degrees of freedom, which gives the surgeon much better control over certain aspects of the procedure, most importantly minimal tissue manipulation and precise suturing. The technological advantages of robotic partial nephrectomy over conventional surgeries may allow novice surgeons a shorter learning curve.

The disadvantage of robotic partial nephrectomy could be the added cost of purchasing and maintaining a surgical robot. But better patient outcome is a notable patient advantage.

Future studies are required to establish robotic partial nephrectomy as a standard surgical management for patients with small renal masses by evaluating the long-term cancer and the functional outcomes.

REFERENCE

1. Shyam Sukumar, Craig G. Rogers. Robot-Assisted Partial Nephrectomy. Journal of Endourology. 2011;25(2):151-7.

CHAPTER

27

Donor Nephrectomy

Vinay Mahendra, Jaydip Bhadra Roy, Tridibes Mondal

INTRODUCTION

Renal transplant is the best treatment modality for patients with end-stage renal disease (ESRD). It ensures good quality of life and increases survival compared to dialysis. Living donor nephrectomy is associated with better graft function resulting in improved patient survival and graft survival compared to deceased donor transplantation. Open donor nephrectomy has been used for more than 60 years until the first laparoscopic donor nephrectomy by Ratner et al. 20 years ago. Thelaparoscopic approach for kidney retrieval has since become more and more popular across the world as it has been shown to provide equivalent graft survival rates with less morbidity to the donor. This has been a crucial development towards addressing the problem of the living donor pool. However, laparoscopic donor nephrectomy has a long learning curve and given the scenario of renal transplant many centers are still continuing with open approach for kidney retrieval. da Vinci robotic system combines robotic techniques and computer imaging to enable microsurgery in a laparoscopic environment.

A surgeon does not need to be a proficient laparoscopic surgeon to be able to do robotic surgery. Many surgeons across the specialties have been able to take up robotic-assisted laparoscopic surgeries with minimal or no experience in laparoscopic surgery. Hence this technique offers an opportunity for many centers to move to minimally invasive donor nephrectomy. This will help to reduce the donor morbidity and thereby go a long way in increasing the living donor pool.

PREOPERATIVE INVESTIGATIONS

The donor evaluation does not need any special evaluation for suitability of robotic donor nephrectomy.

The donor needs to be evaluated by the nephrologist from compatibility point of view and by the recipient surgeon form the operative planning view point. Anesthetist evaluation is done from fitness for surgery.

- CT renal angigram and Tc99m DTPA (or MAG3 renogram): Left side is preferable over the right (longer renal vein) and single artery is preferable over multiple arteries. More than three renal arteries is generally considered as a contraindication for donor nephrectomy. Better functioning kidney stays with donor.

SURGICAL STEPS

The procedure is done under general anesthesia using transperitoneal approach.

- *Position:* Right or left semilateral depending upon the laterality. The legs and the back are cushioned adequately to avoid any injuries due to positioning.
- *Instruments:* Robotic monopolar hook and bipolar maryland.

Port Placement and Docking of Robot

Left Robotic Donor Nephrectomy

Three robotic ports and 1 assistant port. An additional subxiphisternal assistant port is placed in case of early bifurcation of the renal artery or complex venous anatomy.

Right Robotic Donor Nephrectomy

Three robotic ports and 2 assistant ports are placed. 12 mm camera port at the level of umbilicus at the pararectal line. 8 mm robotic port just below the tip of 9th costal cartilage. 8 mm robotic port above the anterior superior iliac spine. 12 mm assistant port in the left groin. 6 mm assistant port in subxiphisternal area (optional on left side) **(Fig. 27.1)**.

The robotic tower is moved at a right angle to the patient from behind the patient for docking **(Fig. 27.2)**.

Surgical Procedure

Camera port is placed using open Hassan technique. The pneumoperitoneum is induced with pressure at 12–15 mm Hg. The two robotic ports and assistant port(s) are placed under vision as stated above. The robotic tower is docked as stated above.

Bipolar Maryland is introduced through the robotic port at the tip of 9th costal cartilage and monopolar hook is

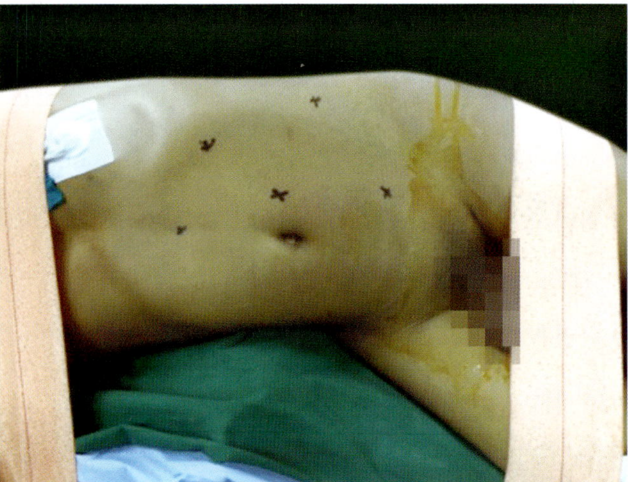

Fig. 27.1: Ports placement for right robotic nephrectomy

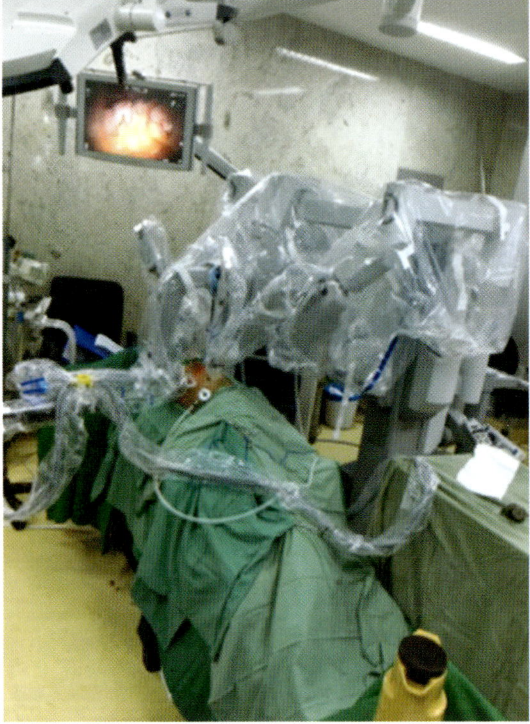

Fig. 27.2: Docking of robotic tower for right nephrectomy

inserted through the robotic port above the anterior superior iliac spine. The assistant port is used for laparoscopic bowel grasper.

The surgery starts with reflection of descending colon and splenic flexure (left side) or ascending colon and hepatic flexure (right side). The subxiphisternal 6 mm port is essential in all the patients undergoing right robotic nephrectomy to retract the liver.

After the reflection of colon the gerota's fascia is divided to expose the kidney and ureter and the ureter is dissected up to the pelvic brim to ensure adequate length. Care is taken to preserve periureteric tissue to avoid denuding the ureter which may compromise the blood supply. It is preferable to stay close to the kidney during this step as it is an avascular plane and the retrieved kidney is also clean thereby reducing the bench dissection and associated cold schema time. In obese patients, it is useful to excise any excess perinephric and retroperitoneal fat. It helps in creating a clean field during hillier dissection thereby useful in harvesting greater length of vessels.

After the ureteric dissection, the gonadal vein is identified on the left side and dissected up to its junction with the renal vein. The renal vein is dissected to ensure adequate length. The lumbar vein, more often than not, needs to be dissected and divided to adequately dissect the renal artery. This step needs to be done carefully as this vein is very friable and can be a source of significant bleeding. The robotic bipolar maryland is a very useful tool to dissect renal vein completely free of the renal artery that is posterior. The suprarenal vein does not always need to be divided without compromising the venous length. In case of early venous bifurcation, the lumbar and gonadal veins usually join the lower tributary and tether it down thereby making it difficult to get a common venous stump. However, once these two veins are carefully dissected and divided the lower tributary is freed and almost always gives a common venous stump once the renal vein is fully mobilized.

On the right side, the renal vein is dissected up to its junction with the inferior vena cava. The lumbar vein is usually not a problem on the right side although gonadal vein sometimes drains either into the renal vein or at the junction of the renal vein and inferior vena cava and one has to be careful avoid injury as this is a source of significant bleeding. It is helpful to dissect the IVC above and below the renal vein. This is an important step as it enables the dissection of renal artery that courses from behind the IVC.

The renal artery is fully dissected by clearing periarterial lymphatics where the robotic hook is very useful to enter the right plane that is crucial for adequate arterial dissection.

In case of early arterial bifurcation or complex renal venous anatomy on the left side, a subxiphisternal port is very useful for medial retraction of peritoneal fold to achieve adequate dissection of the artery up to the aorta.

In case of early bifurcation of the artery on the right side it is helpful to use 30° down telescope which helps in vision behind the IVC and robotic hook and maryland with their endowrist are very useful in dissecting the artery adequately.

Once the above is done, the remaining kidney is fully mobilized with care taken to dissect adrenal glands by entering the avascular plane between the upper pole and the adrenal to avoid any injury and resultant bleeding.

After completing the dissection the kidney is disconnected in the following order when the recipient team is ready:

- Ureter—Hemolok (1)
- Artery—Hemolok (2)
- Vein—Hemolok (1).

After disconnecting the kidney, the robot is undocked and all the ports removed. The kidney is retrieved by hand after making the incision in the groin incorporating the groin port site. Warm ischemia time is counted from the time of first clip on the renal artery.

The groin incision is closed with number 1 vicryl to the rectus sheath and subcuticular monocryl to skin. The camera port is closed using number 1 vicar port closure stitch. 3/0 monocryl is used for remaining ports. A 16 Fr tube drain is inserted in the renal bed.

Role of Assistant

- Traction and contraction during dissection
- Application of hemlock clips on the vessels and ureter
- Undocking of the robot and incision in the groin.

Postoperative Care

Day 0

- Intravenous ringer lactate 100 mL/hour
- Intravenous cefoperazone/sulbactam—two doses postoperative
- Analgesia—Pethidine 50–75 mg intramuscular as and when needed
- Oral liquids started 6 hours after surgery.

Day 1

- Patient is mobilized
- Orally free fluids
- Soft diet once patient passes flatus
- Intravenous fluids and urethral cateter removed.

Day 2

Patient discharged.

Follow-up

After 1 week in outpatients—long-term follow-up with the nephrologist and yearly with renal parameters and urine examination for protein.

DISCUSSION

The apprehensions of increased warm ischemia time were raised when laparoscopic donor nephrectomy was introduced and subsequent studies showed it to be safe and effective with reduction in donor morbidity. The same apprehensions were raised with the advent of robotic donor nephrectomy due to slightly more time being taken to undock the robot. This has not translated into effect on the immediate or delayed graft function and nadir creatinine. The experience till date shows robotic donor nephrectomy to be at least as effective as laparoscopic donor nephrectomy.

The arguments have been made regarding the benefit and cost justification of robotic donor nephrectomy over laparoscopic donor nephrectomy. Although the postoperative recovery is essentially the same in both techniques, the robotic donor nephrectomy enables better dissection in complex vascular anatomy especially early arterial bifurcation on the right side due to increased range of movements offered with the robot. Also, the robotic donor nephrectomy has a less steeplearning curve compared to laparoscopic donor nephrectomy. This is likely to increase the number of minimally invasive donor nephrectomy thereby reducing the donor morbidity and will go a long way in increasing the living renal donor pool.

The only drawback of robotic donor nephrectomy at present is its general availability and the cost which I feel is going to improve with time. In any case, increased focus needs to be put on the morbidity to the donor to ensure early recovery.

BIBLIOGRAPHY

1. Al-Mamari SA, et al. Right robotic nephrectomy. A practical guide. 2014, ISBN 978-3-319-04588-7.
2. Cohen A, Williams D, Bohorquez H, Bruce D, Carmody I, Reichman T. Series of 100 consecutive donors. Multiorgan Transplant Institute, Ochsner Clinic Foundation, New Orleans, LA. Meeting 2013 American Transplant Congress.
3. Ratner LE, Ciseck LJ, Moore RG, Cigarroa FG. Laparoscopic live donor nephrectomy. Transplantation. 2013;60(9):1047-9.

CHAPTER

28

Adrenalectomy

Sohrab Arora, Gagan Gautam

INTRODUCTION

With advancing imaging modalities, adrenal incidentaloma is becoming an increasing presentation in the clinic with a reported incidence as high as 4.4% in contemporary computerized tomography series.[1] The prevalence of adrenal masses increases with increasing age.[2] Therefore, it is expected to become even more common as the population is aging due to higher life expectancy. The first laparoscopic adrenalectomy was performed by Gagner et al. in 1992.[3] Since then, laparoscopy has emerged as the gold standard procedure for adrenalectomy.[4] Piazza et al. performed the first robot-assisted adrenalectomy using the ZEUS/AESOP system in 1999.[5] Subsequently, the da Vinci robot (Intuitive Surgical, Mountain View, California) has been used in multiple series for different indications of adrenalectomy.[6-9] Robot-assisted surgery has the advantages of better ergonomics for the surgeon, more degrees of freedom of the robotic instruments, elimination of tremor and three dimensional vision. For adrenalectomy, it has the advantages of less blood loss, shorter hospital stay with similar outcomes when compared to laparoscopic adrenalectomy.[10] These factors become more important as more adrenal masses are being diagnosed as incidentalomas nowadays. In this chapter, we will review the technique, results and evidence for robot-assisted adrenalectomy with an emphasis on what goes on in the operation theater.

Table 28.1: Indications

1. Benign functional lesions • Adrenal adenoma • Adrenal hyperplasia • Pheochromocytoma • Congenital adrenal hyperplasia • Aldosteronoma
2. Benign nonfunctional lesions • Symptomatic cyst • Myelolipoma – >4 cm – Suspicion of malignancy – Symptomatic
3. Malignancy • Primary adrenal carcinoma • Indeterminate adrenal lesion >5 cm • Indeterminate adrenal lesion 2–5 cm but increasing in size on subsequent scans • Solitary symptomatic metastases

Table 28.2: Contraindications

Absolute	*Relative*
Severe cardiopulmonary disease	Pregnancy (can be done in 2nd trimester)
Uncorrected coagulopathy	Tumor thrombus (reports of excision with robot-assisted surgery)
Invasive carcinoma	Infiltrative tumors
Uncontrolled pheochromocytoma	

PATIENT SELECTION

The indications and contraindications for robot-assisted adrenalectomy are summarized in **Tables 28.1 and 28.2**.

Functioning adrenal lesions should be considered for removal unless there is an absolute contraindication for surgery (except in mild cases of hyperaldosteronism which can be managed medically).[11] It is important to note that some functioning lesions may be completely asymptomatic and present as incidentalomas. In these cases, it is prudent to operate all cases with radiological and biochemical features of pheochromocytoma due to life-threatening complications if left untreated. Even in cases of subclinical Cushing's syndrome, surgery is shown to improve metabolic parameters like diabetes, hypertension, and osteoporosis.[12]

A size cutoff of 6 cm has long been used to distinguish benign from malignant adrenal lesions. The cutoff has since been lowered to 4 cm in the American Association of Clinical Endocrinologists 2009 guidelines.[11] The size cut-off of

4 cm has been shown to have 93% sensitivity of predicting a malignancy but a low specificity of 42%.[13] Therefore, clinical judgement and other radiological features (discussed later) may be used to guide treatment planning in addition to the size criteria.

The indications of partial adrenalectomy are discussed later.

WORK-UP AND PREOPERATIVE PREPARATION

Imaging

Imaging of an adrenal mass is fairly specific and sensitive to ascertain the type of tumor. Adenomas typically have more fat content. On a contrast-enhanced CT scan, adenomas are typically less dense (<10 HU attenuation on a CT scan virtually confirms an adenoma with almost 100% sensitivity). Nevertheless, about 30% of adenomas may be fat poor and have a density of >30 HU causing a diagnostic dilemma.[14] In these cases, the fact that adenomas have a faster washout of contrast is helpful in diagnosis. More than 40% washout at 10 minutes is typical of adenomas.[15] Pheochromocytomas will generally enhance to more than 100 HU on a contrast-enhanced CT.

MRI imaging is also helpful in making a preoperative diagnosis. Adenomas will typically have higher intracellular fat, which results in loss of signal intensity on out-of-phase images in opposed-phase MRI sequences. Pheochromocytoma is a spot diagnosis with a "light bulb sign", very high intensity on a T2 sequence of MRI.[16]

Hormonal Evaluation

Full hormonal evaluation is essential to exclude functional lesions. The complete metabolic workup is beyond the scope of this chapter, but all patients should be tested for plasma free metanephrines, normetanephrines, 24-hour total urinary metanephrines and fractionated catecholamines to rule out pheochromocytoma.[17] Patients should also be screened for cortisol excess. The simplest method would be a low dose (1 mg) dexamethasone suppression test. 1 mg dexamethasone is given the night before and serum cortisol is measured in the morning. If the cortisol level is >5 ug/dL, it indicates subclinical Cushing's syndrome. To rule out aldosteronoma, both serum aldosterone and renin should be measured and an aldosterone:renin ratio of >20 suggests aldosteronoma.[11]

Anesthetic Considerations

The full discussion of anesthetic consideration is beyond the scope of the present chapter but to summarize, patients with raised cortisol levels have metabolic complications like diabetes and hypertension, which should be adequately controlled before surgery. Due to high levels of cortisol, and the resulting immunosuppression, antibiotics should be used in the perioperative period. These patients are also at an increased risk of thromboembolism, therefore, DVT prophylaxis should be given. Adequate, tapering cortisol replacement should be done as the hypothalamus-pituitary axis is suppressed for about 15 months after surgery.[18] For pheochromocytoma, long acting alpha-blockers such as phenoxybenzamine should be started 1–3 weeks before surgery till adequate control of blood pressure. Intra-operatively, invasive hemodynamic monitoring should be considered, and drugs like nitroprusside, nicardipine, nitroglycerin, or phentolamine be used to control intra-operative blood pressure fluctuations.

TECHNIQUE

Approaches

- Robotic lateral transabdominal adrenalectomy
- Robotic posterior retroperitoneal adrenalectomy
- Single port robot-assisted adrenalectomy
- Partial adrenalectomy.

OT Setup and Equipment

Figures 28.1 and 28.2 show right- and left-sided OT setup, respectively. The list of equipment required is given in **Table 28.3**.

Patient Positioning

Patient is placed in a modified lateral decubitus position with the ipsilateral side up **(Fig. 28.3A)** and an angle of 45° from the vertical **(Fig. 28.3B)**. All bony prominences are adequately padded and the patient is secured to the table with tapes.

Port Placement and Docking

Pneumoperitoneum is created with a Veress needle. Insufflation may be done to 20 mm Hg till the placement of the first port and subsequently reduced to 12–15 mm Hg through the surgery. Port placement is done to ensure triangulation at the ipsilateral adrenal area. The camera port (12 mm) is placed at the lateral edge of the rectus muscle superior and lateral to the umbilicus. The distance cephalad from the umbilicus may be more in an obese patient as the umbilicus is situated lower. An 8 mm robotic port is placed 1 cm below the subcostal margin at the lateral edge of rectus. Another 8 mm robotic port is placed superior to the anterior superior iliac spine. The third robotic 8 mm port is placed along the lateral rectus line in the suprapubic region. It should be ensured that the ports are at least 8–10 cm away from each other to avoid clashing of robotic instruments. An assistant port, 12 mm is placed in the midline between the cephalad robotic port and the camera port. This port is used for suction and traction as needed. For the right side, an additional 5 mm port is placed in the epigastrium for retraction of the liver. The right- and left-sided port placement is shown in **Fig. 28.4A and B**, respectively. Robot is docked over the ipsilateral shoulder **(Fig. 28.5)**.

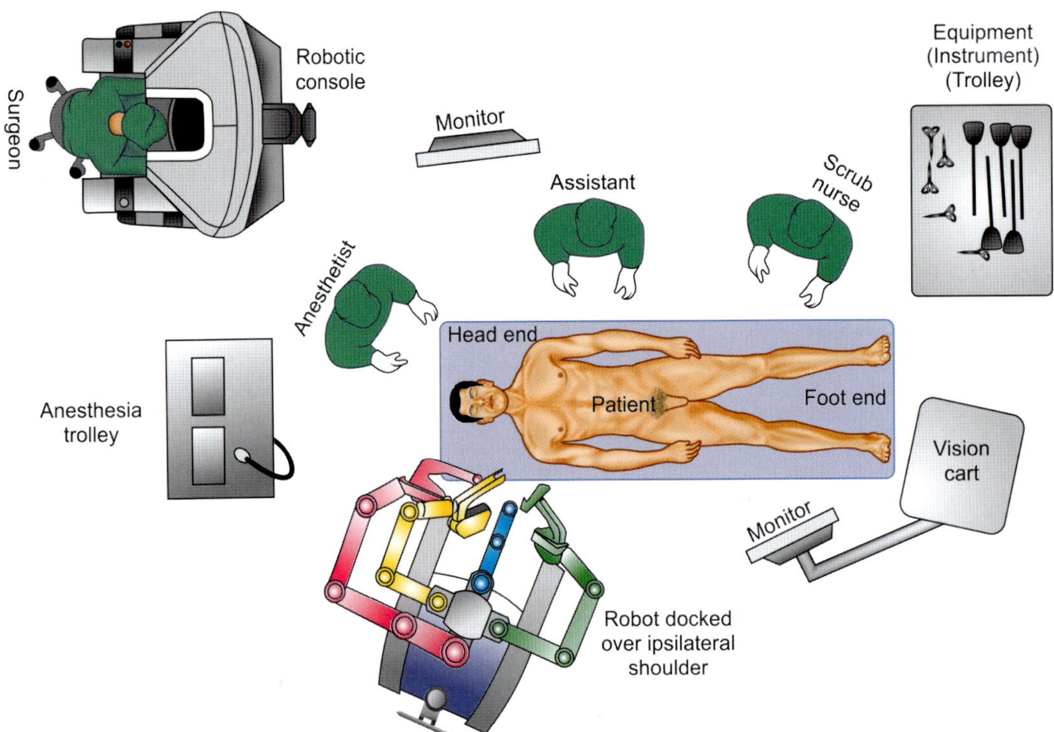

Fig. 28.1: Right-sided OT setup

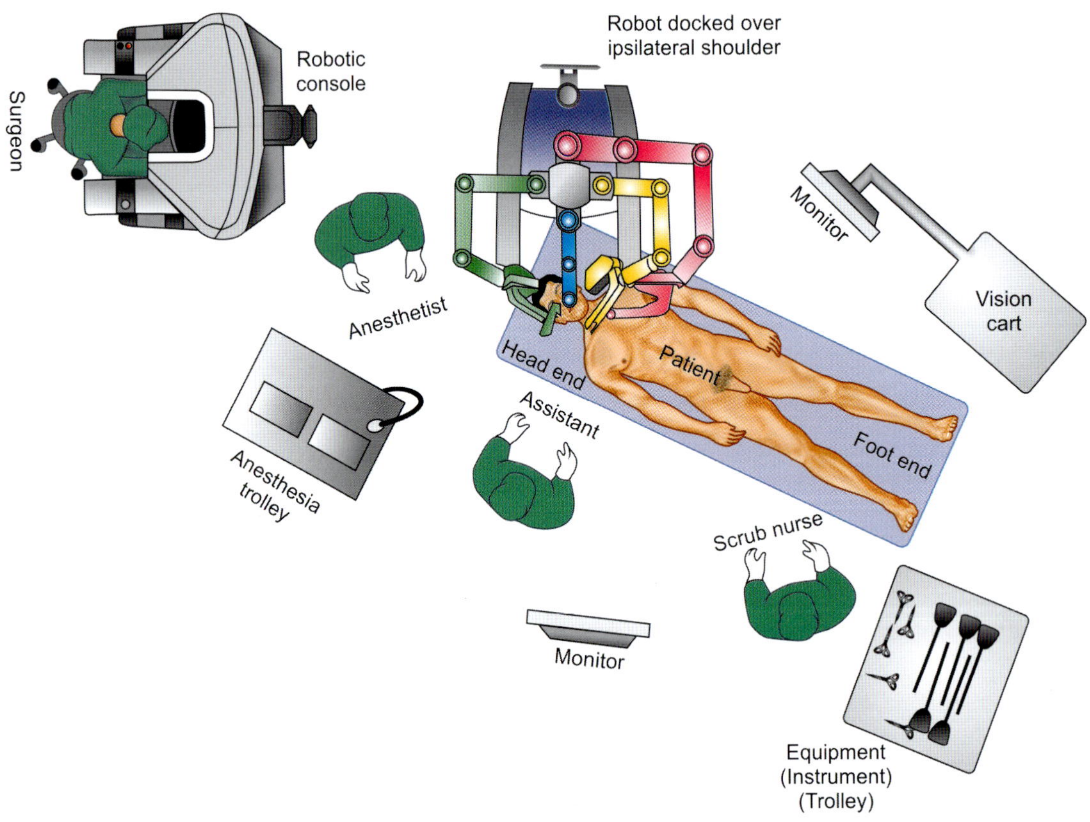

Fig. 28.2: Left-sided OT setup

Technique and Steps

Robotic Lateral Transabdominal Adrenalectomy

Left side

The dissection begins with reflection of colon along the line of Toldt **(Fig. 28.6)**. The scissor with monopolar is a useful instrument during this step as it can be used as a knife and dissector as well. Splenorenal and splenocolic ligaments are divided **(Fig. 28.7)**. This exposes the adrenal gland as the upper pole of the kidney falls away from the working area. A sponge interposition may also be done to increase exposure.[19] The tail of pancreas is also carefully medialized. After adequate exposure of the adrenal gland, the renal hilum is identified and the renal vein is dissected with an intent to expose the adrenal vein which drains into its cranial aspect **(Fig. 28.8)**. Once identified and dissected, the adrenal vein is clipped by the assistant. If the capsule of adrenal is difficult to identify, it is useful to dissect the adrenal vein for 1–1.5 cm towards the adrenal to stay away from the renal hilum which may have aberrant renal veins. Circumferential dissection of the adrenal is then started. Gerota's fascia and perinephric fat of the upper pole of the kidney can be left with the adrenal to avoid handling the adrenal itself. Minimal manipulation of the adrenal should be done and the "patient should be dissected away from the adrenal rather than adrenal from the patient". The arterial supply of adrenal is highly variable and is best controlled with bipolar forceps or clips whenever possible, especially on the cranial side of adrenal gland where one may encounter adrenal branches of inferior phrenic artery. Once the dissection is complete, an endocatch bag is used to extract the specimen from one of the port sites. Routine placement of drain is unnecessary.

Table 28.3: List of equipments required
da Vinci robotic system® with stack containing insufflator, light source and monitors
Sterile drapes for robotic arms
No. 11 scalpel blade
Electrocautery machine with hand piece
2 langenbeck retractors
Veress needle
2 × laparoscopic 12 mm ports
3 × robotic 8 mm ports
Sterile flask filled with warm water to warm the telescope
0° or 30° down scope depending on surgeon preference
Endowrist® prograsp forceps
Endowrist® monopolar scissors
Endowrist® fenestrated bipolar forceps
Laparoscopic suction-irrigation
Laparoscopic atraumatic grasper
5 mm and 10 mm Weck® hem-o-lock clips
10 mm Endocatch® bag
Laparotomy set with 2 × satinsky and 4 × bulldog clamps (Keep ready)
5-0 Prolene® on a round-bodied needle with laparoscopic needle driver (Keep ready)

Right Side

On the right side, minimal reflection of the colon is usually sufficient. After reflecting the colon, the duodenum is carefully kocherized trying to minimize the use of monopolar electrocautery near it, till the right edge of vena cava is exposed. Division of triangular ligament of the liver may be necessary to increase the working space. On the right side, adrenal vein drains directly into the vena cava and is cranial to the insertion of right renal vein. After clipping the adrenal vein, procedure is similar to the left side. In the authors' experience, division of the peritoneal reflection between the adrenal gland and the liver as an initial step and exposure of the psoas between these structures, facilitates the exposure of the adrenal vein and subsequent mobilization of the gland.

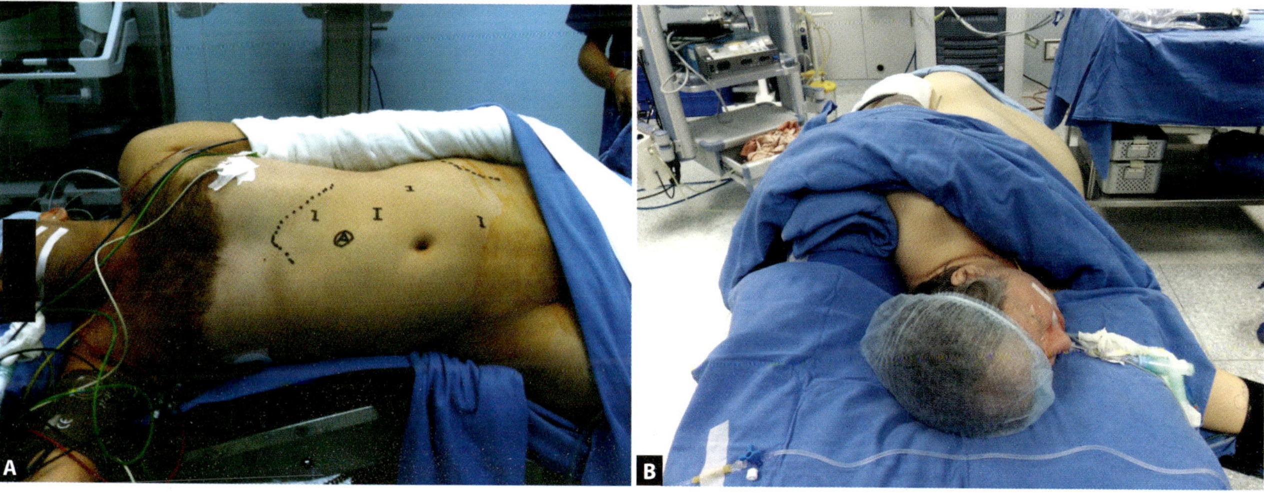

Figs 28.3A and B: Picture showing patient positioned (A) in a modified lateral decubibus position with the ipsilateral side up and (B) an angle of 45° from the vertical

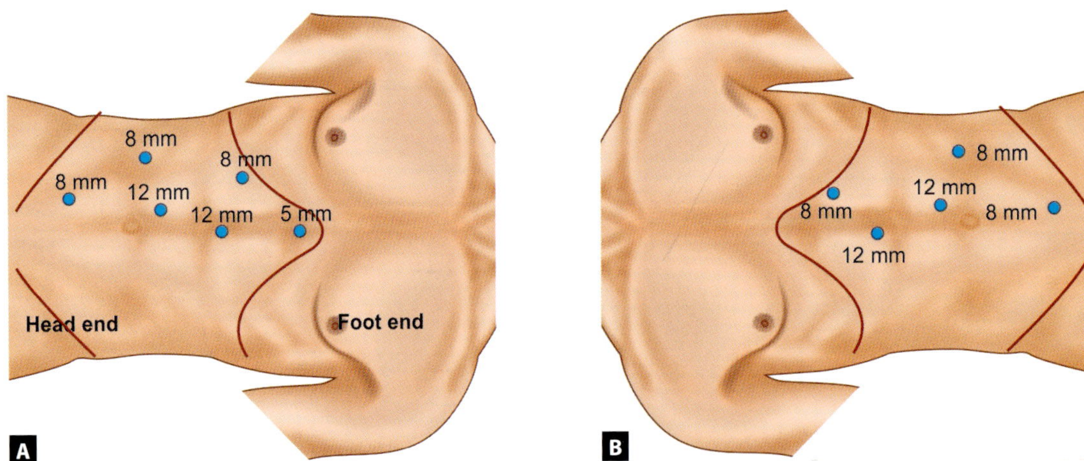

Figs 28.4A and B: (A) Right-sided port placement; (B) Left-sided port placement

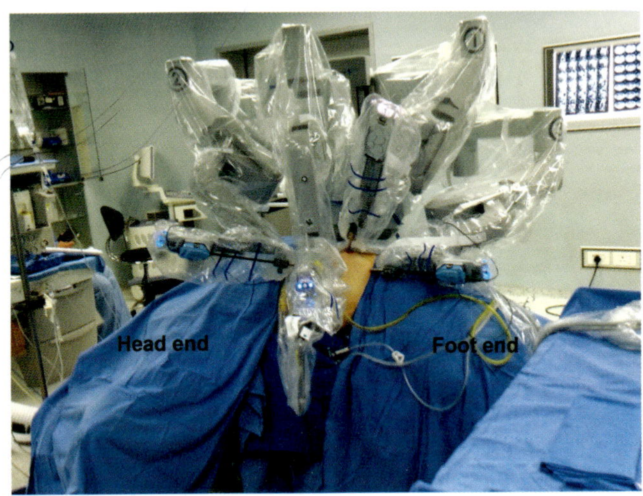

Fig. 28.5: Robot is docked over the ipsilateral shoulder

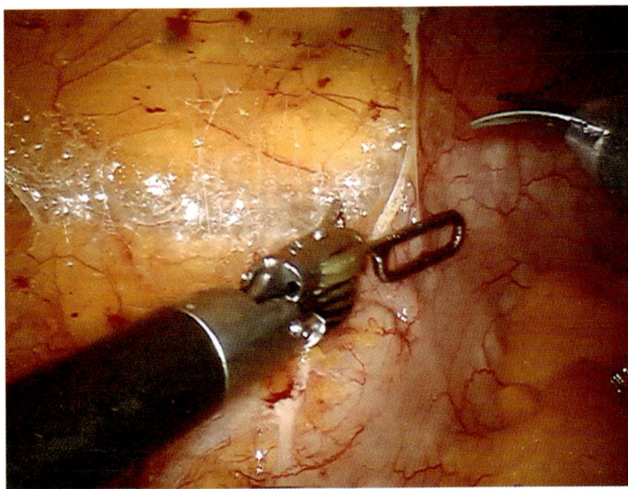

Fig. 28.6: Mobilization of the colon as the initial step in left adrenalectomy

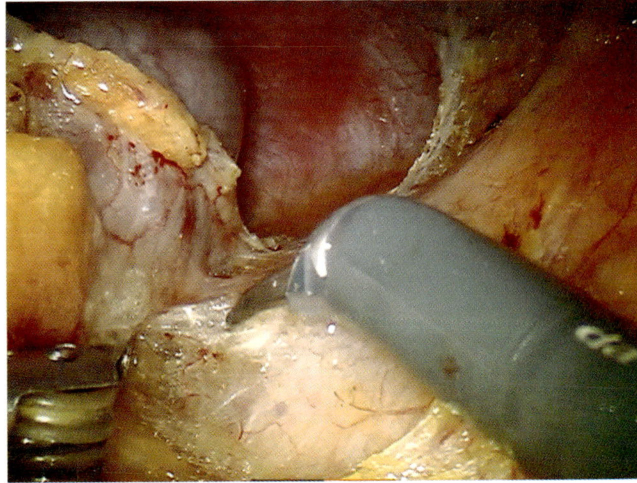

Fig. 28.7: Separation of the adrenal gland from the spleen

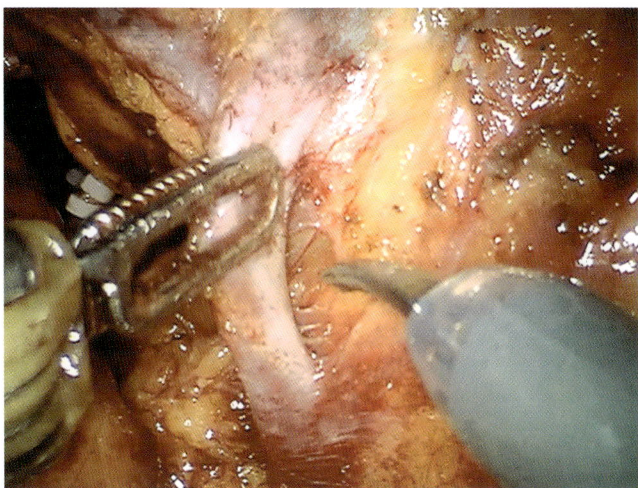

Fig. 28.8: Identification of the left adrenal vein

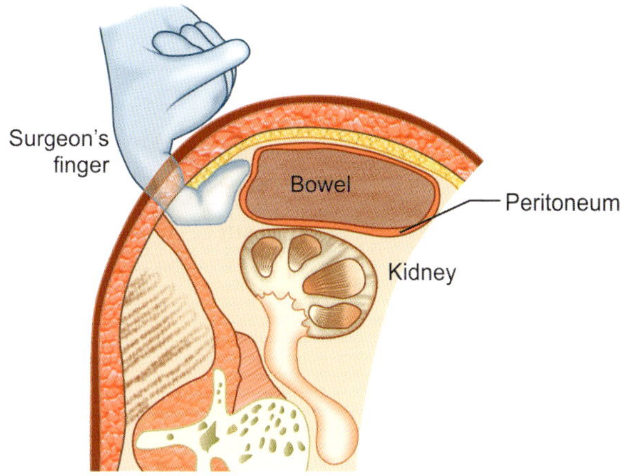

Fig. 28.9: Creating space for balloon in retroperitoneum

Posterior Retroperitoneoscopic Robot-assisted Adrenalectomy

This approach may be beneficial in patients who have had abdominal surgery in the past. It has the advantages of direct approach to the adrenal gland without the need to enter peritoneal cavity, or to mobilize adjacent organs. It may also be beneficial to patients who cannot tolerate peritoneal insufflation with carbon dioxide due to hemodynamic or respiratory considerations.

It may be difficult in tumors more than 6 cm due to the limited working space, and when the distance between the iliac crest and the 12th rib is less than 4 cm. It is also contraindicated in suspected malignancy where invasion of other structures is suspected.[20]

In this approach, in the prone jack knife position, a small incision is made 1.5 cm below the tip of the 12th rib and lumbodorsal fascia is punctured. A finger is then inserted into the retroperitoneum and space is made for the balloon **(Fig. 28.9)**, which is subsequently placed in this space and inflated with 100 mL of saline. After creation of the space, one robotic 8 mm port is placed 5–6 cm medial to the initial incision under finger guidance, at the edge of paraspinous muscles and the other 8 mm port is placed 5–6 cm lateral to the camera port. The camera port is inserted in the end, insufflation done to 20–25 mm Hg, and the robot is docked in an imaginary line leading from the camera port to the target organ. The dissection and retroperitoneal anatomy is beyond the scope of this chapter but is similar to conventional retroperitoneoscopic adrenalectomy. Ludwig Aaron et al. provided the first description of this procedure and reported operative times around 2 hours.[21]

Single-port Robot-assisted Adrenalectomy

Single port laparoscopic surgery had its inherent disadvantages of being cumbersome and ergonomically challenging with loss of triangulation and clashing of instruments. With the advent of robotic surgery, the challenges of single site surgery may be partly overcome. Arman Arghami et al. reported a case series of 16 patients with a mean BMI of 32, who underwent a single port robot-assisted adrenalectomy.[22]

The procedure involves a flexed lateral decubitus position and a single 2.5 cm incision in the ipsilateral middle quadrant. An additional port is placed in the epigastrium on the right side for liver retraction. After docking of the robot, rest of the procedure is similar to laparoscopic adrenalectomy.

The mean operative duration from incision to closure was 3 hours in this series, which was not significantly longer than laparoscopic adrenalectomy. The requirement of narcotics in the postoperative period was less in the single site surgery group. There were three conversions, one of which was due to inability to retract the colon properly.

Partial Adrenalectomy

In solitary adrenal glands and in hereditary cancer syndromes with bilateral adrenal masses (e.g.: Neurofibromatosis-I and Von Hippel Lindau Syndrome), partial adrenalectomy is indicated. Partial adrenalectomy has also been described in unilateral aldosteronoma but is not without problems. Additional nodules are present in the same gland which can lead to treatment failure.[11]

The position and port placement is the same as for total adrenalectomy. Tumor pseudocapsule is identified and the tumor is enucleated with blunt dissection. Intraoperative ultrasound can be used to delineate the tumor but is difficult to use while the actual excision of the mass. A novel method of identifying the tumor by intravenous administration of Indocyanin green dye and near-infrared imaging has been proposed.[23]

POSTOPERATIVE CARE

Besides adequate hydration, appropriate antibiotics and deep vein thrombosis prophylaxis, steroid replacement in cases of clinical or subclinical Cushing's syndrome is important. The patient is ambulated on the next day and normal diet is gradually started on the next day. Patient may be discharged on the first or second postoperative day.

TECHNICAL TIPS AND TRICKS

- Hemostasis is crucial in this surgery as even minor bleeding can cause staining of tissues and darken the operative field, making the identification of planes challenging.
- Identifying and staying away from the adrenal itself is important to avoid entering the adrenal tissue which can cause bleeding and further loss of planes.
- Take care while giving traction in the plane between upper pole of kidney and adrenal. Tributaries of the main renal vein might get injured during this step.
- On the right side, while dissecting the adrenal vein, it is useful to dissect close to the vena cava to avoid small vessel bleeding from the adjacent tissue.
- On the right side, division of the peritoneal reflection between the adrenal gland and the liver as an initial step and exposure of the psoas between these structures, facilitates the exposure of the adrenal vein and subsequent mobilization of the gland.
- Knowing the anatomy of adrenal while operating is helpful. You might be able to anticipate and identify bleeding from:
  - Tributaries of the inferior phrenic vein coursing along the medial side of the adrenal draining into the left adrenal vein.
  - Superior, middle and inferior adrenal arteries arising variably from renal artery, aorta and inferior phrenic arteries.
  - Lumbar veins entering the inferior vena cava on the right side.
- The lateral attachments of adrenal gland may help in stability of the gland and it may be useful to divide them at the end.
- Once the adrenal vein has been clipped and divided, it may be useful to hold the adrenal side of the vein and lift it up. this will help in developing a plane between the adrenal and psoas muscle. Identifying the psoas muscle is a helpful step during circumferential dissection.
- Knowing the color difference between the adrenal and the tail of pancreas is helpful while dissecting on the medial side of the left gland. The adrenal is typically golden yellow.

COMPLICATIONS

The complications of robot-assisted adrenalectomy are similar to laparoscopic adrenalectomy in both the type and frequency. The complication rate is related to the pathology rather than the method of adrenalectomy and is reported variably between 0 and 20% in various studies[10] Most of the complications are minor.[24] The conversion rate is also similar between laparoscopic and robotic approach except in large tumors >5 cm when the conversion is significantly less with robot assisted surgery.[8] The detailed management of complications is beyond the scope of this chapter and is essentially similar to management of complications of laparoscopic adrenalectomy.

EVIDENCE

Systemic review and meta-analysis of randomized controlled trials and retrospective observational studies comparing laparoscopic to robot-assisted adrenalectomy in 2015 revealed that operating time was significantly longer in RA compared with LA (WMD=17.52 minutes; p=.01). RA had significantly less blood loss (WMD= -19.00 mL; p=.02) and shorter length of hospital stay (WMD =-0.35 days; p <.001). There were no statistically significant differences between the two groups in terms of conversion rate or overall complications. There is a significant trend to choose patients with lower BMI and higher incidence of previous surgery for robot-assisted surgery. This may represent a selection bias in the current studies on the subject.[10]

The overall complication rate depends on the pathology in question rather than the method of surgery, and both RA and LA are safe with regard to complications.

Robot-assisted adrenalectomy has a definite learning curve. The difference in operative time between laparoscopic and robot-assisted surgery evens out after 20 cases. Moreover, in obese patients, operative time is longer with LA.[7] The learning curve for robotic adrenalectomy is shorter than laparoscopic adrenalectomy with the curve flattening at around 20 cases for robotic adrenelctomy and 30–40 cases for laparoscopic adrenalectomy.[25]

Robotic surgery is still costly when compared to laparoscopic surgery and that reflects in the literature on adrenalectomy as well.

SUMMARY

Robotic adrenalectomy may offer certain distinct technical advantages as it offers excellent vision and dexterity within a relatively confined space around the adrenal gland. Moreover, it appears to be easier to learn as compared to conventional laparsocopy and hence offers the advantages of extending minimally invasive surgery benefits to a larger proportion of patients. However, there is still a lack of data comparing robotic and laparoscopic adrenalectomy and further well designed studies are the need of the hour. In the future, decreasing costs of equipment, the availability of a larger number of robotic trained surgeons and increasing awareness about the potential advantages of robotic surgery is likely to make robotics a very popular approach for adrenalectomy procedures.

REFERENCES

1. Bovio S, et al. Prevalence of adrenal incidentaloma in a contemporary computerized tomography series. J Endocrinol Invest. 2006;29(4):298-302.
2. Kannan S, Remer EM, Hamrahian AH. Evaluation of patients with adrenal incidentalomas. Curr Opin Endocrinol Diabetes Obes. 2013;20(3):161-9.
3. Gagner M, Lacroix A, Bolte E. Laparoscopic adrenalectomy in Cushing's syndrome and pheochromocytoma. N Engl J Med. 1992;327(14):1033.
4. Smith CD, Weber CJ, Amerson JR. Laparoscopic adrenalectomy: new gold standard. World J Surg. 1999;23(4):389-96.
5. Piazza L, et al. Laparoscopic robot-assisted right adrenalectomy and left ovariectomy (case reports). Chir Ital. 1999;51(6):465-6.
6. Morino M, et al. Robot-assisted vs laparoscopic adrenalectomy: a prospective randomized controlled trial. Surg Endosc. 2004;18(12):1742-6.
7. Brunaud L, et al. Robotic-assisted adrenalectomy: what advantages compared to lateral transperitoneal laparoscopic adrenalectomy? Am J Surg. 2008;195(4):433-8.
8. Agcaoglu O, et al. Robotic versus laparoscopic resection of large adrenal tumors. Ann Surg Oncol. 2012;19(7):2288-94.
9. Pineda-Solis KH, Medina-Franco and Heslin MJ. Robotic versus laparoscopic adrenalectomy: a comparative study in a high-volume center. Surg Endosc. 2013;27(2):599-602.
10. Tang K, et al. Robot-assisted versus laparoscopic adrenalectomy: a systematic review and meta-analysis. J Laparoendosc Adv Surg Tech A. 2015;25(3):187-95.
11. Zeiger MZ, Quan-Yang Duh GBT, Hamrahian AH, Angelos DEP, Fishman E, Kharlip J. American association of clinical endocrinologists and american association of endocrine surgeons medical guidelines for the management of adrenal incidentalomas. Endocrine practice, 2009. pp. 1-20.
12. Toniato A, et al. Surgical versus conservative management for subclinical Cushing syndrome in adrenal incidentalomas: a prospective randomized study. Ann Surg. 2009;249(3):388-91.
13. Angeli A, et al. Adrenal incidentaloma: an overview of clinical and epidemiological data from the National Italian Study Group. Horm Res. 1997;47(4-6):279-83.
14. Hamrahian AH, et al. Clinical utility of noncontrast computed tomography attenuation value (hounsfield units) to differentiate adrenal adenomas/hyperplasias from nonadenomas: Cleveland Clinic experience. J Clin Endocrinol Metab. 2005;90(2):871-7.
15. Caoili EM, et al. Adrenal masses: characterization with combined unenhanced and delayed enhanced CT. Radiology. 2002;222(3):629-33.
16. Elsayes KM, et al. Adrenal masses: mr imaging features with pathologic correlation. Radiographics. 2004;24(Suppl 1):S73-86.
17. Lenders JW, et al. Biochemical diagnosis of pheochromocytoma: which test is best? JAMA. 2002;287(11):1427-34.
18. Doherty GM, et al. Time to recovery of the hypothalamic-pituitary-adrenal axis after curative resection of adrenal tumors in patients with Cushing's syndrome. Surgery. 1990;108(6):1085-90.
19. D'Annibale A, et al. Robotic adrenalectomy: technical aspects, early results and learning curve. Int J Med Robot. 2012;8(4):483-90.
20. Callender GG, et al. Posterior retroperitoneoscopic adrenalectomy. Adv Surg. 2009;43:147-57.
21. Ludwig AT, et al. Robot-assisted posterior retroperitoneoscopic adrenalectomy. J Endourol. 2010;24(8):1307-14.
22. Arghami A, et al. Single-port robotic-assisted adrenalectomy: feasibility, safety, and cost-effectiveness. JSLS. 2015;19(1):e2014 00218.
23. Manny TB, Pompeo AS and Hemal AK. Robotic partial adrenalectomy using indocyanine green dye with near-infrared imaging: the initial clinical experience. Urology. 2013;82(3):738-42.
24. Brandao LF, et al. Robotic versus laparoscopic adrenalectomy: a systematic review and meta-analysis. Eur Urol. 2014;65(6):1154-61.
25. Guerrieri M, et al. The learning curve in laparoscopic adrenalectomy. J Endocrinol Invest. 2008;31(6):531-6.

CHAPTER

29

Urolithiasis: Expanding the Horizons of Robotic Surgery

Siddharth Yadav, Prabhjot Singh, Prem Nath Dogra

INTRODUCTION

Upper urinary tract stones frequently require surgical intervention. The standard surgical treatment has evolved over the past century, from open surgery in beginning of 20th century to minimally invasive treatment, and is ever advancing. The description of nephrolithotomy by Brodel's and pyelolithotomy by Kelly in 1902 marked the era of surgical management of stone disease and these remained the most commonly performed procedures for almost a century. Although these open procedures allowed for intact removal, a large incision, significant bleeding and difficulty in managing peripheral calculi were major drawbacks. These forced technologic advances and 'Endourology' was born—a term coined by Arthur Smith to describe closed controlled manipulation of genitourinary tract. Rupel and Brown in 1941 were the first to perform nephroscopy to remove stones during open surgery, but it was Fernstrom and Johansson in 1976 who first described percutaneous renal collecting system access and stone removal under radiologic control and marked the era of endourology. Similarly, ureteric stones were also initially managed by open surgery but with technologic advances and development of smaller rigid and later flexible ureteroscopes, currently even the stones in intrarenal collecting system can be approached endoscopically.

Endourologic procedures (percutaneous nephrolithotomy (PNL) for renal and ureterorenoscopy (URS) for ureteric calculi) are now well-established as gold standard management of large calculi with acceptable morbidity. Endoscopic management of complex renal calculi (very large size, staghorn configuration, minimal hydronephrosis) poses greater challenge. Besides being time consuming, the inherent need to fragment these large renal stones increases the risk of sepsis and residual fragments, and because the burden is high one may require multiple punctures and multiple sittings.[1] Similarly, ureteroscopy for large (>1.5 cm) impacted ureteric calculi, especially in juxtavesical location, although minimally invasive, is time consuming, fraught with complications and up-migration of fragments into the kidney. Due to the ingrowing of the impacted stone into the ureteral wall, fragmentation with any energy source invariably damages the ureteral wall causing stricture formation in the future. Thus, although endoscopic management appears to be appealing but is neither safe nor effective for this particular category of patients, and intact removal without fragmentation is the ideal treatment. With the advent of laparoscopy the concept of intact stone removal, established in the era of open surgery, was revisited.[2] Laparoscopy provided for intact removal, which ensured complete clearance preventing recurrence, its minimally invasive approach limited the postoperative morbidity and the functional and cosmetic results approached that of PNL or URS. But the technical difficulty associated with intracorporeal suturing and limited range of motion of instruments limited its role to large stone in extrarenal pelvis. Introduction of surgical robot, with its endowrist instruments with 7 degrees of freedom and magnified 3D vision, broadened the applicability of minimally invasive approach to renal and ureteric stones.[3] Robotic assisted laparoscopy made it possible to replicate the results of open pyelolithotomy, extended pyelolithotomy and ureterolithotomy while maintaining the benefits of minimal invasive approach.[4]

ROBOTIC STONE SURGERY

Preoperative Preparation and Precautions

Robotic assistance has been well-described for reconstructive procedures such as pyeloplasty and partial nephrectomy but its indications and patient selection for stone surgery is still evolving. The major benefit of robotic assistance is observed in patients with either large renal stones in small pelvis or with staghorn stones or in large impacted ureteric stones (>1.5 cm) **(Figs 29.1 and 29.2)**. Such patients are best treated robotically as pure laparoscopic approach will be technically demanding and there may be a need for multiple punctures or multiple sittings with PNL and high chance of stricture formation if URS is chosen. Caution must be exercised in patients with either compact system with complete staghorn or with multiple small secondary calculi as there are high chances of residual calculi requiring adjuvant procedures **(Figs 29.3 to 29.5)**.

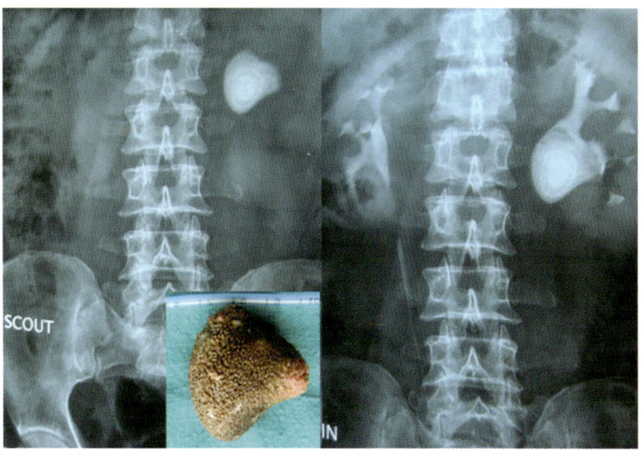

Fig. 29.1: Plain and 10 minute films of intravenous pyelogram showing solitary 4 cm left renal calculus in extrarenal pelvis. Inset – stone removed in completely after pyelolithotomy

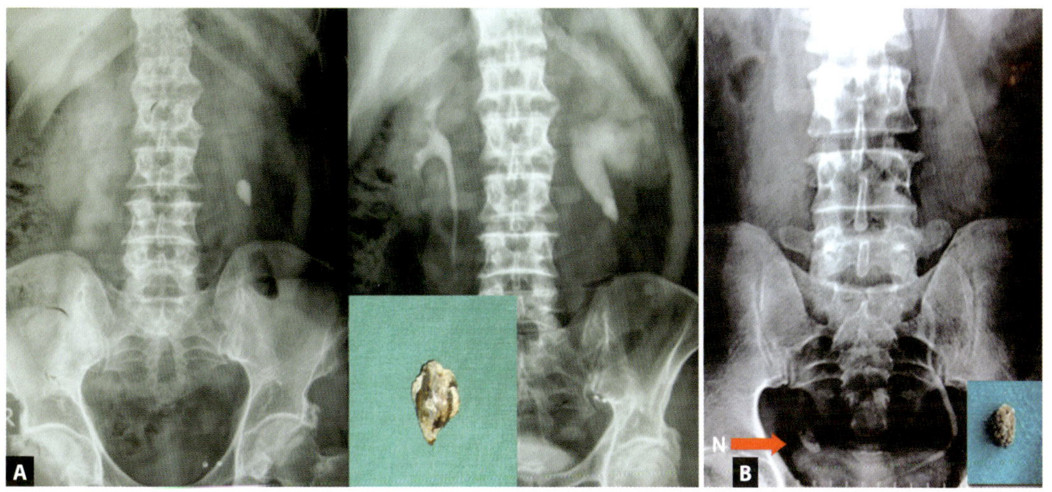

Figs 29.2A and B: (A) Plain and 20 minute films of intravenous pyelogram showing large impacted left upper ureteric calculus. Inset-calculus removed completely after ureterolithotomy; (B) A 20 minute film of intravenous pyelogram showing large impacted juxtavesical right ureteric calculus. Inset–stone removed intact

Robotic renal and ureteric procedures are commonly performed via transperitoneal approach although retroperitoneoscopic approach has also been described in the literature.[5,6] The principles of both have been adapted from principles of laparoscopic renal surgery.[2,7] Retroperitoneoscopic approach theoretically avoids peritoneal contamination with infected urine and bowel handling, but the limited working space makes surgery extremely challenging and is rarely preferred. There are many published articles mentioning use of transperitoneal approach for all renal and ureteric surgeries without any major adverse affect.[8,9]

Preoperative evaluation is essentially same as for other modalities of treatment.

ROBOTIC RENAL STONE SURGERY

The patient position, port placement and initial approach to kidney for robotic pyelolithotomy and extended pyelolithotomy is similar to that for robotic/laparoscopic pyeloplasty or partial nephrectomy. Availability of commonly used robotic and laparoscopic equipment and that specific to stone surgery required as per each case must be checked beforehand. Five commonly used robotic EndoWrist instruments should be ready on the patient cart, which include, Maryland forceps, curved scissors, 2 needle drivers and a ProGrasp forceps. Equipment for basic laparoscopic assistance should also be available and that for open conversion should be kept on standby. If there are secondary

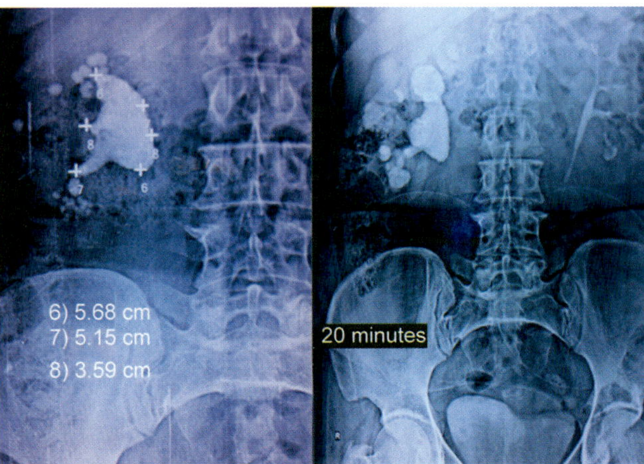

Fig. 29.3: Plain and 20 minute films of intravenous pyelogram showing 5 cm sized right renal pelvic calculus with multiple secondary calculi. In such cases there is likely hood of residual stones despite intraoperative use of flexible nephroscopy

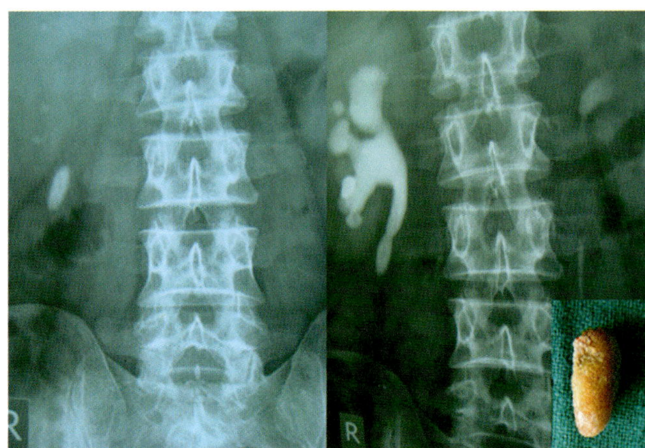

Fig. 29.4: Plain and 15 minute films of intravenous pyelogram showing large impacted right upper ureteric calculus with 2 secondary renal calculi. Such cases will require adjuvant procedures for renal calculi usually SWL. Inset–ureteric stone removed after ureterolithotomy

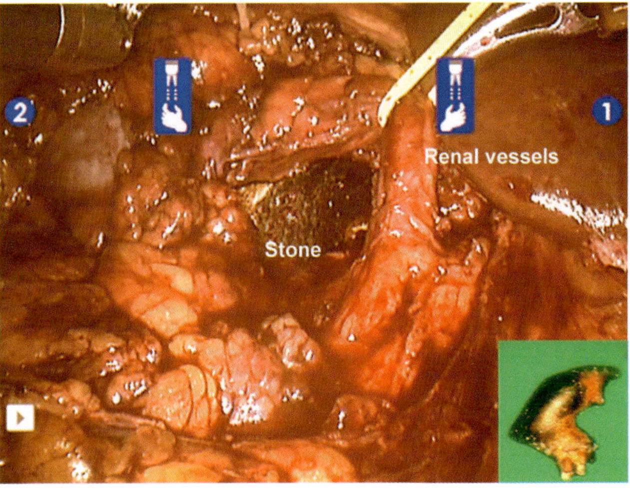

Fig. 29.5: Intraoperative image of robotic anterior pyelolithotomy showing how renal vasculature which lies anterior to renal pelvis can be handled for pyelolithotomy. Inset removed staghorn stone

calculi, intraoperative ultrasound probe as well as flexible scopes should be kept ready. To retrieve the stone, either proprietary endocatch bag or homemade bag of adequate size should be available. Appropriate size double J stent should be available.

Anesthesia

All procedures are performed under general anesthesia and antibiotics are administered at the time of induction. Orogastric tube may be placed after induction to decompress the stomach and removed before reversal. Patients are catheterized after induction before turning lateral and bag tubing is clamped to facilitate stent placement.

Positioning and Port Placement

After induction and per urethral catheterization the patient is turned into modified lateral position (45–60° with operative side up). There is no need to elevate the kidney bridge or to place a roll **(Figs 29.6A and B)**. While making the position the patient's abdomen is brought at the edge of the table so that there is enough space for the instrument play without any hindrance. Pressure points are padded, the dependent leg is flexed and a cushion is placed between the two legs as well as on the back. Caution must be exercised with the nondependent arm, which is placed on arm rest and turned towards the head of the patient at the shoulder joint. This will prevent the robotic arm hitting the patient's arm during surgery.

After prepping and draping, pneumoperitoneum is created using Veress needle which is placed in ipsilateral iliac fossa or the hypochondrium. As the patient is in lateral position, the small bowel falls towards the umbilicus. This increases the chances of injury if Veress is placed at the umbilicus. Authors use the Da Vinci S - 4 arm system which has a 12 mm stereoscopic camera and the port placement technique used at our institute has been previously described.[3] We usually use a 0° telescope through a 12 mm port placed at the level of the umbilicus on the lateral edge of belly of rectus muscle. Two 8 mm robotic ports are placed, first at the midpoint between xiphoid and umbilicus, 1-inch lateral from midline towards the ipsilateral midclavicular line, second one is placed in ipsilateral iliac fossa on anterior axillary line. Both ports should be at-least 8 cm away from the camera port and form a wide isosceles triangle to avoid clashing of robotic arms and adequate triangulation. A 12 mm assistant port is placed in midline between the camera port and the 1st robotic port, which is used for suction-irrigation, suture delivery and clip application. For right sided procedures, another 5 mm port can be placed in midline, cranial to 1st robotic port, for liver retraction **(Figs 29.6A and B)**.

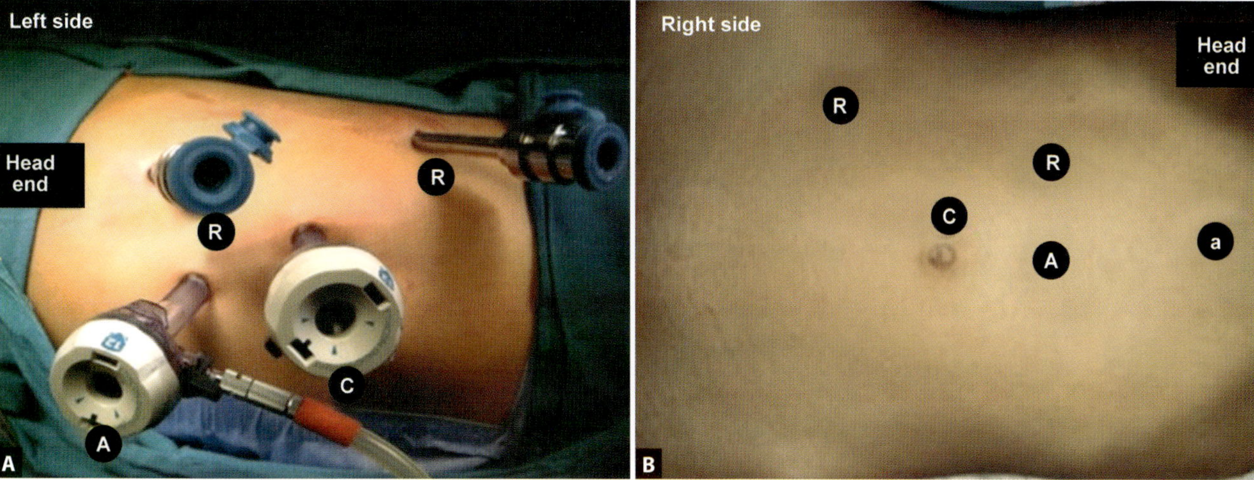

Figs 29.6A and B: Patient positioning and port placement for renal pelvic stones
Abbreviations: R, robotic port; C, camera port; A, assistant's port; a, liver retractor port

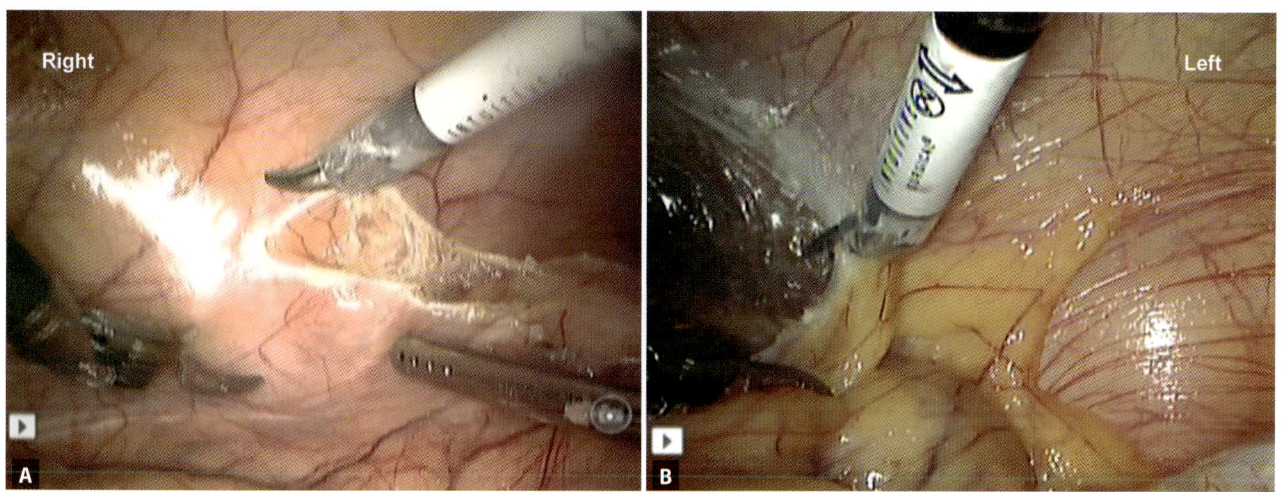

Figs 29.7A and B: Intraoperative photographs showing colon reflection. Peritoneum is incised at white line of Toldt's to gain access to retroperitoneum

STEPS OF SURGERY

Colon Mobilization and Dissection of Ureter and Renal Pelvis

After docking the robot, surgery is begun with robotic scissors in right arm with attached monopolar cautery and Maryland forceps in left arm with bipolar cautery. On right side, the dissection is started by incising line of Toldt and reflecting the ascending colon. On the left side, if the individual is thin and mesocolic fat is sparse, the dilated renal pelvis can be seen as a bulge through the mesocolon, and a window is created in mesocolon to reach to the pelvis. Otherwise, like on the right side, the descending colon is reflected **(Figs 29.7 and 29.8)**. One must avoid renal mobilization, which may flip the kidney medially, obstructing vision and adequate access to the pelvis.

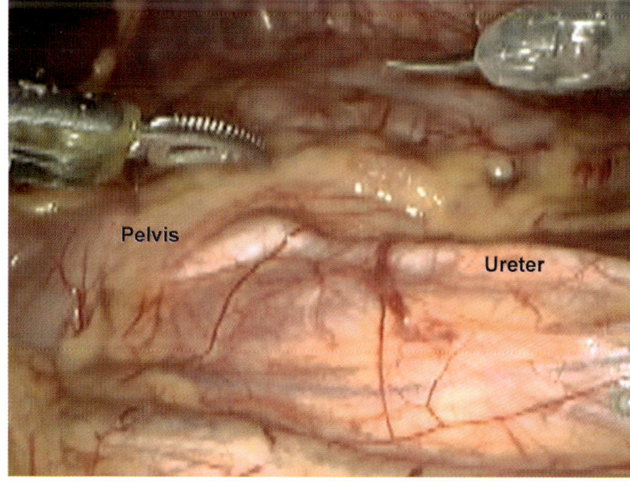

Fig. 29.8: Dilated renal pelvis and ureter can be identified through the mesocolon in a thin patient on the left side which allows for transmesocolic approach

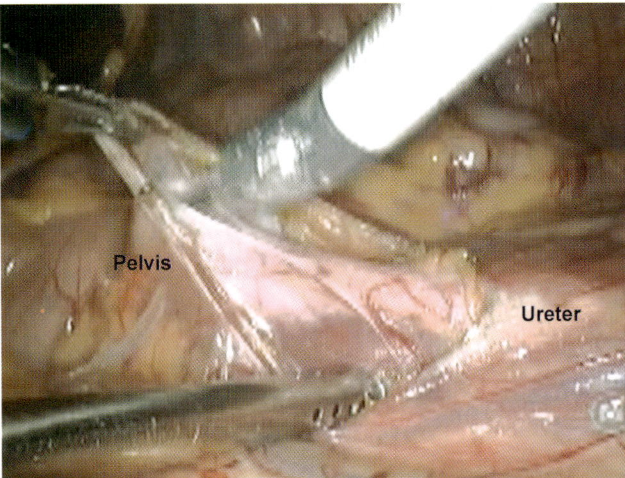

Fig. 29.9: Peripelvic dissection at the UPJ via transmesocolic approach on the left side. After identification of ureter it is traced to renal pelvis which is dissected free

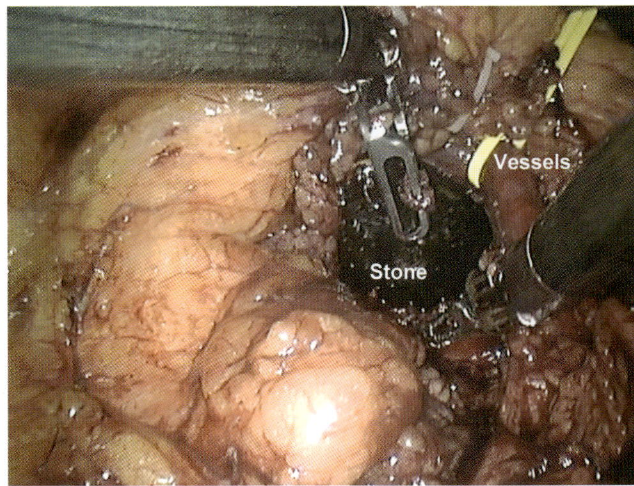

Fig. 29.10: Intraoperative photograph of pyelolithotomy. After pyelotomy to deliver the stone, it is held in the ProGrasp forceps in left arm and the mucosa is dissected off with Maryland in right arm

After colon reflection, the retroperitoneal tissues below the lower pole of the kidney are dissected to identify the ureter which is then followed till its insertion into renal pelvis **(Fig. 29.8)**. The renal pelvis is then dissected off the fat, which may be sometimes difficult because of inflammatory peripelvic adhesions in response to the stone **(Fig. 29.9)**. Care must be taken of the renal vessels, which are usually present at cranial end of the renal pelvis, and should be carefully separated and preserved. Sometimes, an anterior branch of renal vessels or an aberrant vessel may cross anterior to renal pelvis.

Pyelolithotomy and Extended Pyelolithotomy

After adequate mobilization of the renal pelvis, a V shaped pyelotomy is made. Depending on the pelvic anatomy (intrarenal pelvis), size of the stone and its configuration (location of maximal bulk) and the location of vasculature, it may be required to extend the pyelotomy either into superior or inferior major calyx (extended pyelolithotomy). For this, blunt dissection is performed in the Gilvernet's plane to expose the infundibula facilitating extension of the pyelotomy into it. Care must be taken during superior calyceal infundibulotomy where the renal vasculature is at the risk of injury. Once the incision is of adequate size, the pelvic mucosa is dissected off from the stone using scissors or Maryland forceps in right arm. The ProGrasp forceps or robotic hook in left arm is used to rotate and manipulate the stone to deliver through the pyelotomy **(Fig. 29.10)**. The laparoscopic assistant can also use a suction to retract the renal pelvic wall or use a grasper and help in stone retrieval. A see-saw type movement of the stone helps in easy delivery and prevents tearing of the renal pelvis. Once delivered, stone is either placed in paracolic gutter or is bagged.

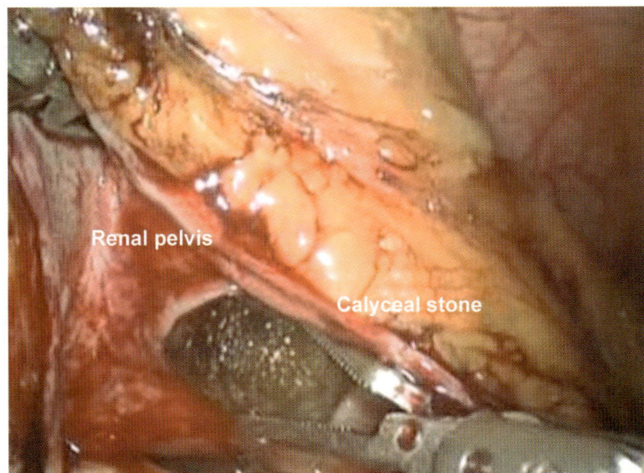

Fig. 29.11: Removal of calyceal stones: Large secondary calculi can be picked up with Maryland forceps

Removal of Calyceal Calculi

Once the pelvic stone is removed, the secondary calyceal stones can be taken care of. The larger stones can be removed under direct vision by steering the camera close and removing the stone with Maryland or ProGrasp forceps **(Fig. 29.11)**. Smaller ones can be flushed using suction irrigation device. It is mandatory to keep a count of number of stones as the docked robot prevents intraoperative use of fluoroscopy. Alternatively intraoperative ultrasonography can be utilized to assess the location and number of residual stones. Intraoperative rigid/flexible scope via assistant's 12 mm port with saline irrigation can also be used. Smaller stones should be immediately bagged to prevent migration into

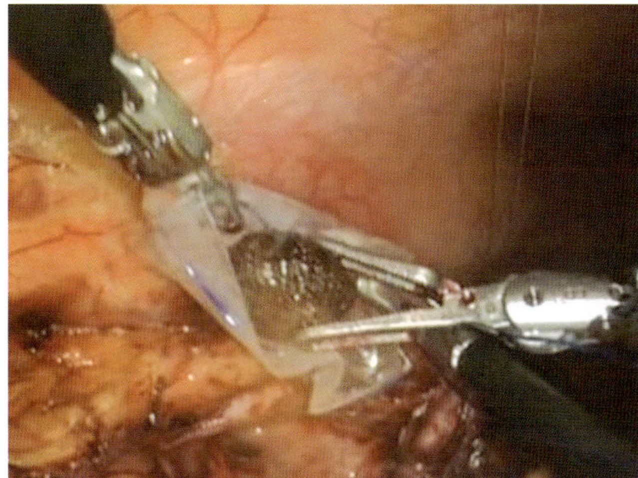

Fig. 29.12: Securing the stones: Removed stones are immediately secured in a homemade bag to prevent migration into abdominal cavity

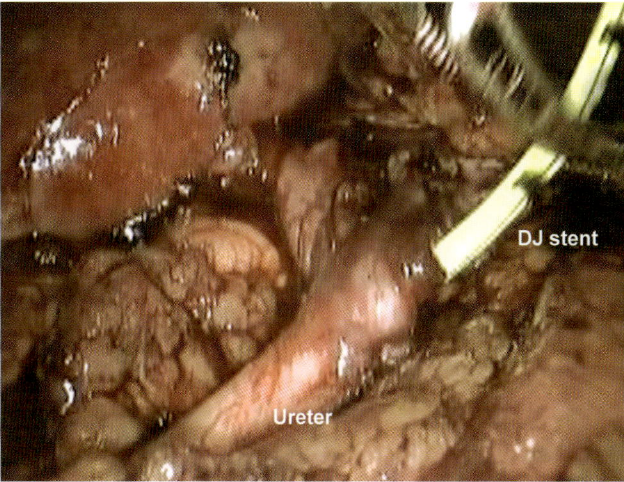

Fig. 29.13: Antegrade DJ stenting: The stent over its guidewire is pushed into the ureter, floppy side first, till its distal loop reached the bladder when the guidewire is withdrawn

abdominal cavity. Either a homemade bag or proprietary endocatch 10 mm entrapment device can be deployed via assistants 12 mm port for this purpose **(Fig. 29.12)**.

Antegrade Double J Stenting

Once stones are cleared, the DJ stent is placed antegradely. This saves time by avoiding separate cystoscopy and retrograde placement. The stent over the guidewire is delivered into the operative field via assistant's port, floppy end first **(Fig. 29.13)**. The assembly is advanced into the ureter until only the proximal part is left which is placed into pelvis after removing the guidewire. Once the guidewire is removed, small drops of urine seen emanating from proximal coli of stent confirms the position of distal loop into the bladder. The Foleys catheter tube can now be unclamped.

Repair of Pelvic and Infundibular Incision, Placement of Drain and Retrieval of Bagged Stone

The incision in closed with 3-0 or 4-0 vicryl suture on a round body needle cut to length of 6 inches in a continuous fashion **(Fig. 29.14)**. Care must be taken to use adequate length of suture while using continuous technique for longer incisions. Peripelvic fat may be approximated over the suture line. The mobilized colon is repositioned and reattached to abdominal wall using clips or sutures to avoid contamination of peritoneal cavity if there is urinary leak. A 14 Fr drain is placed intraperitoneally in paracolic gutter via lateral most 8 mm robotic port and kept on gravity drainage. The bagged stones are removed by marginally enlarging 12 mm assistant port thus avoiding a separate incision. All midline and 10 mm or larger port sites are closed with port closure vicryl suture undervision avoiding peritoneal contents.

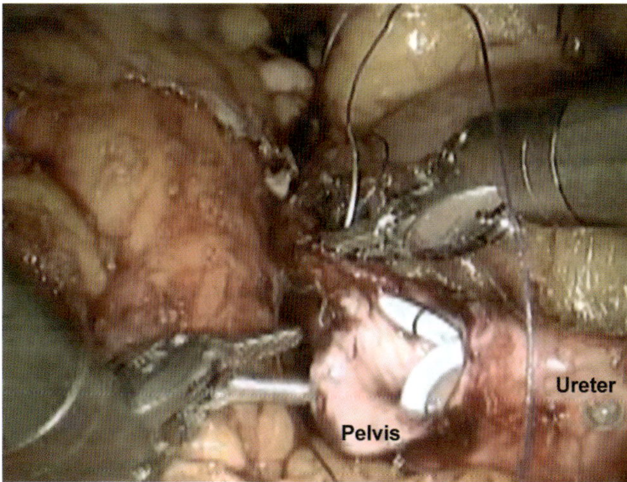

Fig. 29.14: Closure of pyelotomy: A 3-0 vicryl suture 6 inches in length is used to close the pyelotomy in continuous watertight fashion

ROBOTIC URETEROLITHOTOMY

The patient positioning and port placement for ureterolithotomy vary according to location of stone within the ureter. The general equipment for robotic and laparoscopic assistance is similar to that for renal stone surgery but the intraoperative ultrasonography or the flexible nephroscope are usually not required. A small homemade bag should be adequate to retrieve even the largest of the ureteric stones. Double J stents (6 Fr and 4.8 Fr) and corresponding guidewires should be available. The location of ureteric stone must always be confirmed on X-ray of KUB region obtained on the morning of surgery to avoid intraoperative surprises.

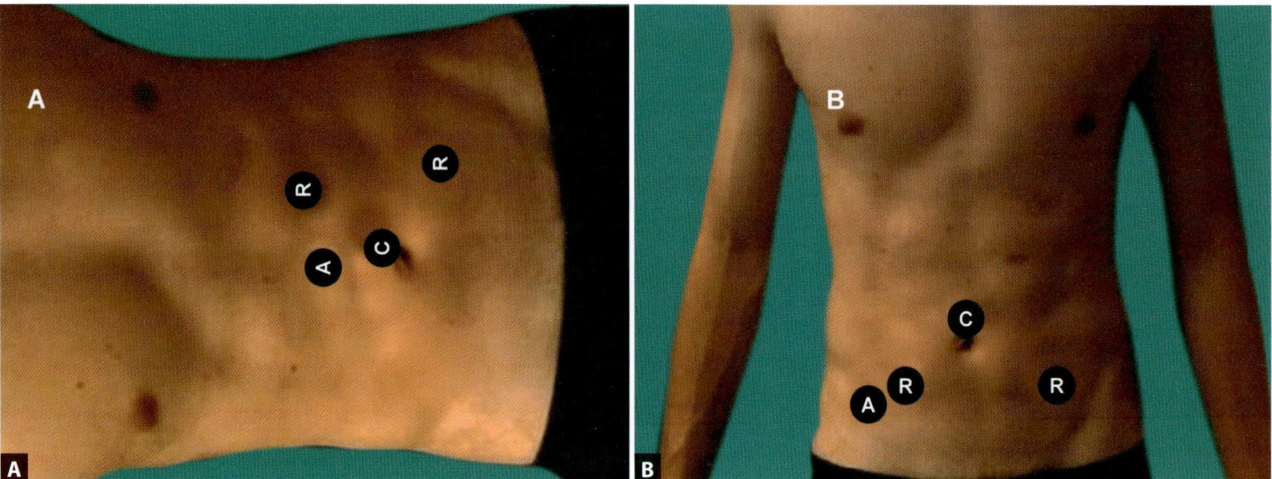

Figs 29.15A and B: Port placement for upper (A) and juxtavesical (B) left ureteric calculus
Abbreviations: R, robotic port; C, camera port; A, assistant's port

Positioning and Port Placement

The position of patient and port placement for upper ureteric stone is same as that for renal stone surgery. For mid ureteric stones the camera and other ports are placed a little lower down (towards ipsilateral iliac fossa) as compared to that for upper ureteric stone but in similar configuration. For lower ureteric stones, position and ports placement are same as that for robotic radical prostatectomy.[9] The patient is placed in the Trendelenburg position. The 12 mm camera port is placed just above the umbilicus and two 8 mm robotic working ports are placed below the camera port in midclavicular line on each side. A 12 mm assistant port in placed in the right iliac fossa just above the anterior superior iliac spine **(Figs 29.15A and B)**.

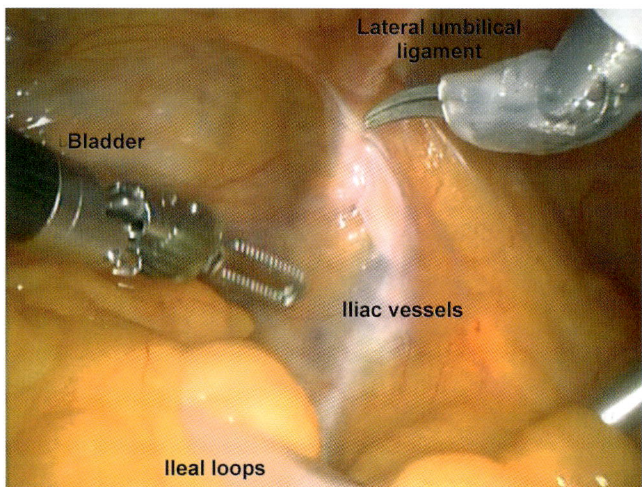

Fig. 29.16: The dissection to localize the juxtavesical stone begins deep in the pelvic cavity over the area of common iliac vessels

STEPS OF SURGERY

Colon Mobilization, Dissection of Ureter and Localization of Stone

For upper and midureteric stones the colon is mobilized after incising white line of Toldt's, similar to that for renal stones **(Fig. 29.7)**. In the retroperitoneum the ureter is identified and is traced towards the stone which can be easily seen as a bulge in the ureter. For proximal ureteric stones care must be taken to avoid upmigration of stone into renal pelvis during dissection.

In lower ureteric or juxtavesical stones the dissection is not as difficult as in laparoscopy or open surgery. The peritoneum is incised over the pelvic brim where the ureter crosses the common iliac vessels and is traced down up to the level of the stone **(Figs 29.16 and 29.17)**.

Ureterolithotomy and Antegrade DJ Stenting

Once the ureter is mobilized adequately, a longitudinal ureterotomy is made over the stone with scissors and stone is visualized. The ureteric mucosa is separated off the stone using scissors. Maryland or ProGrasp forceps is used to deliver the stone, which is either bagged or placed into paracolic gutter or can even be retrieved with the help of a grasping forceps through the 12 mm assistants port **(Fig. 29.18)**. After securing the stone, DJ stent is placed. The stent is railroaded over guidewire such that the floppy tip of guidewire comes out of the distal end of DJ stent. This assembly is delivered to the surgeon, who places the floppy tip of guidewire into distal end of ureterotomy and pushes the stent towards the bladder till its loop lies in the bladder and the guidewire is withdrawn completely. Now the hard end of guidewire is passed from the proximal end opening and brought out through the side holes close to the ureterotomy site. The assistant, with the help of a grasper, grasps the lower end of the stent along with the ureter so as to prevent inadvertent slipping of the distal end while surgeon pushes the floppy tip and the proximal

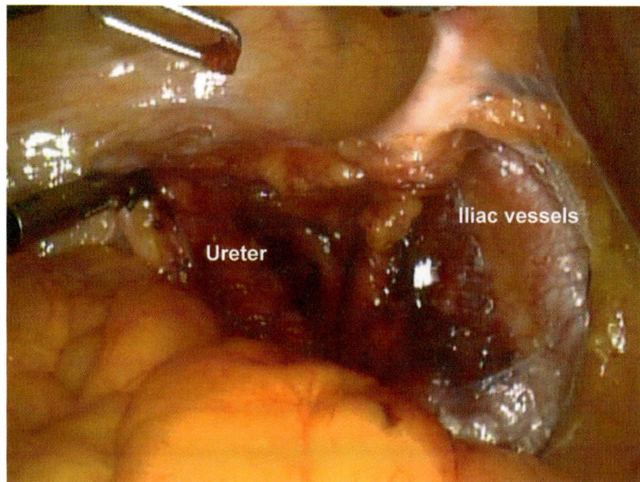

Fig. 29.17: intraoperative image depicting proximity of juxtavesical ureter to external iliac vessels

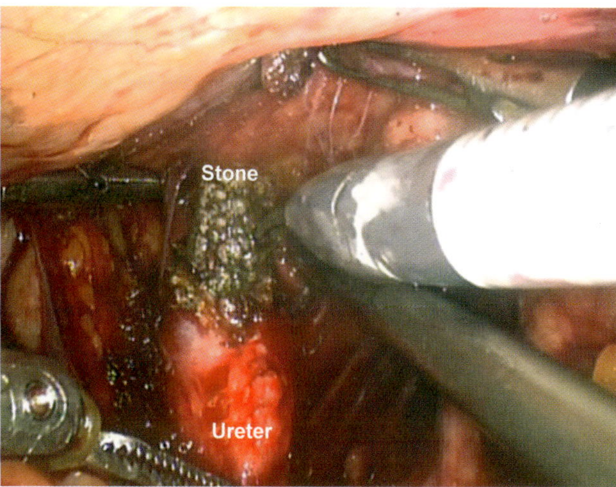

Fig. 29.18: Intraoperative image showing delivery of juxtavesical ureteric stone. After longitudinal urethrotomy, robotic scissors is used to dissect the mucosa off the stone, facilitating its delivery

end of stent inside the proximal ureter. When the stent is positioned, the guidewire is withdrawn **(Figs 29.19A to C)** and the ureterotomy is closed in a continuous manner using round body 3-0 or 4-0 vicryl suture **(Fig. 29.20)**. Colon is repositioned and the drain is placed as described. The bagged stone is removed after de-docking from the 12 mm assistant port, which may be enlarged if required.

POSTOPERATIVE CARE

Patients usually require injectable analgesics in the postoperative period, which are shifted to orals as tolerable, usually the next day. We commonly use either diclofenac or paracetamol depending on renal function tests. Antibiotics are usually given for 1st 24 hours after surgery but can be continued longer as there is higher risk of sepsis associated with staghorn stone surgery.[1] Catheter is removed the next morning until and unless indicated otherwise. Drain can be removed 24 hours after catheter removal, if 24 hours output is less than 30 mL. Position of the double J stent is confirmed on plain X-ray KUB obtained on the next day of surgery. The reported mean hospital stay is 3.8–6.5 days for laparoscopic pyelolithotomy and 2 days for robotic pyelolithotomy or ureterolithotomy.[2-4,7,9] The usual hospital stay at our center is 36–48 hours.

OUTCOMES, COMPLICATIONS AND MANAGEMENT

Robotic renal pelvic or ureteric surgery is relatively safe with a low 2–11% reported complication rate.[8-10] The spectrum of complications associated with laparoscopic and robotic stone surgery is very different from that from PNL or URS. Whereas sepsis and postoperative bleeding are noted with PNL these are rare with laparoscopic or robotic surgery.[1,4] Conversion to open surgery is rare in carefully selected cases and range from 0–2%.[2,7,11] There is low risk of sepsis and renal parenchymal injury (0–2.3%).[2,11] A unique complication not noted with PNL is postoperative urine leak which is reported to be 6.2–12.5% in laparoscopic surgery but is not seen with robotic procedures.[3,4,9,11-13] Most of these complications can be managed conservatively. In case of increased drain output or long suture line or intraoperative pelvic tear the Foleys catheter can be kept longer to avoid urine leak allowing for healing of the suture line.

The use of robotic extended pyelolithotomy for treatment partial staghorn calculi was first described by Badani et al. in 2006.[3] They operated 12 patients and noted complete clearance in all with mean console time of 108 mins and mean blood loss of 100 mL and noted no major intraoperative or postoperative complication. They found robotic extended pyelolithotomy is safe effective and renal parenchymal sparing approach comparable to PNL for partial staghorns. Nayyar et al. in 2007 operated upon 3 patients with partial staghorn in intrarenal pelvis with secondary calculi in 2 patients and noted complete clearance in all 3 with mean operative time of 85 minutes and mean blood loss of less than 50 mL and there were no complications.[4] Dogra et al. shared their experience of robotic ureterolithotomy in 16 patients with juxtavesical ureteric stones of mean size 2.2 cm. Their mean console time was 20.3 minutes and no major complications were noted. According to authors, for large impacted ureteric stones, complete clearance without any complication is impossible with ureteroscopy and there is associated high chance of stricture formation. Robot reproduces results of open surgery with minimal invasion and complication in terms of stricture formation in these patients. Thus robotic assisted laparoscopy is safe and effective

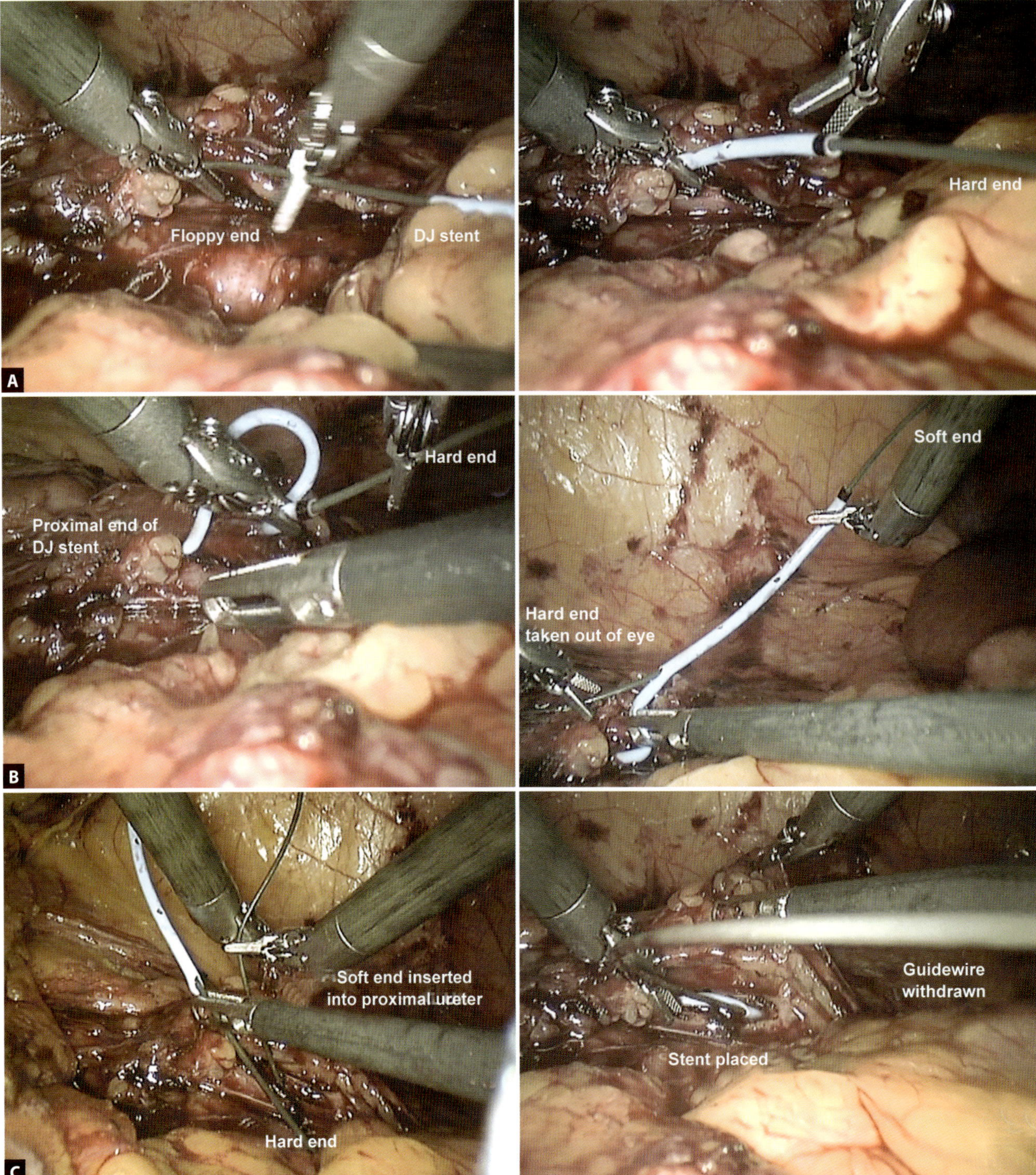

Figs 29.19A to C: The technique of antegrade DJ stenting after ureterolithotomy. (A) Guidewire is placed through the DJ stent such that its floppy end comes out of distal end of stent. The floppy end of guidewire along with the stent is pushed into distal end of ureterotomy till it reaches the bladder and then guidewire is withdrawn; (B) Hard end of guidewire is reinserted into the end of the proximal loop of DJ stent and taken out of its lumen from one of its eye close to the ureterotomy. The assistant grasps the lower end of the DJ stent along with the ureter to prevent inadvertent slippage; (C) Soft end of guidewire along with the proximal end of DJ stent is then pushed into proximal ureter to reach the renal pelvis. Once the stent is placed the guidewire is withdrawn

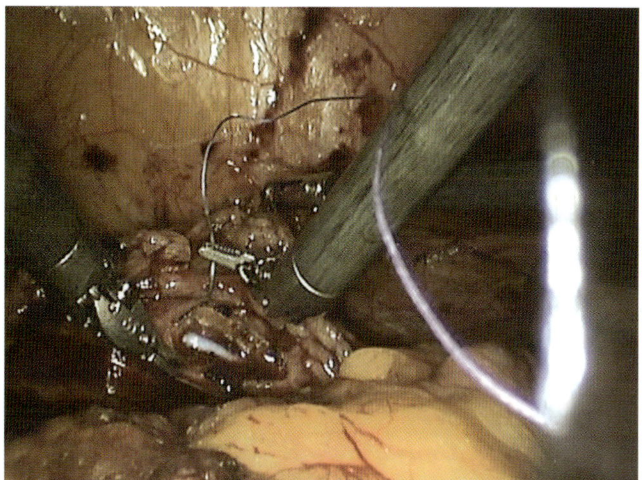

Fig. 29.20: Closure of longitudinal ureterotomy with 3-0 vicryl suture in continuous watertight fashion over a DJ stent

approach in armamentarium of urologist for management of large and complex renal and ureteric calculi.

With robotic assistance, the treating urologist is able to tackle complex renal and ureteric calculi effectively, with minimal complications. This parenchyma sparing, minimally invasive approach allowing for intact removal with low chances of sepsis serves as additional approach for stone disease and broadens the horizon of robotic surgery.

REFERENCES

1. Kreydin EI, Eisner BH. Risk factors for sepsis after percutaneous renal stone surgery. Nat Rev Urol. 2013;10:598-605.
2. Gaur DD, Trivedi S, Prabhudesai MR, Gopichand M. Retroperitoneal laparoscopic pyelolithotomy for staghorn stones. J Laparoendosc Adv Surg Tech A. 2002;12:299-303.
3. Badani KK, Hemal AK, Fumo M, et al. Robotic extended pyelolithotomy for treatment of renal calculi: a feasibility study. World J Urol. 2006;24:198-201.
4. Nayyar R, Wadhwa P, Hemal AK. Pure robotic extended pyelolithotomy: cosmetic replica of open surgery. J Robotic Surg. 2007;1:207-11.
5. Hu JC, Treat E, Filson CP, McLaren I, Xiong S, Stepanian S, et al. Technique and outcomes of robot assisted retroperitoneoscopic partial nephrectomy: A multicenter study. Eur Urol. 2014;66; 542-49.
6. Hemal AK, Menon M. Robot-Assisted Extended Pyelolithotomy and Ureterolithotomy; In: Su LM; Atlas of robotic urologic surgery; New York: Humana Press; 2011. pp. 173-86.
7. Goel A, Hemal AK. Evaluation of role of retroperitoneoscopic pyelolithotomy and its comparison with percutaneous nephrolithotripsy. Int Urol Nephrol. 2003;35:73-6.
8. Hemal AK, Nayyar R, Gupta NP, Dorairajan LN. Experience with robotic assisted laparoscopic surgery in upper tract urolithiasis. Can J Urol. 2010;17:5299-305.
9. Dogra PN, Regmi SK, Singh P, Saini AK, Nayak B. Lower Ureteral Stones Revisited: Expanding the Horizons of Robotics. Urology. 2013;82:95-9.
10. Khan F, Ahmed K, Lee N, Challacombe B, Khan MS, Dasgupta P. Management of ureteropelvic junction obstruction in adults. Nat Rev Urol. 2014;11:629-38.
11. Meria P, Milcent S, Desgrandchamps F, Mongiat-Artus P, Duclos JM, Teillac P. Management of pelvic stones larger than 20 mm: laparoscopic transperitoneal pyelolithotomy or percutaneous nephrolithotomy? Urol Int. 2005;75:322-6.
12. Sinha R, Sharma N. Retroperitoneal laparoscopic management of urolithiasis. J Laparoendosc Adv Surg Tech A. 1997;7:95-8.
13. Holman E, Toth C. Laparoscopically assisted percutaneous transperitoneal nephrolithotomy in pelvic dystopic kidneys: experience in 15 successful cases. J Laparoendosc Adv Surg Tech A. 1998;8:431-5.

CHAPTER

30

Pyeloplasty

Manu Gupta

INTRODUCTION

Pelvi-ureteric junction (PUJ) obstruction is a common urology pathology known to exist since modern medicine has been documented. Pyeloplasty remains one of the most commonly performed urology operations. It has been traditionally done by the open flank technique. In the last two decades, laparoscopy has almost replaced the open technique. With the introduction of the da Vinci robot in 1998, there has been a paradigm shift in the way PUJ obstruction has been approached surgically.

DIAGNOSIS OF PELVI-URETERIC JUNCTION (PUJ) OBSTRUCTION

A detailed history and physical examination is necessary, paying particular attention to symptoms and timing. Laboratory studies should include renal function tests and urinalysis. Anatomic and functional imaging of the upper urinary tract is mandatory to making the correct diagnosis and treatment plan.

Intravenous pyelography is useful in evaluating anatomy of the renal pelvis and ureter. More recently computed tomography is preferred because it allows for visualization of the renal pelvis and ureter, associated calculi, as well as any extrinsic obstructions including crossing vessels or tumors. Radionuclide diuretic renography is helpful to confirm the diagnosis, quantify the degree of obstruction, and compare split renal function. Retrograde pyelograms may be useful to delineate the anatomy at the time of surgery, especially in children.

INDICATIONS FOR ROBOT-ASSISTED SURGERY

The leading causes for any kind of laparoscopy or robotic assisted pyeloplasty are same to that of open surgeries. That consists of conditions like characteristic features of PUJ blockage (pain in flank), repeated infections, stones, or increasing loss of kidney functions. Other associated causes include increased deterioration of hydronephrosis or severe blockage, as reported by activity/time curve generated by nuclear medicine renal imaging procedures.

TREATMENT

Surgical procedure like dismembered pyeloplasty is considered as the gold standard of treatment for conditions like UPJ obstruction, however there are other surgical procedures which had evolved with aim to reduce the morbidity related to open surgical procedure. More than 95% success rate is reported for open pyeloplasty in many modern cases which is judged as higher benchmark to compare with newly implemented lesser invasive procedures.[1-4]

Other options are open surgical intubated ureterotomy with endopyelotomies which may be antegrade or retrograde where cautery wire balloon procedure or under direct vision procedure with laser, cold knife or cautery may be used. There is decreased morbidity in comparison to open pyeloplasty, the rate of success of endopyelotomy is noted to be around 60–80%, and patients who are well selected had mild to moderate hydronephrosis without any report of crossing vessels.[5-7] Endopyelotomy is considered as most suitable for recurrent obstruction following the prior UPJ treatment where its rate of success reported around 40–60%. Dismembered pyeloplasty is considered as successful and versatile surgical procedure which helps the operating surgeon to handle many issues intraoperatively like crossing vessels, any renal pelvis that is big or redundant, repair adjustments and high insertion. Good results were noted in conditions where formal reconstruction of UPJ has led to laparoscopy procedure, it was reported by Schuessler et al.[8] and also Kavoussi and Peters in 1993.[9] Both had reported higher success rate around 100% with minimum loss of blood and without any complications but the operative procedure duration ranged between 3 hours to 7 hours. Jarrett et al.[10] had observed around 96% success rate with initial 100 patients operated at Johns Hopkins. Mean duration of hospital stay reported as 3.3 days and reported morbidity was low when compared to open pyeloplasty procedures. Even though the duration of operative time got reduced with experienced surgeons but the duration of mean operative time was noted as 4.2 hours. Many surgeons with higher experience in laparoscopic procedures had tried to decrease the morbidity of the surgical procedure further. Many pediatric case series had also observed that pyeloplasty performed by laparoscopy could be done safely among children with success rates as high as 90%, with marked improvement in duration of hospital stay and use of any narcotic.[11]

ROBOT-ASSISTED PYELOPLASTY

By using the AESOP robot Partin et al. had successfully completed 17 cases of laparoscopic urologic procedures including three pyeloplasties which was noted as very first use of robotic assistance.[12]

In July 2000, FDA had approved the da Vinci® Surgical System which was manufactured by Intuitive Surgical Inc. (Mountain View, California, USA) to perform laparoscopic surgical procedures. It is considered as a type of master slave surgical robot that provides comfortable console for surgeon, portable side cart for patient which integrates one arm of camera and two arms of robotic instruments. This unique robotic instrument is having 7 degrees of freedom in its 'wrists' by which exaggerated movements due to the long fulcrum effect is eliminated during pelvic laparoscopic procedures. In comparison to typical instruments used in laparoscopy, the robotic arm usually moves towards the same direction of surgeon's hand. This improved depth perception allows for more rapid and precise fine movements like suture placement. The comfortable sitting position at the surgeon console helps to reduce surgeon fatigue, a significant factor in laparoscopic cases with long operative times that require focus and concentration for accurate intracorporeal suturing. Sung et al. observed that the most significant contribution to decreased operative time appears to be a decreased anastomotic suturing time.[13] Then the subsequent reports had repeatedly shown better results with significant reduced operative times which was nearly comparable to pyeloplasty procedures done by open method and using standard laparoscopy. Recently, few case series that are preliminary had also reported that the procedure could be effectively carried out in many children with same advantage in operative times as compared to conventional laparoscopic pyeloplasty procedure.

OPERATION THEATER ERGONOMICS

The position of the patient is maintained in the flank position with affected part or side of the body being up. The patient side cart reaches the back of patient from the side of shoulder facing the umbilicus at around angle of 45°, as depicted in **Figure 30.1**. After docking, the arms of robot would reach over the flank and then turn back toward the upper quadrant. The monitor of operation assistant can be placed alongside to the patient side cart.

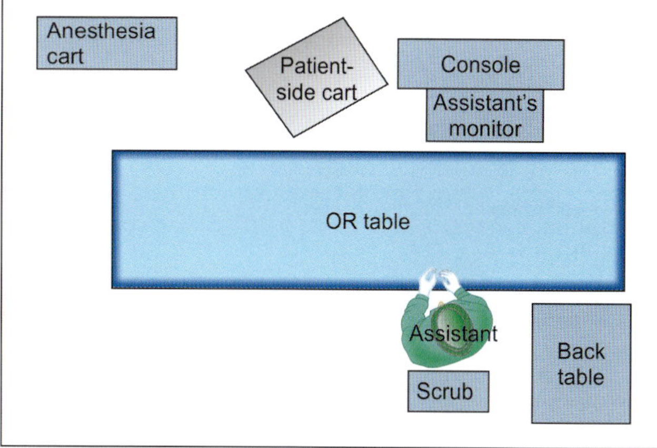

Fig. 30.1: Operating room set-up and robot positioning for left-sided pyeloplasty

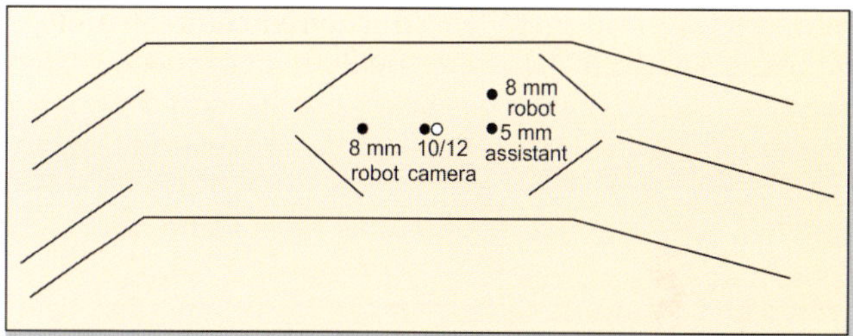

Fig. 30.2: Trocar placement for left-sided robotic-assisted laparoscopic pyeloplasty
Source: http://www.dcurology.net/robotic/pdfs/pyeloplasty.pdf

TECHNIQUE

After adequate general anesthesia, the patient is positioned in the flank position and the pressure points were cautiously padded to provide protection from any kind of neuromuscular injuries. At the beginning, by using Veress needle the access into the peritoneum is obtained in the area of umbilical or paramedian location. Applying the conventional approach of triangulation, the trocars are positioned as displayed in **Figure 30.2**. A trocar of 10–12 mm size is introduced at umbilicus area for camera and a robotic port of 8 mm size is inserted at least 8 cm superiorly in midline. Another robotic port of 8 mm size is introduced at least 8 cm lateral in midclavicular line and distant from the port containing camera. An assistant port of 10–12 mm size is inserted between the port having camera and inferior port of 8 mm size, minimum 8 cm distant from each so that any interference with robot is prevented. For initial dissections and exposure a separate laparoscopy set-up is used exclusively. The positioning docking of the robot is done thereafter. Mobilization of the colon is done towards medial side along the white line of Toldt and then the exposure of the anterior surface of Gerota's fascia is performed. Focus and attention is then provided to identify the lower pole of kidney, psoas muscle, vein from gonad and ureter. After identification of the ureter it is usually retracted upwards and then dissected from the blood vessels like gonadal vein. To preserve and maintain the blood supply to ureter utmost care is taken, as it gets dissected towards the pelvis of kidney. The dissection of tissues pursued to expose the inferior part of the kidney pelvis and any blood vessels crossing are also identified. If at the same time there is requirement of laparoscopic pyelolithotomy, then smaller longitudinal pyelotomy may be done to help removal of stone using a flexible type of nephroscope.

The PUJ is transected precisely, ensuring that the two ends once anastomosed are not in tension. The pyeloplasty anastomosis is then completed using a double armed running suture of 4-0 monocryl on RB-1 needles. A double J stent is inserted before the anastomosis is completed. 3/16″ round closed-suction drain is brought out through the lateral port and secured. The colon is secured back to the lateral peritoneum. Fascial defects 10 mm or larger are closed. Patients are given parenteral antibiotic prophylaxis and monitored in the hospital for 3 days at our center. The drain is generally removed when output is less than 100 mL per 24 hours. Usually the stent is removed at 6 weeks. Follow-up includes a radionuclide renal scan at 3 months and again at 1 year.

RESULTS

There are numerous series documenting robotic assisted laparoscopic pyeloplasty to be comparable and sometimes superior to simple laparoscopic pyeloplasty. Patel had reported the initial large series of fifty cases where it was concluded that the procedure provides excellent short-term efficacy and minimum morbidity and also it is easy and quick method to learn.[14] Schwentner et al. had published their 5 years of experience with 92 operated cases of dismembered Anderson-Hynes robotic surgical procedures.[15] They reported durable outcomes without any late complication which substantiated the precession of robotic assisted procedures like intracorporeal suturing and the afterward quality of pelviureteric anastomosis. Mufarrij et al. described the initial multi-institutional experiences, reporting the various outcomes among 140 cases which included primary or secondary ureteropelvic junction obstruction with or without accompanying procedure for extraction of stone and also cases with solitary kidney.[16]

In the largest series published in 2012, Sivaraman et al. operated with success on 168 patients using the transmesocolic approach. The average operative time was 135 minutes, with a complication rate of <7%.[17]

DIFFERENT SURGICAL TECHNIQUES

Retroperitonial Approach

A retroperitoneoscopic access path for minimal invasive pyeloplasty has been proposed because it permits a quicker access to the kidney pelvis. But, the unique anatomical position, highly delicate maneuvering and comparatively limited work space represent some of the recognized challenges. Many of retroperitoneoscopic case series involving both adult and pediatric population had been published.[18-19]

Transmesocolic Approach

Shadpour et al. had first compared the left sided transmesocolic laparoscopic pyeloplasty with standard surgical procedure on same side in a randomized prospective study.[20] The clinical study had enrolled 64 cases (both adult and pediatric) randomized them into two groups (transmesocolic vs standard procedure) of 32 cases. The patient groups were alike in terms of gender, age distribution, initial kidney function, body mass index (BMI). The average duration of operation was 23% lower in the transmesocolic group, mostly due to the reduced time interval from placement of trocars to incision of the ureteropelvic junction. The mean duration of hospitalization was also reported as less for the transmesocolic group patients (mean: 2.9 vs 3.6 days; $p < 0.001$). In both groups the success rate was reported as 96.9%.

Based on the reported evidences in various publications, the transmesocolic surgical robotic approach for ureteropelvic junction obstruction repair could be considered suitable whenever feasible as it offers few significant benefits of no higher risk, given a meticulous patient selection, much of it based on the intraoperative observations.

Alternative Procedures

Nondismembered pyeloplasty surgical procedures that do not need a total disconnection of renal pelvis and the ureter, so they would seem to be technically much direct and unsophisticated. It was the rationale behind introduction of Fenger-plasty to laparoscopy, which includes a longitudinal surgical incision in the narrower portion of the ureteropelvic junction, followed by a transverse surgical closure that permits preservation of blood supplies to the proximal ureter which comes out from the pelvis. By placing few interrupted sutures the number of knot tying and suturing in laparoscopy can be decreased. The standard reason for Fenger-plasty is shorter stenosis along with a minimally dilated renal pelvis. Janetschek et al. in 2000 had published the first larger series of cases of laparoscopic Fenger-plasty, which they believed it to be the preferred mode of surgical procedure at their center for the treatment of ureteropelvic junction obstruction at that time.[21]

Ahlawat et al. had reported the laparoscopic 'postanastomotic dismembered' procedure which had partial division of dilated renal pelvis at the beginning and ureteral spatulation without dismembering the ureteropelvic junction.[22] Mesrobian had reported 'bypass pyeloplasty' procedure which is suitable for cases with high insertion of ureter, which involves 1-2 cm wide side to side anastomosis made between dilated and elastic part of ureter just distal to the ureteropelvic junction obstruction and the inferior and dependent part of the hydronephrotic pelvis of kidney.[23]

Use of Stents

Cystoscopiy and retrograde stent placement is generally performed shortly before the pyeloplasty and it provides scope for doing a retrograde pyelogram to rule out any abnormity of the urerter.

However, other than the need of repositioning of patients, a collapsed renal pelvis may be observed due to a preplaced stent there by making it difficult to identify of the transition point in between the normal part of ureter and distended renal pelvis. Sometimes the proximal part of stent may cause interference with intracorporeal suturing. To avert these challenges, antegrade stenting at the time of pyeloplasty was advised.

While making sure of sufficient drainage and thereby reducing the chances of formation of any urinoma, ureteral stents may not be absolutely free from some risks and possible complications.[24] Many times a secondary procedure is needed for removing stent, which, in the pediatric patients, is performed under anesthesia.

Stentless pyeloplasty was initially reported as achievable and safe in the pediatric publications.[25] From the surgical and technical point of view, stentless surgical procedures can stop the debate over inserting the stents in either antegrade or retrograde fashion. Shalhav et al. had first reported stentless laparoscopic pyeloplasty in adult patients.[26] But, they still advised about the placement of a stent in cases of solitary kidney, at the time of difficult ureteral anastomosis, major bleeding during repair of ureteropelvic junction obstruction and in a thicker noncompliant ureter in presence of chronic inflammations. Recently, Kumar and Mandhani had reported about16 cases (10 pediatric and 6 adults) selected for stentless laparoscopic pyeloplasty by transperitoneal approach.[27]

DISCUSSION

Laparoscopic pyeloplasty is no doubt an excellent procedure. Its only drawback is a very steep learning curve. The access of robots surgical field and the popular introduction of da Vinci Surgical System has helped in the preference of laparoscopic surgeries for many open surgeons who were not trained in standard laparoscopy in past. Switching to the robotic assisted procedure has helped in reduction of duration of operation times even by many laparoscopic surgeons with experience. The easiness of suturing, speed and accuracy are considered as significant benefits of the robot assisted procedures versus standard laparoscopic technique. These significant benefits of the robot may result in much broader applications and acceptance of the laparoscopic surgical procedures. Despite reports of large series of cases primarily reported from few select institutions or centers, there is growing evidence, which supports similar success rates between open procedures, laparoscopic procedure and robotic assisted laparoscopic pyeloplasty. There are few pediatric centers that had also been pioneers in robotic assisted surgical procedures have demonstrated the appropriateness, safety and efficacy of the procedure in children. There are certain arguments like higher cost and steeper learning curve against the usage of robots in surgery when it is compared with open procedures or endourologic techniques. Additionally, the robot is considered bulky due to the space occupied and for optimal results a team of dedicated personals required to keep the duration of operation time reasonable. Lastly, there is lack of haptic feedback or lesser kinesthetic communication which restricts tactile sensations for the operating surgeon, which may be an issue initially. The experience and knowledge obtained from cases of robotic assisted laparoscopic prostatectomy has also helped significantly to improve our capability to perform the robotic assisted laparoscopic pyeloplasty procedure.

CONCLUSION

The use of da Vinci robot for surgical procedures like reconstruction of ureteropelvic junction had been reported as appropriate, much safer and highly effective. Many clinical studies had reported large series of cases where there is reduction of operative time and decrease in learning curve when compared to standard laparoscopic pyeloplasty, while providing best outcome. Robotic surgery is also associated with few challenges, mainly increased cost. Robotic assisted laparoscopic pyeloplasty is our preferable method for management of PUJ obstruction.

REFERENCES

1. Persky L, Krause JR, Boltuch RL. Initial complications and late results in dismembered pyeloplasty. J Urol. 1977;118:162.
2. Notley RG, Beaugie JM. The long-term follow-up of Anderson-Hynespyeloplasty for hydronephrosis. Br J Urol. 1973;45:464.
3. Nguyen DH, Aliabadi H, Ercole CJ, Gonzalez R. Nonintubated Anderson-Hynes repair of ureteropelvic junction obstruction in 60 patients. J Urol. 1989;142:704.
4. Sovion M, Livine PM, Savir A. Long-term follow-up of patients after pyeloplasty for ureteropelvic junction obstruction. Isr J Med Sci. 1990;26:144.
5. Meretyk I, Meretyk S, Clayman RV. Endopyelotomy: Comparison of ureteroscopic retrograde and antegrade percutaneous techniques. J Urol. 1992;148(3):775-82.
6. Nakada SY, Pearle MS, Clayman RV. Acucise endopyelotomy: Evolution of a less-invasive technology. J Endourol. 1996;10(2): 133-9.
7. Van Cangh PJ, Nesa S. Endopyelotomy. Prognostic factors and patient selection. Urol Clin North Am. 1998;25(2):281-8.
8. Schuessler WW, Grune MT, Tecuanhuey LV, Preminger GM. Laparoscopic dismembered pyeloplasty. J Urol. 1993;150(6): 1795-9.
9. Kavoussi LR, Peters CA. Laparoscopic pyeloplasty. J Urol. 1993; 150(6):1891-4.
10. Jarrett TW, Chan DY, Charambura TC, Fugita O, Kavoussi LR. Laparoscopic pyeloplasty: The first 100 cases. J Urol. 2002; 167(3):1253-6.
11. Tan HL. Laparoscopic Anderson-Hynes dismembered pyeloplasty in children. J Urol. 1999;162(3 Pt 2):1045-7.

12. Partin AW, Adams JB, Moore RG, Kavoussi LR. Complete robot-assisted laparoscopic urologic surgery: A preliminary report. J Am Coll Surg. 1995;181(6):552-7.
13. Sung GT, Gill IS, Hsu TH. Robotic-assisted laparoscopic pyeloplasty: A pilot study. Urology. 1999;53(6):1099-103.
14. Patel V. Robotic-assisted laparoscopic dismembered pyeloplasty. Urology. 2005;66:45-9.
15. Schwentner C, Pelzer A, Neururer R, et al. Robotic Anderson-Hynes pyeloplasty: 5-year experience of one centre. BJU Int 2007;100:880-5.
16. Mufarrij PW, Woods M, Shah OD, et al. Robotic dismembered pyeloplasty: a 6-year, multi-institutional experience. J Urol. 2008;180:1391-6.
17. Sivaraman A, Leveillee RJ, Patel MB, et al. Robot-assisted laparoscopic dismembered pyeloplasty for ureteropelvic junction obstruction: a multi-institutional experience. Urology. 2012;79:351-5.
18. Shoma AM, El Nahas AR, Bazeed MA. Laparoscopic pyeloplasty: a prospective randomized comparison between the transperitoneal approach and retroperitoneoscopy. J Urol. 2007;178:2020-4.
19. Abuanz S, Gamé X, Roche JB, et al. Laparoscopic pyeloplasty: comparison between retroperitoneoscopic and transperitoneal approach. Urology. 2010;76:877-81.
20. Shadpour P, Nayyeri RK, Daneshvar R, Salimi H, Radfar H. Prospective clinical trial to compare standard colon-reflecting with transmesocolic laparoscopic pyeloplasty. BJU Int. 2012;110: 1814-8.
21. Janetschek G, Peschel R, Bartsch G. Laparoscopic Fengerplasty. J Endourol. 2000;14:889-93.
22. Ahlawat R, Gautam G, Khera R, Kaushik VB, Ghosh P. Laparoscopic pyeloplasty using the postanastomotic dismemberment method: technique and results. J Endourol. 2009;23:89-99.
23. Mesrobian HG. Bypass pyeloplasty: description of a procedure and initial results. J Pediatr Urol. 2009;5:34-6.
24. Damiano R, Oliva A, Esposito C, De Sio M, Autorino R, D'Armiento M. Early and late complications of double pigtail ureteral stent. UrolInt. 2002;69:136-40.
25. Smith KE, Holmes N, Lieb JI, et al. Stented versus nonstented pediatric pyeloplasty: a modern series and review of the literature. J Urol 2002;168:1127-30.
26. Shalhav AL, Mikhail AA, Orvieto MA, Gofrit ON, Gerber GS, Zorn KC. Adult stentless laparoscopic pyeloplasty. JSLS. 2007;11:8-13.
27. Kumar V, Mandhani A. Laparoscopic stentless pyeloplasty: an early experience. Indian J Urol. 2010;26:50-5.

CHAPTER 31

Ureteric Reimplantation

Vipin Tyagi

INTRODUCTION

The reconstruction of distal end of ureter in the form of ureteric reimplantation by laparoscopy is a demanding procedure. The robotic assistance for laparoscopic ureteric reimplantation (RALUR) not only provides outcomes at par with gold standard of open ureteric reimplantation but also have significant less morbidity.

INDICATIONS

Reimplantation of the ureter is required to be done for congenital and acquired pathology of the distal ureter **(Table 31.1)**.

The congenital disorders are normally managed in pediatric age group and the acquired are the problems of adulthood.

Table 31.1: Indications for uretric reimplantation

Congenital	*Acquired*
• VUR	• Trauma to lower or mid ureter-latrogenic/ accidental
• Megaureter	• Lower ureteric stricture – GUTB – Iatrogenic
• VUJ obstruction	• Uretero-vaginal fistula

Following are the contraindications of RALUR:

- *Patient not fit for insufflations:* Primary heart or lung disease.
- Previous abdominal surgery, which prevent safe access to the abdomen.
- *The long ureteric stricture:* It is a relative contraindication and depends on the competence of the surgeons.
- Patient not affordable.
- Pediatric patients whose abdomen cannot accommodate the big robotic arms.

TYPE OF URETERIC REIMPLANTATION

- Intravesical.
- Extravesical
  - Simple ureteric reimplantation
  - Ureteric reimplantation with psoas hitch
  - Ureteric reimplantation with boari flap.

The intravesical method for ureteric reimplantation is mainly used in the children's with VUR with adequate bladder capacity. The choice of only ureteric reimplantation (UR) or UR with psoas hitch or boari flap depends on the length of ureter involved. The aim is to provide a tension free ureter to urinary bladder anastomosis. The robotic assistance provides more abilities to perform more of psoas hitch or boari flap whenever required.

PREOPERATIVE EVALUATION AND PREPARATION

The aims of preoperative evaluation are:

- To measure the length of defective ureter
- *Evaluation of bladder volume:* This is more of importance in planning for intravesical approach or for UR with boari flap.
- Evaluation of kidney function and drainage pattern.
- Evaluation for general fitness of the patient for the robotic approach.

Appropriate imaging includes USG, VCUG, renal scan, IVP, CT scan, antegrade nephrostogram and RGP used as per the underlying indication for UR and the clinical condition of the patient.

There is no need for any specific preparation for RAUR. Surgeon may have surgical surprises at the time of surgery in the form of longer ureteric stricture, so the surgeon should be expert in use of all type of surgical variations if required.

The patient usually admitted on the day of surgery. Prophylactic antibiotics should be administered at the time of induction of anesthesia.

OPERATING ROOM CONFIGURATION AND PATIENT POSITIONING

Place the patient on the OT table with split leg position or with stirrups. Split the leg about 30° away from each other and then rotate them down ward in relation to the table. This allows the robot to be moved sufficiently close to the patient. Carefully secure the patient to the table so that an exaggerated head down position can be used to move the bowel content away from bladder **(Fig. 31.1)**.

In addition, it is recommended to be careful to ensure that the head of the patient is turned to the side to avoid the robotic arms.

In children take special care in order to avoid the injury from the robotic arms. Although new Xi davinci system with small and light robotic arms is of advantage in childrens.

It is always important to assign the best possible position of the patient as robot once docked cannot be moved.

The foley catheter is placed in sterile fashion and placed within the field to allow access during the procedure. I prefer to place three way Foleys in order to have smooth filling and emptying of the urinary bladder during the course of surgery.

TROCAR PLACEMENT

After insufflation, the trocars are placed as shows in **Figure 31.2**.

The camera post is placed supra-umbilical so as to have good working space. The two robotic ports are placed under direct vision at the lower border of umbilicus in midclavicular line. If performing a unilateral re-implantation then the ports can be skewed so that ipsilateral port is placed more cephlalod then contralateral side to improve the working distance to that side and maximize triangulation towards the region of interest.

In pediatric patients it will be great idea to move all the ports cranially in order to have sufficient working space.

I use two robotic arms, but for convenience using the third arm is not a bad idea. The instruments used are either Maryland grasper or bipolar forcep on the left and scissor on the right. I do the whole UR with using a single needle holder but when required do not hesitate to use second needle holder in order to take the advantage of being ambidextrous.

Steps of extravesical UR:

- After the placement of the port, the sigmoid colon is mobilized with incision along while line of Toldt on the left side, but on right side there may be no need of bowel mobilization.
- Ureter is identified at level of bifurcation of common iliac vessels with inspection of the vermiculate motion of ureter.
- Peritoneum is incised over the ureter and ureter is dissected along with the peri-ureteric fat and lifted of the vessels.
- The ureter is dissected distally till vesicoureteric or till the strictured ureter. It is vital to take case of the vas in the males. Also superior vesical pedicle is identified and secured by bipolar energy or clips.
- Proximally ureter in mobilized as per the length of the stricture with adequate freedom of movement with minimal tension when lifted towards the bladder.
- Transect ureter above the strictured area and distal part of ureter should be secured either by clip or suture.
- The bladder is filled with 200cc–300cc of saline.
- Bladder is dropped down by incising the anterior and contralateral peritoneum and by entering into retzius space with sharp and blunt dissection.
- In case of only ureteric re-implantation, bladder mobilization is enough for tension free re-implant.
- The psoas hitch may require the clipping of contralateral vesical pedicle
- In case of boari flap the contralateral vesical pedicle should be divided in order to achieve additional bladder mobility.

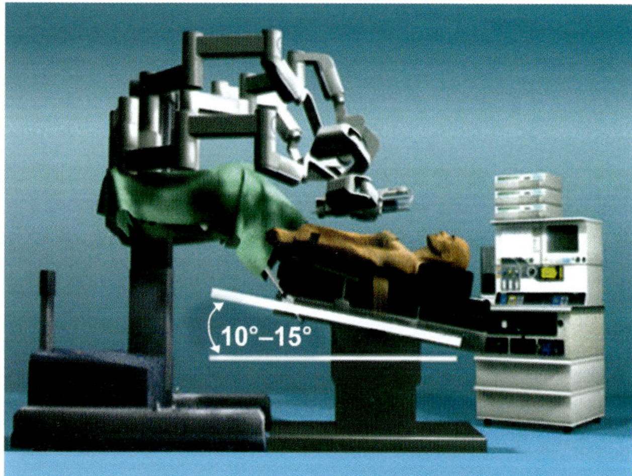

Fig. 31.1: Picture of operating room

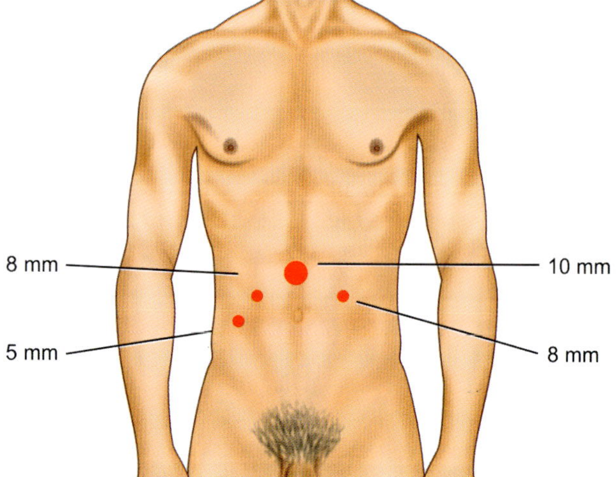

Fig. 31.2: Port position for ureteric reimplantation

- In case of only ureteric re-implantation with the hook cautery or scissors the detrusor is incised making sure not to enter the mucosa. Mucosa start appearing like a blue doom.
- I use of vicryl 3.0 to take a stay suture across the mucosa and fixed it to the anterior wall of the abdomen, so as to prevent retraction of mucosa once the mucosa is cut.
- A long detrusor incision is given as compared to mucosa opening in order to make a tunnel by detrussoraphy after reimplant.
- The ureter is spatulated posteriorly.
- Ureter then anastomosed to the bladder mucosa with vicryl or PDS40 in continuous or interrupted manner over a stent, choice depends on surgeons preference.
- The needle of suture, which was already placed into the mucosa, is passed below the detrusor at the distal end and reinserted from detrusor towards mucosa, so as to slide the mucosa beneath the detrusor. In some cases mainly with VUR, I take double needle PDS/or two vicryl tied together to achieve sliding of mucosa beneath the detrusor.
- Detrussoraphy done over the ureteroneocystostomy with vicryl 3.0 in interrupted manner so as to make a tunnel of length of 4 or 5 times of the diameter of the ureter.
- The care is to be taken to avoid tight closure of detrusor over the ureter so as to avoid constriction of the ureter.

PSOAS HITCH

In psoas hitch the bladder dome is secured to the psoas minor tendon or the psoas major muscle using several absorbable sutures followed by ureteric reimplant in above described manner.

BOARI FLAP

After the mobilization of the urinary bladder and division of contralateral pedicle, a posterolateral bladder flap is outlined based on the vascular supply. Following should be the characteristic of the flap

Flap length should equal the estimated ureteral defect plus an additional 3-4 cm.

Ratio of flap length to base width should not be greater than 3:1 to help minimize flap ischemia.

The flap is pexed to the psoas minor tendon and ureter is delivered through a small opening created in the posterior flap and a tension free mucosa to mucosa anastomosis is performed followed by tubularized anteriorly.

Intravesical

Under cystoscopic guidance 2 sutures are placed transabdominally through the rectus fascia and into bladder, to keep the bladder tented to abdominal wall during the surgery.

Camera port is placed below the umbilicus at the dome of bladder

Two robotic working arms are placed at edge of rectus muscles on each side.

After placement of the port saline is emptied and CO_2 is filled in to the bladder.

Intravesical ureteric reimplantation is the done in standard manner.

POSTOPERATIVE MANAGEMENT

After the surgery it is essential to have unobstructed urinary drainage. The drain output monitoring is also important for any disruption or excessive leak.

Patient is usually started orally on next day morning and usually discharged on second postoperative day with foleys catheter and drain.

Foleys is removed on 4th or 5th POD and if next day drain output is not in excess drain should be removed.

We usually take out the DJ Stent after 3-4 weeks and then follow-up the patients every 3-6 months for any obstruction after repair to maximum 2 years.

COMPLICATIONS

Robotic assisted laparoscopic ureteric reimplantation is subjected to the same complications as of laparoscopic complications.

There are enough evidences to state that robotic assistance had results in decrease in the complications as compared to the simple laparoscopic approach.

SUMMARY

Any minimally invasive surgical technique carry the necessary burden of proving that the benefits of improved cosmesis and decreased analgesia is not predicated on compromised safety and efficacy of the procedure.

Laparoscopic ureteric reimplantation is like any other pelvic surgery is having a steep learning curve and thus sometimes it is not proved to be as effective as the open methodology.

Robotic assistance with all its advantages not only able to give the cosmesis and less morbidity but also provides the efficacy.

The long-term durability and safety of the repair has to be supported with concrete scientific evidences.

Points of importance, which is related to robotic surgery:
- It is always important to assign the best possible position of the patient as robot once docked cannot be moved.
- In small children better to move all the ports cranially to have better space.
- Try to have small movements at the time of suturing so as to avoid breakage of sutures.
- Do not compromise the ideal principle of suturing.

Index

Page numbers followed by *f* refer to figure and *t* refer to table

A

Abdominal wall 84*f*
Abdominoperineal resection 52
Adhesiolysis 128
Adnexectomy 121
Adrenal gland 176*f*
Adrenal lesions 172
Adrenal vein, left 177*f*
Adrenalectomy 172
- complications of robot-assisted 178
- left 176*f*
- partial 177
- posterior retroperitoneoscopic robot-assisted 177
- robot-assisted 178
- single-port robot-assisted 177

African-American women 88
Airway pressure 18
American Association of Gynecologic Laparoscopists 90, 93
American Society for Metabolic and Bariatric Surgery 27, 33
American Society of Anaesthesiologists 157
Androgen-deprivation therapy 152
Anesthesia 17, 20, 48, 64, 72, 88, 115, 182
- general 72
- induction of 105
- influence of general 56
- intraoperative management 17
- preoperative preparation 17

Anesthetic challenges 128
Anesthetic considerations 173
Anorectal dysfunction 95
Antegrade double J stenting 185, 185*f*, 186
Aortic bifurcation 107
Aortic surgery, status of robotic 77
Aortoiliac surgery, robotic 77
Apparent diffusion coefficient 150
Arterial blood 19
Arterial pressure, mean 19

B

Bagged stone 185
Bean bag 105
Bile duct 11
- common 57, 58
- resection 57
- tumors, robotic surgery for 55

Biliary imaging 11, 12
Birt-Hogg-Dubé syndrome 162
Bladder volume, evaluation of 195
Bleeding
- excessive 66
- vessels, small 166

Blood
- flow 12
- loss
  - estimated 94
  - techniques to reduce 83
- vessels, anatomy of 12

Boari flap 195, 197
Body mass index 47, 157
Bowel
- distension 128
- grasper 30*f*
- marking 35

Bronchus, division of 70
Bulky machine parts 18

C

Calyceal calculi, removal of 184
Calyceal stones, removal of 184*f*
Camera port 183
- placement 143*f*

Cancer specific mortality 152
Cancer tissues, removal of 55
Capnothorax, deleterious effects of 21*t*
Carbon dioxide 19
Cardiac arrhythmias 66
Cardiac status 17
Cardiopulmonary complications 160
Caroli's disease 55
Cell histologic types 105
Central venous pressure 19, 21
Cerebral blood flow 21
Cerebral circulation 19
Cerebral edema 128
Cerebral perfusion pressure 19
Cervical cancer 111, 114
- robotic surgery in 114

Cervical cerclage 98
Cervical spine pathology 17
Cholangiocarcinoma 55
Choledochal cysts 55
Circumferential resection margin 47
Clermont-Ferrant manipulator 106
Colon reflection 183*f*
Colorectal disease 40
- robotic surgery for benign 40

Common bile duct 12
Common iliac
- artery 151
- vessels 186*f*

Congenital disorders 195
Coronary artery bypass 14
Cushing's syndrome 172
Cyst wall
- dissection on 120*f*
- incision on 120*f*

Cystic duct 12, 57
Cystoplasty, robotic augmentation 136
Cystostomy 128
- closure 129

D

da Vinci robotic surgery set-up 4*f*
da Vinci robotic system 49*f*
da Vinci SI robotic surgery system 164*f*
da Vinci SI surgical system integrated fluorescence 10*f*

da Vinci surgery, complications to 123
da Vinci surgical robot, robotic console of 163
da Vinci surgical
  disadvantages of 93
  system 29
Denonvilliers fascia 145
  incision of 145*f*
Dermoid cystectomy, robotic 122
Diabetes 172
Docking 29*f*, 69
Donor nephrectomy 169
  robotic 171
Dorsal vein complex 159
Dorsal venous complex, ligation of 144*f*
Double-docking technique 43
Double-pinch maneuver 144
Duodenal switch, part of 27

E

Ectopic ureters 135
  cases of 135
Endobronchial ultrasound 68
Endometrial biopsy 111
Endometrial cancer 101, 105, 111
  robotic staging surgery for 105
Endometrioma
  radical treatment for 122
  robotic cystectomy of 121
Endometriosis 96
Endometrium, carcinoma 111
Endopelvic fascia, incision of 143*f*
Endoscopic robotic-assisted procedures, total 14
Endowrist instrument tips 92
Ergonomics 6
Esophageal
  cancer 74
  surgery, robotic-assisted 74
Esophagectomy 72
  first robotic-assisted 73
  robot-assisted 21, 72
European Medicines Agency 10
Exercise 7
External iliac
  artery 151
  vein 151
Extrafascial hysterectomy, total 111
Extrahepatic tumors 55
Eye edema 128

F

Fallopian tubes 106
Femoral arteries, exposure of 76
Femoral nerve injuries 153
Fibroid 81
  retrieval 86
Fissures, dissection of 70
Fistula, closure of 128
Flank drain 166
Flank, pain in 190
Fluorescent cholangiogram 12
Fluorescent lymphatics 103*f*
Foley's catheter 68, 110, 196
Follicle-stimulating hormone 124
Food and Drug Administration 10, 105
Foot switch panel 163

G

Gastric band, laparoscopic adjustable 27
Gastric bypass
  advantages of robotic Roux-en-Y 33
  robot-assisted Roux-en-Y 33, 35*f*
  Roux-en-Y 34
Gastric calibration tube 29, 30
Gastric pouch 37*f*
  formation 35
  small 36*f*
Gastrojejunal anastomosis 36
Gastrojejunostomy 37*f*
  creation of 37
  first technique 35
  layer of 36
Gastrolysis using umbilical tape 29*f*
Gel mattress on operating table 106*f*
Genitofemoral nerve 153
Gerota's fascia 191
Glomerular filtration rate 20
Great vessels, injury to 66
Green cartridge 30*f*
Gynecologic surgery
  port placement for 107*f*
  robotic 93
Gynecological cancers 101
Gynecology 79
  robotics in benign 92

H

Heart rate 21
Hemicolectomy, robotic right 40, 41
Hemi-nephroureterectomy 136
Hemorrhage 167
Hepatectomy
  extended right 58
  left 58
  robot-assisted right extended 57*f*
Hepatic duct, common 12
Hepaticojejunostomy, Roux-en-Y 58
Hepatitis C 55
Hepatocellular carcinoma 14
Hepatolithiasis 55
High-intensity focus ultrasound 90
Hilar access 166
Hormonal evaluation 173
Hybrid technique 43
Hypertension 172
Hysterectomy 89, 93, 109, 112
  placement of arms for 108*f*
Hysterotomy 84

I

Ileocystoplasty, comparison of open and robotic 137*t*
Ileus 113
  postoperative 160
Iliac lymphadenectomy, common 113*f*
Iliac spine, anterior superior 173
Iliac vessels, external 187*f*
Immunofluorescence 10
  in robotic surgery 12*t*
Indocyanine green 10, 58, 101, 113
  dye 102*f*
Infundibulopelvic ligaments 84
Instrument placement 108
Internal iliac artery 151
International robotic cystectomy consortium 161
Intra-abdominal access 141
Intracranial pathology 17
Intracranial pressure 21
Intracranial tension 19
Intraductal tumors 55
Intraocular pathology 17
Intrathoracic
  esophageal mobilization 73
  pressure 21
Intrauterine manipulation, role of 82
Intravenous
  pyelogram 181*f*
  pyelography 190

Ipsilateral iliac fossa 186
Ipsilateral shoulder 176*f*

J

Jejunojejunal anastomosis 37
Jejunojejunostomy
  creation of 37*f*
  first technique 37
Joint pathology 17
Juxtavesical stone 186*f*
Juxtavesical ureter, proximity of 187*f*

K

Kidney 19*f*
  functions, loss of 190
  insertion, incision for 22*f*
  perfusion 20
  removal of part of 162*f*

L

Laparaotomy, conversion to 89
Laparoscopic assisted robotic procedure, port placement in 49*f*
Laparoscopic hysterectomy
  robotic-assisted 93
  total 93
Laparoscopic instruments 34
Laparoscopic procedure 52
Laparoscopic pyeloplasty 193
  left-sided robotic-assisted 191*f*
Laparoscopic radical prostatectomy, robot assisted 142*f*
Laparoscopic rectal surgery 51
Laparoscopic right colectomy 41
Laparoscopic Roux-en-Y gastric bypass 33
Laparoscopic supracervical hysterectomy 93
Laparoscopic surgery 48*t*, 51*t*
Laparoscopic ureteric reimplantation 197
Laparoscopy
  diagnostic 35
  robot-assisted 112
Lesions, identification of 14
Limb hypoperfusion 20
Liver
  disease, chronic 55
  flukes infestation 55
  retractor port 183
  surgery, robot-assisted 21
  transplantation 59
Lobe resection, caudate 58
Lobectomy
  position for 69*f*
  robotic 70
Lumen endotracheal tube, double 72
Lung
  cancer
    early stages of 14
    primary 68
  condition 17
  resection 68
    right 7*f*
Lymph node 13, 52
  evaluation 113
  group of 151*f*
  identification 12
  involvement 148
  status 101
Lymphadenectomy 101, 115*f*
  completion of 70
Lymphatic channels 12
Lymphedema 113
Lymphocele 153
Lymphocyst 113
Lymphotropic nanoparticle-enhanced magnetic resonance imaging 150
Lynch syndrome II 55

M

Mass forming tumors 55
Master arms 163
Mediastinal diseases 63
Mediastinal surgery 19*f*
Memory' foam 105
Mesenteric artery, inferior 111
Mesenteric defects, closure of 37
Methylene blue 10, 11
Minimal access laparoscopic surgery 40
Minimally invasive
  renal transplantation, robot-assisted 20
  surgery 90, 133
Molecular weight heparin, low 30
Mucinous cystadenomas 119, 120
Muscle fatigue 8
Muscular load and disorders 6
Musculoskeletal pain 6
Musculoskeletal system 6
Myasthenia gravis 63, 66
Myasthenic crisis 66
Myoma 85*f*
  bed 85*f*
  capsule 84*f*
  enucleation of 89
  pull on 85*f*
Myomectomy 81, 86
  robotic assisted 81
  steps of 89
Myometrial invasion, deep 109
Myometrium, normal 85*f*

N

Nausea 166
Nauseating sensation 159
Nephrectomy
  partial 136, 162
  robotic partial 165
Nephro-ureterectomy 136
Nerve
  identification 12, 13
  injury 20, 153
  palsy 113
  preservation 53*t*
  to rectum, relation of 50*f*
Neurovascular bundle 159
  preservation of 146*f*
Non-organ sparing technique 160
Nonsteroidal anti-inflammatory drugs 20

O

Obesity 17
Obturator
  artery 151
  node 151
  sentinel node, right 103*f*
Occupation myalgia 6
Ocular considerations 19
Oophorectomy 121
Operation room, challenges in 7
Operation theater ergonomics 191
Optic nerve 22*f*
Organ-sparing technique 160
Osteoporosis 172
Ovarian cancer 122
Ovarian cyst
  dissection for 120*f*, 121*f*
  removal of 120*f*, 121*f*

Ovarian cystectomy 117, 121*f*
robotic 120
Ovarian lesions
benign 117
malignant 117
Ovarian surgery, suturing in 123
Ovarian torsion 122
Ovarian tumors, malignant 122

P

Palliative surgery 59
Para-aortic lymphadenectomy 109, 111, 112
Para-aortic node dissection 109
Parathyroid identification 12
Parenchymal perfusion, assessing 11*f*
Peak airway pressure 21
Pediatric pyeloplasty, robotic assisted 134*t*
Pediatric robotic program 133
Pediatric urology 131, 133
Pelvic 111, 112
and infundibular incision, repair of 185
cavity 186*f*
lymphadenectomy 109, 115, 152
complete 101
complications with 152
extent of 151
indications of 150
right 113*f*
robot-assisted 153
role of 148
nodal dissection 109
pain, chronic 93
retroperitoneal structures, left 113*f*, 115*f*
surgery
robotic 20
types of 98
Pelviureteric junction 190
diagnosis of 190
obstruction 134
Pericardiophrenic neurovascular bundle 14
Periductal infiltrating tumors 55
Perigastric dissection 36
Peripelvic dissection 184*f*
Peritoneal cytology 111
Phrenic nerve 65
injury 66
Physical activity 7
Pneumoperitoneum 76
Port locations, anatomy of 83*f*
Port placement 73, 88, 106, 169, 173, 182, 186
left-sided 176*f*
locations of 159*f*
right-sided 176*f*
Pouch ileo-anal anastomoses 43
Pouch of Douglas 89
Pregnancy, ovarian tumors in 122
Prostate
cancer 148
lymphatic drainage of 148, 149*f*
specific antigen 150, 151
membrane 149
transurethral resection of 144
Psoas hitch 195, 197
Pull-spread-toggle technique 84
Pulmonary resections, robotic surgery for 71
Pulmonary vein preparation, robotic 70
Pyelolithotomy 184
extended 184
robotic anterior 182*f*
Pyeloplasty 134, 190, 191
left-sided 191*f*
robot-assisted 191
robotic 136
technique 191
treatment 190
Pyelotomy, closure of 185*f*

R

Radical cystectomy
robotic 157, 158
robotic-assisted 161
Radical cystoprostatectomy 157
Radical hysterectomy, robot-assisted 114
Radical prostatectomy 141
component of 148
robot assisted 143*f*, 148, 153, 154
Radical trachelectomy, robotic 114
Reconstruction procedures 159
Rectal cancer 53
laparoscopic surgery in 47
robotics in 50
Rectopexy 43
Rectum, carcinoma 47
Rectus sheath 143*f*
Renal access 166
Renal anomalies, complex 136
Renal disease, end-stage 169
Renal failure, acute 113
Renal function 17
Renal insufficiency 167
Renal mobilization 167
Renal pelvic stones, port placement for 183*f*
Renal pelvis 183, 190
dilated 183*f*
Renal stone surgery, robotic 181
Renal vein, longer 169
Renorrhaphy 167
Retroperitoneum, balloon in 177*f*
Retroperitonial approach 192
Retrosacral facia 45
Right nephrectomy, docking of robotic tower for 170*f*
Robot 176*f*
and surgery 1
docking 35
docking of 169
itself 18*t*
placement of 7*f*
positioning 191*f*
Robotic arms 22*f*, 47, 65, 108*f*, 163
heavy 18
pinching with 144*f*
Robotic augmentation ileocystoplasty 137*t*
Robotic colectomy 41
Robotic donor nephrectomy
left 169
right 169
Robotic esophagectomy
ports for 73*f*
positioning for 72*f*
Robotic instruments 34, 128
Robotic lobectomy, ports for 69*f*
Robotic myomectomy 83*f*
challenges in 88
Robotic nephrectomy, ports placement for right 170*f*
Robotic ovarian cystectomy, complications of 123
Robotic partial nephrectomy 165*f*
steps in 165*t*
Robotic pelvic surgery 19*f*
Robotic port 183
placement 119*f*
Robotic procedure 52
Robotic pyeloplasty in children 135*t*
Robotic radical cystectomy, earlier 157

Robotic rectal surgery 51
Robotic route 113
 comparison of 115
Robotic surgery 3, 10, 31, 48*t*, 51*t*, 178, 197
 advantages of 122
 applications in 14
 current advantages 4
 future of 5
 horizons of 180
 imaging in 12
 pain after 159
 past 3
 present 3
 set-up, current 4
 technique 4
 transoral 20
Robotic system 68
 current 4
Robotic technology 137
Robotic tenaculum 84, 85*f*
Robotic thymectomy 66
 port placement for 65*f*
Robotic ureterolithotomy 185
Ryles tube aspiration 49

S

Sacrocolpopexy 95
Salpingo-oopherectomy
 bilateral 111
 robotic 120
Sclerosing cholangitis, primary 55
Segmentectomy 14
Sentinel lymph node 101
 imaging 150
 technique of 101
Sentinel node biopsy 113
Serous cystadenoma 119
Serum lactate dehydrogenase 88
Sexual and urinary functions 50
Sexual dysfunction symptoms 95
Sexual function 51*t*
Shoulder braces 106*f*
Sigmoid colectomy 42
Single-docking technique 43
Skin closure 109
Sleeve gastrectomy 27
 instruments for robot-assisted 28*f*
 port position for robot-assisted 29*f*
 robot-assisted 27, 28*f*
Solitary kidney 192
Solitary myoma 82*f*
Spinal needle 84*f*
Spleen 176*f*
Stable remission, complete 63
Stents, use of 193
Stomach 30*f*
Stone
 localization of 186
 securing 185*f*
 surgery, robotic 180
Straight-stick surgery 92
Stroke 113
Supraumbilical incision 143*f*
Surgery
 general 11, 25
 indications for robot-assisted 190
 robot-assisted 6, 18
 robotic staging 105
 steps of 48, 69, 73, 89, 128, 183
Suspension stitch, anterior 144*f*
Suturing techniques 85
Swift coag 108
Symptomatic fibroids 94

T

Teratoma, mature 122
Thoracic surgery 61
 robotic-assisted 20
Thoracoscopic esophagectomy 74
 robot-assisted 74
Thoracoscopic exploration 70
Thoracoscopic surgery, video-assisted 66
Thromboembolic deterrent 105
Thymectomy 64*f*
Thymus 63
 robotic surgery for 63
Tissue perfusion 12
Transabdominal adrenalectomy, robotic lateral 175
Transabdominal cervical cerclage 98
Transhiatal esophagectomy 73
Transhiatal robotic esophagectomy 74
Transmesocolic approach 192
Transoral robotic surgery 21*f*
Transthoracic esophagectomy 73
Transthoracic robotic esophagectomy 74
Transverse colectomy 41
Trendelenburg position 158*f*
 effect of 128
Trocar placement 141, 191*f*, 196
Tubal reanastomosis 94
Tubal sterilization 94
Tumor 11
 common benign 88
 identification of 167
 node metastases 105
 resection 167

U

Ulcerative colitis 40
Umbilical artery, obliterated 109
Umbilicus 196
Ureter 183*f*, 190
 dissection of 183, 186
 distal end of 195
 retrocaval 135
 surgery, upper 19*f*
Ureteral injury 153
Ureteral stricture identification 14
Ureteric calculus, left upper 181*f*
Ureteric procedures 181
Ureteric reimplant 197
Ureteric reimplantation 136, 195
 for refluxing 135
 port position for 196*f*
 simple 195
 type of 195
Ureteric stricture
 long 195
 lower 195
Ureterolithotomy 186
Uretero-vaginal fistula 195
Urethra, transection of 146*f*
Uretric reimplantation, indications for 195*t*
Urinary bladder 197
 cancer 157*f*
 catheterization of 159
Urinary catheter 166
Urinary diversion, complications of 161
Urinary fistula 167
Urinary function 51*t*
Urinary retention 113
Urinary tract stones, upper 180
Urine leak 161
Urogynecology 125
Urolithiasis 180
Urology, adult 139

Uterine
  artery 103*f*
  bleeding, abnormal 93
  fibroids 88
  manipulation 83*f*, 106
Uterus, anterior wall of 82*f*

V

Vaginal hysterectomy, laparoscopic-assisted 93
Vaginal vault opening 112*f*
Vascular imaging 12
Vascular injury 160
Vascular surgery 61, 76
Vein thrombosis, deep 160
Vena cava, inferior 58
Venous drainage, dependent part 20
Veress needle 84*f*
  insufflation 143*f*
Vesicovaginal fistula 97, 127
  repair of 127
Vicryl suture 185
Visual display units 6
Visual loss, postoperative 19
von Hippel-Lindau disease 162
von Hippel-Lindau syndrome 177

W

Waldeyer facia 45